Geriatric Emergency Medicine

Editor

CHRISTOPHER R. CARPENTER

CLINICS IN
GERIATRIC MEDICINE

www.geriatric.theclinics.com

February 2013 • Volume 29 • Number 1

ELSEVIER

1600 John F. Kennedy Blvd., Suite 1800. Philadelphia, Pennsylvania 19103-2899

http://www.theclinics.com

CLINICS IN GERIATRIC MEDICINE Volume 29, Number 1
February 2013 ISSN 0749–0690, ISBN-13: 978-1-4557-7094-6

Editor: Yonah Korngold

Clinics in Geriatric Medicine (ISSN 0749-0690) is published quarterly by Elsevier Inc., 360 Park Avenue South, New York, NY 10010-1710. Months of issue are February, May, August, and November. Business and Editorial Offices: 1600 John F. Kennedy Blvd., Suite 1800, Philadelphia, PA 191023-2899. Periodicals postage paid at New York, NY, and additional mailing offices. Subscription prices is $257.00 per year (US individuals), $448.00 per year (US institutions), $131.00 per year (US student/resident), $334.00 per year (Canadian individuals), $559.00 per year (Canadian institutions), $355.00 per year (foreign individuals) and $559.00 per year (foreign institutions). Foreign air speed delivery is included in all *Clinics* subscription prices. All prices are subject to change without notice. POSTMASTER: Send address changes to *Clinics in Geriatric Medicine,* Elsevier Health Sciences Division, Subscription Customer Service, 3251 Riverport Lane, Maryland Heights, MO 63043. Telephone: 1-800-654-2452 (U.S. and Canada); 314-447-8871 (outside U.S. and Canada). Fax: 314-447-8029. E-mail: journalscustomerservice-usa@elsevier.com (for print support) or journalsonlinesupport-usa@elsevier.com (for online support).

Reprints. For copies of 100 or more, of articles in this publication, please contact the Commercial Reprints Department, Elsevier Inc., 360 Park Avenue South, New York, New York 10010-1710. Tel.: (212) 633-3812; Fax: (212) 462-1935, email: reprints@elsevier.com.

Clinics in Geriatric Medicine is covered in *MEDLINE/PubMed (Index Medicus), EMBASE/Excerpta Medica, Current Contents/Clinical Medicine (CC/CM),* and the *Cumulative Index to Nursing & Allied Health Literature.*

Printed and bound by CPI Group (UK) Ltd, Croydon, CR0 4YY

Transferred to digital print 2012

Contributors

GUEST EDITOR

CHRISTOPHER R. CARPENTER, MD, MSc, FACEP, FAAEM
American College of Emergency Physicians Geriatric Section Chair, Associate Professor, Department of Emergency Medicine, Director of Evidence Based Medicine, Washington University in St Louis, St Louis, Missouri

AUTHORS

VICTORIA M. ADDIS, MD
Department of Ophthalmology, MedStar Washington Hospital Center, Washington, DC

ABDULLAH ALZAHRANI, MD
Senior Resident and Assistant Clinical Instructor, Department of Emergency Medicine, SUNY Downstate College of Medicine, Brooklyn, New York

ROBERT S. ANDERSON JR, MD
Attending Physician Emergency Medicine and Geriatric Medicine, Maine Medical Center, Assistant Professor of Emergency Medicine, Assistant Professor of Internal Medicine, Tufts University School of Medicine, Portland, Maine

MICHAEL C. BOND, MD, FACEP, FAAEM
Assistant Professor, Residency Program Director, Department of Emergency Medicine, University of Maryland School of Medicine, Baltimore, Maryland

STEPHANIE BONNE, MD
Instructor in General Surgery, Washington University in St Louis, St Louis, Missouri

KENNETH H. BUTLER, DO, FACEP, FAAEM
Associate Professor, Associate Residency Program Director, Department of Emergency Medicine, University of Maryland School of Medicine, Baltimore, Maryland

CHRISTOPHER R. CARPENTER, MD, MSc, FACEP, FAAEM
American College of Emergency Physicians Geriatric Section Chair, Associate Professor, Department of Emergency Medicine, Director of Evidence Based Medicine, Washington University in St Louis, St Louis, Missouri

JEFFREY M. CATERINO, MD, MPH
Associate Professor, Department of Emergency Medicine, The Ohio State University, Columbus, Ohio

HEATHER K. DEVORE, MD
Clinical Instructor, Department of Emergency Medicine, MedStar Washington Hospital Center, Georgetown University, Washington, DC

JEFFREY DUBIN, MD, MBA
Assistant Professor of Clinical Emergency Medicine, MedStar Washington Hospital Center, Georgetown University School of Medicine, Washington, DC

ZAYD ELDADAH, MD, PhD, FACC
Director of Cardiac Arrhythmia Research and Interim Co-Director of the Electrophysiology Laboratories, MedStar Washington Hospital Center, Assistant Professor of Medicine, Georgetown University School of Medicine, Washington, DC; Adjunct Assistant Professor of Medicine, Johns Hopkins University School of Medicine, Baltimore, Maryland

JOEL GERNSHEIMER, MD
Director, Division of Geriatric Emergency Medicine, Visiting Associate Professor, Department of Emergency Medicine, SUNY Downstate College of Medicine, Brooklyn, New York

SARAH A.M. HALLEN, MD
Attending Physician Geriatric Medicine, Assistant Medical Director, Acute Care for Elderly Unit, Internal Medicine Geriatrics Rotation Director, Department of Internal Medicine, Maine Medical Center, Clinical Instructor of Internal Medicine, Tufts University School of Medicine, Portland, Maine

JIN H. HAN, MD, MSc
Assistant Professor of Emergency Medicine, Department of Emergency Medicine, Associate Research Director, Center for Quality Aging, Vanderbilt University School of Medicine, Nashville, Tennessee

CAROLINE N. HARADA, MD
Birmingham Veterans Affairs Medical Center; Department of Medicine, Division of Gerontology, Geriatrics and Palliative Care, University of Alabama Birmingham, Birmingham, Alabama

MILES P. HAWLEY, MD, MBA
Assistant Professor, Department of Emergency Medicine, The Ohio State University, Columbus, Ohio

LAURA E. HEITSCH, MD
Assistant Professor, Division of Emergency Medicine, Washington University School of Medicine, St Louis, Missouri

ULA HWANG, MD, MPH
Associate Professor, Department of Emergency Medicine; Brookdale Department of Geriatrics and Palliative Medicine, Mount Sinai School of Medicine, New York; Geriatric Research, Education and Clinical Center, James J. Peters Veterans Affairs Medical Center, Bronx, New York

NAMIRAH JAMSHED
Assistant Professor of Clinical Medicine, MedStar Washington Hospital Center, Georgetown University School of Medicine, Washington, DC

CHAD KESSLER, MD, MHPE
Section Chief, Emergency Medicine, Jesse Brown VA Hospital; Clinical Associate Professor, Departments of Emergency Medicine, Medical Education and Internal Medicine, Associate Program Director, Combined Internal Medicine/Emergency, Medicine Residency, University of Illinois-Chicago, Chicago, Illinois

SANGEETA LAMBA, MD
Associate Professor of Emergency Medicine and Surgery, Director of Medical Education, Director of Palliative Care, Department of Emergency Medicine, UMDNJ-New Jersey Medical School, Newark, New Jersey

ALEXANDER X. LO, MD, PhD
Assistant Professor, Department of Emergency Medicine, University of Alabama Birmingham, Birmingham, Alabama

SUMI MISRA, MD
Assistant Professor, Division of General Internal Medicine and Public Health; Section Chief, Palliative Medicine, Veterans Administration Medical Center, Vanderbilt University Medical Center, Nashville, Tennessee

MARK G. MOSELEY, MD, MHA
Associate Professor, Department of Emergency Medicine, The Ohio State University, Columbus, Ohio

JOHN N. MOUSTOUKAS, MD, MBA
Department of Emergency Medicine, University of Illinois-Chicago, Chicago, Illinois

PETER D. PANAGOS, MD, FACEP, FAHA
Associate Professor, Division of Emergency Medicine, Department of Neurology, Washington University School of Medicine, St Louis, Missouri

CLEO PAPPAS, MLIS
Assistant Information Services Librarian, Associate Professor, University of Illinois at Chicago - Library of the Health Sciences, Chicago, Illinois

TIMOTHY F. PLATTS-MILLS, MD
Assistant Professor, Department of Emergency Medicine; Department of Anesthesiology, University of North Carolina at Chapel Hill, Chapel Hill, North Carolina

MARK ROSENBERG, DO, MBA
Assistant Professor, Clinical Emergency Medicine, New York Medical College, Valhalla, New York; Chairman, Emergency Medicine; Chief, Geriatric Emergency Medicine; Chief, Palliative Medicine; St. Joseph's Regional Medical Center, Paterson, New Jersey

DOUGLAS J.E. SCHUERER, MD
Trauma Director, Barnes-Jewish Hospital; Associate Professor of Surgery, Washington University in St. Louis, St. Louis, Missouri

RICHARD SINNERT, DO
Research Director and Professor of Emergency Medicine, Department of Emergency Medicine, SUNY Downstate College of Medicine, Brooklyn, New York

MICHAEL E. SUMMERFIELD, MD
Residency Program Director, Department of Ophthalmology, MedStar Washington Hospital Center, Georgetown University, Washington, DC

SCOTT T. WILBER, MD, MPH
Associate Professor of Emergency Medicine, Director, Department of Emergency Medicine, Emergency Medicine Research Center, Summa Akron City Hospital, Northeastern Ohio Medical University, Akron, Ohio

MEREDITH C. WILLIAMS, MD, MBA
Section of Emergency Medicine, Department of Medicine, University of Chicago, Chicago, Illinois

Contents

Palliative Medicine and Geriatric Emergency Care: Challenges, Opportunities, and Basic Principles 1

Mark Rosenberg, Sangeeta Lamba, and Sumi Misra

> Patients with serious or life-threatening illness are likely to find themselves in an emergency department at some point along their trajectory of illness, and they should expect to receive high-quality palliative care in that setting. Recently, emergency medicine has increasingly taken a central role in the early implementation of palliative care. This article presents an overview of palliative care in the emergency department and describes commonly encountered palliative emergencies, strategies for acute symptom management, communication strategies, and issues related to optimal use of hospice service in the emergency department.

Evolving Prehospital, Emergency Department, and "Inpatient" Management Models for Geriatric Emergencies 31

Christopher R. Carpenter and Timothy F. Platts-Mills

> Alternative management methods are essential to ensure high-quality and efficient emergency care for the growing number of geriatric adults worldwide. Protocols to support early condition-specific treatment of older adults with acute severe illness and injury are needed. Improved emergency department care for older adults will require providers to address the influence of other factors on the patient's health. This article describes recent and ongoing efforts to enhance the quality of emergency care for older adults using alternative management approaches spanning the spectrum from prehospital care, through the emergency department, and into evolving inpatient or outpatient processes of care.

Transitions of Care for the Geriatric Patient in the Emergency Department 49

Chad Kessler, Meredith C. Williams, John N. Moustoukas, and Cleo Pappas

> This article reviews and summarizes more than 200 studies regarding key issues surrounding the transition of elderly patients to or from the emergency department (ED), with particular attention paid to the relationship between the ED and nursing homes. Transfers of care often occur with incomplete information, which results in increased morbidity, recidivism, and cost. Transitions of elderly patients could be improved by standardizing hand-offs processes, improving discharge planning for elderly patients, developing metrics for transfers of care and geriatric care quality, and finding sustainable sources of research funding.

Acute stroke is a devastating disease that affects almost 800,000 Americans annually. Worldwide, the incidence of stroke is rapidly increasing. Although stroke can affect all age groups, patients over age 80 are at much higher risk for ischemic stroke. Despite this, there are disparities in thrombolytic treatment rates, and as well as outcomes, between elderly stroke patients and their younger counterparts. This article discusses what is currently known about the elderly stroke patient for a greater understanding of the disease burden, research limitations and potential treatment options.

Elder abuse and neglect is estimated to affect approximately 700,000 to 1.2 million elderly people a year with an estimated annual cost of tens of billions of dollars. Despite the large population at risk, its significant morbidity and mortality, and substantial cost to society, elder abuse continues to be underrecognized and underreported. This article aims to increase the awareness of elder abuse by reviewing the demographics, epidemiology, and risk factors of elder abuse, followed by a discussion of screening tools and ways to increase awareness and reporting.

This article summarizes the current literature regarding the structural and functional changes of the aging kidney and describes how these changes make the older patient more susceptible to acute kidney injury and fluid and electrolyte disorders. It discusses the clinical manifestations, evaluation, and management of hyponatremia and shows how the management of hypernatremia in geriatric patients involves addressing the underlying cause and safely correcting the hypernatremia. The current literature regarding evaluation and management of hypercalcemia in older patients is summarized. The management of severe hypercalcemia is discussed in detail. The evaluation and management of acute kidney injury is described.

CLINICS IN GERIATRIC MEDICINE

Preface

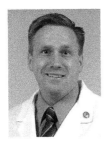

Christopher R. Carpenter, MD, MSc, FACEP, FAAEM
Guest Editor

Aging baby-boomers present an unprecedented challenge to the house of twenty-first century medicine, including the contemporary emergency department. This challenge was recognized over 2 decades ago when the first Geriatric Task Force in emergency medicine convened to highlight the issues that a generation of physicians now confronts. Ultimately, the Task Force combined efforts with Geriatricians to yield clinicians and researchers focused on improving emergency care for older adults. These challenges extend well beyond the traditional science of medicine to include ethical, logistical, and fiscal concerns that clinicians in overbooked offices or overcrowded emergency departments around the world face every day. Technological advances merge an increasingly expensive and fragmented health care system with an aging population larger than history has ever seen.

The foundation for efficient and cost-effective care of geriatric adults rests on collaborative protocols and reliable transitions of care. When health is compromised by acute disease, or by chronic disease decompensation that exceeds the individual's capacity to recover independently, emergency department care often provides the initial stage toward recuperation. Sitting at the crossroads between the inpatient and the outpatient world, the emergency department provides ready access to lab and imaging studies that might take weeks to obtain in other settings. One key challenge for the modern physician is to balance the incessant and expensive advancement of technology with the likelihood of return to health while effectively communicating diagnostic and therapeutic options with patients and caregivers. To accomplish these objectives, geriatric adult health care providers must understand the art and science across a broad spectrum of medical specialties, including emergency medicine.

Effective and reliable health care of the older adult requires a village. In this issue of *Clinics in Geriatric Medicine*, authors provide an up-to-date evidence-based review of common geriatric presenting complaints in today's emergency department. The perspectives include Medicine and Surgery specialists, as well as emergency physicians. The range of issues spans a vast range of complaints and pathology in the emergency department, from the elderly patient with nonspecific complaints like dizziness or weakness to the frail trauma victim. Evolving management models are also explored. For example, one article defines and reviews new concepts like the

Clin Geriatr Med 29 (2013) xiii–xiv
http://dx.doi.org/10.1016/j.cger.2012.10.010
0749-0690/13/$ – see front matter © 2013 Elsevier Inc. All rights reserved.

geriatric-specific emergency department and Hospital at Home care, both of which provide options to restructure the health care delivery system. The role of observation medicine is also reviewed. The concept of transitions of care is defined with pragmatic ideas to enhance the exchange of information between patients, providers, and other stakeholders during the tenuous management of acute disease. Another article explores the opportunity and appropriate settings in which to provide palliative care in the emergency department. This issue provides these discussions and significantly more, from a group of clinicians and investigators dedicated to the continual advancement of geriatric care.

This issue is dedicated to clinicians of all specialties who alleviate suffering in geriatric patients every day throughout the months and years that become a career. Geriatric adults represent a "canary in the coal mine" for our health care system because if we as a profession can effectively care for this challenging population we will undoubtedly provide exceptional management for the nonelderly. Personally, I owe a tremendous debt to each author group for providing thoughtful and well-referenced reviews on particularly challenging topics. All of these author groups were carefully selected based on their clinical expertise, passion for geriatrics, and research profile. I would also like to thank Yonah Korngold and the Elsevier staff for their unyielding guidance and support throughout the various stages of development of this issue. I acknowledge my family and Washington University colleagues who provided me with time and a listening ear as many ideas were formulated and refined. Most importantly, I thank the readers of *Clinics in Geriatric Medicine*, without whom none of these ideas would matter. Carpe diem.

Christopher R. Carpenter, MD, MSc, FACEP, FAAEM
American College of Emergency Physicians Geriatric Section Chair
Associate Professor, Emergency Medicine
Director of Evidence Based Medicine
Washington University in St Louis
Campus Box 8072
660 S. Euclid Avenue
St Louis, MO 63011, USA

E-mail address:
carpenterc@wusm.wustl.edu

Palliative Medicine and Geriatric Emergency Care
Challenges, Opportunities, and Basic Principles

Mark Rosenberg, DO, MBA[a],*, Sangeeta Lamba, MD[b],
Sumi Misra, MD[c]

KEYWORDS

- Palliative care • Geriatrics • Emergency medicine • Elderly • Hospice care

KEY POINTS

- Hospice and palliative medicine, a subspecialty of emergency medicine, concentrates on life-threatening illnesses, whether curable or not.
- Palliative care is not the same as end-of-life (EOL) care.
- Arrival of a patient under hospice care to an emergency department (ED) does not automatically equate to hospice care termination nor does it imply that patient seeks aggressive interventions.
- Challenges to implementation of pre-existing advance planning documents exist, including an unanticipated change in health status, interfamily conflicts, and issues with institutional protocols.
- Many eligible patients, if considered for hospice, are enrolled too late in the course of disease to realize the full benefit of hospice.

OPENING REMARKS

Before starting this article, it is important to have some perspective. **Figs. 1–3** define the terms and summarize necessary concepts of care. On initial presentation of a disease, such as lung cancer or heart failure, the goal of care is curative but patients also receive noncurative symptom management. In cancer, this noncurative management may include nausea relief and relief of constipation. This noncurative symptom management is palliative. Palliative care is the relief of symptoms and pain that interfere with quality of life.

The authors have nothing to disclose.
[a] Department of Emergency Medicine, St Joseph's Regional Medical Center, 703 Main Street, Paterson, NJ 07503, USA; [b] Department of Emergency Medicine, UMDNJ-New Jersey Medical School, MSB C-642, 185 South Orange Avenue, Newark, NJ 07101, USA; [c] Division of General Internal Medicine and Public Health, Veterans Administration Medical Center, Vanderbilt University Medical Center, Nashville, TN 37232, USA
* Corresponding author.
E-mail address: rosenbem@sjhmc.org

Clin Geriatr Med 29 (2013) 1–29
http://dx.doi.org/10.1016/j.cger.2012.09.006
0749-0690/13/$ – see front matter © 2013 Elsevier Inc. All rights reserved.
geriatric.theclinics.com

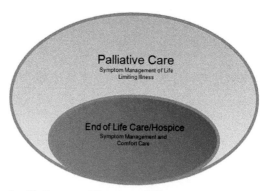

Fig. 1. The sphere of palliative care. (*Courtesy of* Rosenberg M, Patterson NJ. Geriatric palliative care…is it possible? LSMA 2010.)

Fig. 1 shows that as the disease progresses and curative treatment is less or no longer effective, the goal of care moves from curative to noncurative or palliative. When no curative treatment is available, then palliative care is the only treatment that is left to give. The disease course leads to death. This frequently is referred to as advanced end-stage disease. At this point, palliative care or hospice care remains as a treatment choice. Also at this point, life-prolonging interventions may be considered as prolonging suffering. Understanding a patient's goals of care is important in all aspects of care but of utmost importance in this case. This is the point when all additional curative treatment is not life prolonging and may actually cause more unwanted symptoms.

The important point to make is the role of the emergency physician. Along the continuum that is shown in **Fig. 2**, a patient may present to an ED. The physician role is part curative, such as infection management, and part palliative, such as managing nausea. This article discusses symptom management but is not limited to physical symptoms and includes psychosocial as well as ethical issues.

Fig. 3 further defines the disease trajectories. As discussed in this article, there are 4: sudden death, terminal illness, organ failure, and frailty. All dying falls into these 4 domains. Palliative care is focused on all but sudden death.

- The best example of terminal illness is cancer. Patients undergo curative and noncurative treatment as they approach either death or cure.
- In the case of organ failure, examples include renal failure and heart failure. The classic pattern of dying is prolonged with frequent exacerbations and symptom

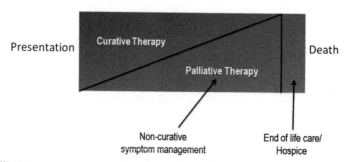

Fig. 2. Palliative care continuum. (*Courtesy of* Rosenberg M, Patterson NJ. Geriatric palliative care…is it possible? LSMA 2010.)

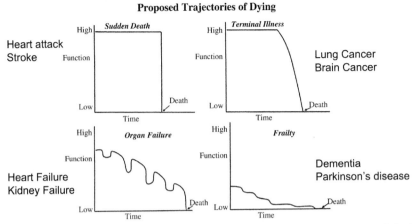

Fig. 3. Theoretic trajectory of dying. (*Reproduced from* Lunney JR, Lynn J, Hogan C. Profiles of older decedents. J Am Geriatr Soc 2002;50:1108–12; with permission.)

resolution but, eventually, the disease is progressive and life limiting. Each time the disease exacerbates, patients may present to an ED.

- Dementia and Parkinson disease are examples of frailty.

The dying trajectory is one of prolonged decline. Symptom management and prognostication, which is the prediction and communication of disease progression, are key to the long-term management of these patients. An example is the Seattle Heart Failure Model that can help predict survival in heart failure. There is even a smartphone application for many of these predictive tools.

An emergency physician may not need to know all the predictive tools but must be able to identify those patients who can benefit by a transition of care to a palliative service or hospice. For example, a 75-year-old man with class 4 heart failure has a 35% chance of dying in 1 year. It is important to realize that this patient is dying from his disease. Over the next year, this patient is likely to visit an ED multiple times. Identifying a disease trajectory and setting up appropriate palliative interventions is beneficial to the patient and helps with starting advance directives and other care planning. At minimum, an ED physician can help identify the patients who may benefit from discussion of palliative needs and make the transition of care to the appropriate resources. (Patients may see their ED physician more than they see their primary care physician in the last year of life.)

One last perspective: 100% of geriatric patients die. All die from one of these trajectories and all but sudden death has a role for palliative care. When President George Washington died of epiglottis, there were no hospitals. Most people died at home, usually without a nurse or physician present. When physicians were present, they had little therapy to offer (eg, Dr Benjamin Rush at Washington's bedside was bloodletting him because bloodletting was the cure for all "moist, wet diseases"). Today, there are vast hospitals with a diagnostic and therapeutic armamentarium that our ancestors never dreamed possible, but overtesting and overdiagnosis are bankrupting our nation and patients too often die away from home and family in cold, sterile hospitals. This is neither financially sustainable nor idyllic for patients. Palliative care offers an opportunity to find the sweet spot—if health care providers accept the philosophy and if appropriate patients can be identified at the right time in the course of their disease process and health care pathway.

INTRODUCTION
Defining Palliative Care

The World Health Organization defines palliative care as "care which improves the quality of life of patients and families who face life-threatening illness, by providing pain and symptom relief, spiritual and psychosocial support from diagnosis to the end-of-life and bereavement."[1] Hospice and palliative medicine, a subspecialty of emergency medicine, concentrates on life-threatening illnesses, whether curable or not.[2] These may include terminal illness (eg, cancer), organ failure (eg, congestive heart failure), and frailty (eg, Parkinson disease). Palliative medicine represents the "physician component of the interdisciplinary practice of palliative care."[3]

Palliative care is not the same as EOL care.[4,5] EOL care, a component of a palliative care program, is the care provided during the last likely hospitalization. It is impossible to know when a person is dying, hence the difficulty in defining EOL, leaving the concept to regulatory interpretation rather than scientific evidence.[6] EOL care, however, usually encompasses a chronic disease with a progressive downward trajectory.[6] Palliative care should not be confused with hospice care, in which patients have less than a 6-month life expectancy.

Older adults with chronic illnesses often present to an ED several times in their last year of life. The ability to change the existing paradigm of care for chronic disease is an opportunity for palliative medicine—specifically, palliative care in EDs—to alter the in-house trajectory of care. Research supports the use of palliative care interventions early in the disease trajectory to promote quality of life as well as reduce costs associated with treatments.[7–9] There is not a great deal of palliative care research related to quality of life and many of the available studies have weak methodology.[9] Yet studies have consistently demonstrated that palliative care consultations and interventions result in reduced symptoms, greater emotional support, and improved patient and family satisfaction.[10]

There are many variables to consider when determining savings associated with palliative interventions in the acute care setting. For example, was the patient admitted to an ICU for several days before a palliative consult and subsequent change in treatment plan to a floor bed? Other considerations include physician practice patterns, timing of consultations, and length of stay, suggesting that the presentation of clinical outcome data with cost-saving data may be the best approach.[11] With that said, researchers are concluding that hospital-based palliative care is associated with significant hospital cost savings.[10,12] Penrod and colleagues[8] compared palliative care admissions with regular hospital admissions and had significant findings. The investigators[8] reported a savings of $464 per day for total direct hospital costs associated with palliative care patients compared with those patients receiving standard care ($P<.001$) and a decrease in ICU use of 43.7% for palliative care patients.

Making the Case for Palliative Care Integration

Emergency medicine providers already offer many interventions that are aspects of palliative care. For example, discussions with family and loved ones to help direct the plan of care, symptom management, and pain control are essential to palliative care medicine. Additional benefits of providing palliative care interventions while in an ED include the ability to manage diagnostics and interventions,[12,13] improved satisfaction for patients and their families,[14] improved outcomes, reduced length of stay,[4,13,14] less use of intensive care compared with similar patients receiving usual care,[8,12] cost savings,[4,8,12,13] and direct referrals to hospice as appropriate.[12]

Patients with advanced and end-stage disease present to EDs every day, emphasizing the need for palliative care and EOL care in EDs.[7,15–17] The older adults in this cohort represent a complex and vulnerable population. EDs function as a safety net for these patients by offering a solution to the large gap in outpatient services. EDs provide access to multidisciplinary teams for assessments, plan of care, and interventions 24 hours a day, 365 days a year.[18] Research focusing on patients who were at EOL found that these patients often did not receive the care they anticipated.[7,18,19] They may present to an ED for assistance with pain management or other symptom relief with full intentions of being discharged. Once registered in an ED, EOL patients may find themselves overwhelmed by the chaotic environment and admitted to the hospital. Emergency physicians need to consider an alternate approach to treatment rather than the typical response of life-prolonging interventions.[18] In this situation, clinical protocols[20] may be used to facilitate palliative care interventions in the plan of care for the chronically ill elderly presenting to EDs.

Types of Programs

There are many ED palliative care delivery systems, based on provider experiences and the needs of the patient community. In general, there are 3 recurring models of palliative medicine/care in this area: ED–palliative care partnerships, ED palliative care champions, and ED hospice partnerships.[18] An advocate of the palliative care program is needed (preferably an ED physician) who possesses the ability to work behind the scenes educating, recruiting, addressing barriers, and promoting inclusion and continuity of the program within the individual hospital structure. It is essential to know the staff and community as well as nuances of the hospital in terms of leadership, internal politics, and resources before designing an ED-based palliative care program.

RECOGNIZING UNMET PALLIATIVE NEEDS IN THE EMERGENCY DEPARTMENT

Elderly patients with serious, advanced illnesses comprise a particularly vulnerable population in EDs.[15,21–23] A recent longitudinal study of patients older than 65 years examined the pattern of ED use in their last months of life[23]: 75% (4518 decedents) visited an ED in the last 6 months of life and 51% in the last month, and repeat visits to an ED were common.[23] This is not unique to the United States; a recent Australian study of patients with a known poor prognosis disease, such as cancer, also revealed that 70% of the cohort (1071) had at least 1 ED visit in the last few months of life.[24] These visits may, therefore, present an opportunity to initiate early goals of care discussions that may help tailor future care plans.[23,25–27] Many system-related, patient-related, and provider-related barriers to recognizing and addressing palliative needs in the ED elderly exist, however, for example, time-constraints, curative disease–focused approach to patient care, patient self-report limited by cognitive disabilities, lack of access to family or primary providers, chaotic environment, and lack of 24/7 availability of interdisciplinary support staff.[3,13,15,23,28,29]

It is well recognized that identifying unmet palliative needs in EDs is vital.[15,25,30] A geriatric competencies for emergency medicine residents consensus group identified palliative care competencies with respect to elders, including (1) rapidly establishing, documenting, and managing elders' goals of care for those with serious life-threatening conditions; (2) assessing and managing pain and key nonpain symptoms; and (3) understanding how to access hospice care and how to manage elders in hospice care in ED.[30] Clinical practice guidelines for quality palliative care in EDs also highlight that "The ED use explicit criteria to identify patients with unmet needs for palliative care."[31]

Prognostication

Predicting and anticipating the needs of patients in the near future requires determining a prognosis. Patients and families desire information about life expectancy so that they are able to plan for the future. The 5 D's of determining prognosis (prognostication) have been discussed in the literature and are related to outlining (1) disease progression, (2) death, (3) disability and discomfort, (4) drug side effects, and (5) dollars (cost of care).[32] Clinicians often find 2 aspects of prognostication challenging: the formulation and the communication of prognosis.[32] Prognostication remains an essential first step, however, that leads to triggering a palliative needs assessment in the elderly. Many palliative prognostic scores and scales that identify patients with life-limiting prognoses exist.[32–35] One such scale, the Palliative Performance Scale, takes into consideration the following domains (range 0–100%): (1) ambulation (bed bound to fully mobile), (2) activity and evidence of disease (no evidence of disease to extensive disease), (3) self-care (full to total assistance), (4) intake (normal to mouth care/sips), and (5) level of consciousness (fully alert to coma). Approximately 10% of patients with a score of 50% or less are expected to survive 6 months or more.[32,33] Although such prognostication tools exist, support tools for ED palliative care consultation and reliable ED screening methods that identify patients (including the elderly) in need of palliative care services early have not yet been widely evaluated or adopted.[7,25,29,36] Prognostication remains challenging in the ED setting when often the event is a terminal crisis can only be recognized retrospectively.[7,26,37]

Identifying Palliative Care Needs

Some early identification programs proactively seek to identify the elderly at high risk for unmet palliative care needs through screening pathways, ED checklists, and standardized assessment tools.[25,36,38–41] Examples include automatic triggering of palliative team consultation for preselected populations, such as those with admissions for placement of a gastrostomy tube[39]; a case management approach[22]; or Screen for Palliative and End-of-life Care Needs in the ED for use in ED cancer patients.[40] The Center to Advance Palliative Care convened a consensus panel of experts that selected criteria by which patients at high risk for unmet palliative care needs can be identified (**Table 1**).[39] Similar checklists (with proper education) may assist hospital staff engaged in day-to-day patient care in identifying the majority of patients with such needs and addressing concerns.[39,42–44]

COMMUNICATION

Effective Communication when Caring for Seriously Ill ED Patients

Optimal communication with shared decision making has been identified by patients and families as a crucial aspect of medical care, especially at EOL.[45–48] Effective communication facilitates improved satisfaction with care and a reduction of anxiety and distress, often with even brief interactions.[49–51] Although most patients and family members want to receive support and hope from clinicians, they also value clear and honest information about the medical condition and prognosis.[52,53] Yet studies, mostly in ICU and inpatient environments, reveal that up to one-third of families of critically ill patients are dissatisfied with the lack of communication or conflicting information from different clinicians.[54–56] EDs may have a disadvantage in communicating with patients and families due to the inherently fast-paced environment. If ED physicians identified the need for palliative care, however, a palliative care team can support the patient and family decision-making process. This transition is best initiated in EDs so goals of care and appropriate treatment are delivered.

Table 1
Criteria for initiating a palliative care assessment at initial patient evaluation

A potentially life-limiting or life-threatening condition[a] AND

Primary criteria[b]	
1. The surprise question	*You would not be surprised if the patient died within 12 mo...*
2. Bounce-backs	More than one ED visit or hospital admission for same condition within past several months
3. Difficult-to-control symptoms	Moderate-to-severe physical or psychological symptom intensity
4. Complex care requirements	Functional dependency; complex home support for ventilator/antibiotics
5. Functional decline	Feeding intolerance or unintended decline in weight (eg, failure to thrive)

Secondary criteria[c]
1. Admission from long-term care facility
2. Elderly patient, cognitively impaired, with acute hip fracture
3. Metastatic or locally advanced incurable cancer
4. Chronic home oxygen use
5. Out-of-hospital cardiac arrest
6. Current or past hospice or palliative care intervention
7. Limited social support (eg, family stress, caregiver distress, chronic mental illness)
8. No history of completing an advance care planning discussion/document

[a] Any disease or condition that is known to be life-limiting (eg, dementia, chronic renal failure, metastatic cancer, or cirrhosis) or that has a high chance of leading to death (eg, sepsis, multiorgan failure, or major trauma). Serious medical conditions for which recovery to baseline function is routine (eg, community-acquired pneumonia in an otherwise healthy patient) are not included.
[b] Primary criteria: global indicators that represent the minimum standard of care that hospitals should use to screen patients at risk for unmet palliative care needs.
[c] Secondary criteria: indicators of a high likelihood of unmet palliative care needs that should be incorporated into a systems-based approach to patient identification if possible.
   Data from Weissman DE, Meier DE. Identifying patients in need of a palliative care assessment in the hospital setting: a consensus report from the center to advance palliative care. J Palliat Med 2011;14:1–5; and Quest TE, Bryant EN, et al. Palliative Care emergency department screening tool. A technical assistance resource from the IPAL-EM Project, Center to Advance Palliative Care. Available at: http://ipal-live.capc.stackop.com/downloads/ipal-em-palliative-care-ed-screening-tool. pdf. Accessed July 20, 2012.

The ED setting poses further significant challenges due to patient-related, physician-related, time-related, and environment-related factors.[3,34] Three communication-related domains that are pertinent to caring for seriously ill elderly patients in EDs are as follows: (1) goals of care and patient-centered decision making, (2) advance care planning, and (3) transitioning patients to palliative care. Typically, these goals are initiated in the ED and are achieved as a process over a day or 2 with multiple coordinated conversations with the patient, family, and essential palliative care team members.

Goals of care and patient-centered decision making
A patient-centered decision making approach requires a shared understanding of patient values and goals so as to tailor suitable treatment plans.[19] Because goals may evolve with a change in health status or one patient goal (relief of pain and suffering) may take precedence over another (cure of disease), often these

discussions with the need to occur in real time in the ED setting[57] with a palliative care advocate. Goals of care discussions are road maps that assist clinicians in clarifying where patients want to go and what they want to avoid so that treatments align with their objectives.[57–59] **Box 1** lists some key elements when negotiating goals of care.

Box 1
Goals of care discussions with the elderly patient in the emergency department

1. Communicating prognosis (key step so the patient/family have a basis to make future plans/ decisions)
   a. Answer 2 key questions: "What is wrong with patient? What will happen to him/her?"
   b. Frame discussion as, "Hoping for the best while preparing for the worst."
2. Eliciting patient values (open-ended questions are suggested)
   a. "What is most important to you in your life right now?"
   b. "What kind of results are you hoping for?"
   c. "What do you hope to avoid at all costs?"
   d. "Have you been with someone who had a particularly good death or a particularly bad death? Please tell me about it."
3. Using appropriate language when describing goals of care
   a. Avoid negative statements ("Do you want us to stop aggressive care?")
   b. Frame appropriately
      i. "We want to ensure that you receive the kind of treatment you want."
      ii. "Let us discuss how we can work toward your wish to stay home."
4. Reconciling goals of care
   a. Sometimes a time-limited trial of therapy is needed to help patient/family cope/decide. If so,
      i. Outline the proposed treatment plan.
      ii. State what the goals are that you are hoping the treatment plan will achieve.
      iii. Clarify how you will recognize and determine that these goals are being met.
      iv. What period of time will be used to see if the treatment plan "works or does not work"?

Unrealistic goals may need limits set without implying abandonment.

"I understand your goal is not to be a burden to your family and you want an assisted death. Unfortunately, I cannot do that. I can however help with the distressing symptoms and alternative ways to help you not be a burden."

5. Recommending a care plan based on the established goals
   a. Any therapies that do not help meet the goals should be discussed for potential discontinuation.
   b. Appropriate diagnostic plans and disposition plans are best formulated/discussed with goals in mind.

Data from Arnold R. Critical Care communication (C3) Module III: determining goals of care. Available at: www.capc.org/palliative-care-professional-development/Training/c3-module-ipal-icu.pdf; and Weissman DE, Quill TE, Arnold RM. The family meeting: end of life goal setting and future planning. Fast Facts and Concepts 2010:227. Available at: http://www.eperc.mcw.edu/fastfact/ff_227.htm.

In general, instead of the yes-and-no answers, it is more important to ascertain the *whys* behind patient decisions and it is best to first ascertain overall big-picture patient goals and then discuss specific treatments.[59,60]

Eliciting goals is particularly challenging when patients lack decision-making capacity.[58,59,61] Capacity is determined "based on the process of the patient's decision making rather than the final decision itself."[62(p423)] Capacity surrogate proxy decision makers need guidance from a clinician to determine what the patient would have wanted given the clinical scenario and available information. It may be necessary to remind family or proxy that they should do their best to communicate the patient's wishes, not their own, although concordance may not always be feasible.[63,64] The ED environment may not be conducive to determining capacity and the process should be guided by the specific policies of the institution. Temporizing measures and/or a transition of care from an ED may provide the opportunity to establish goals of care, determine capacity, or guide a capacity surrogate through the decision-making process.

Advance care planning

Advance care planning is usually a longitudinal process whereby patients, in consultation with health care providers and family/caregivers, make decisions about their future health care, should they become incapable of participating in medical treatment decisions.[64,65] Advance planning documents usually fall into 2 categories: (1) instructional directives that usually provide guidance regarding single focused events, for example, do-not resuscitate, do-not hospitalize, or do-not intubate directives, and (2) proxy directives, which are those that involve the designation of a surrogate or substitute decision maker. Although completion of this process is important to document patient wishes, mere completion of such directives may not improve EOL care.[16,19,34,66–68] As discussed in the Translating Research Into Action for Diabetes (TRIAD) studies,[69,70] living wills and advanced directives are frequently misinterpreted because of a lack of understanding of intent and terminology. Many states are initiating new physician orders for life-sustaining treatment to help clarify the patient wishes and goals of care.

The availability of these documents in a crisis is variable; the applicability can be unclear and especially challenging in rapidly deteriorating elderly ED patients, often creating conflict, anxiety, and uncertainty.[16,19,34,66–68] Therefore, real-time rapid goals of care discussions are usually needed in the ED setting.[34] Again, prognostication is a key initial step and it is known that patients often vary their choices when informed about the likelihood and severity of outcomes, including those related to functional and cognitive disability.[71,72] In general, it may be best not to use mechanistic terms (put on breathing machine) and approach advance directives in the context of the whole person–big picture as opposed to isolating discussions around cardiopulmonary resuscitation.[34,58] The discussion and documents should be based on goals of care, not specific management decisions, such as "I do not want to be ventilator dependent" versus "do not put on breathing machine."

Transitioning an elderly patient to palliative care

Transition of elderly patients into palliative care may be one of the most confusing and traumatic transitions for patients and their loved ones.[73] A family may face conflict due to the time needed to cope and adjust and due to the intrinsic nature of the transitions, the timing of the transition, and the lack of information surrounding this transition.[73] In a discipline where the training focus is on life-prolonging care, the shift of a patient to comfort care may pose a philosophic challenge for ED clinicians as well, such that support to family may be lacking at the time that they most need it.[4,16,34,74] Therefore, when the issues are complex and difficult to manage, the ability to engage interdisciplinary staff (clergy, social worker, hospice case manager, and so forth) and/or consultation with a specialist palliative care clinician may be particularly helpful. Even if these services are not available in an ED, it is likely that some or all services are available in the hospital. Identifying the need and conveying the need is the domain of the ED team.

The availability to transfer a patient directly from an ED to a hospice or palliative care service or in-patient palliative unit may also assist in ease of transition to palliative care.[34] Another significant and stressful transition for patients is when they are already in palliative or hospice care and seek care in a different setting (like the ED). Lack of communication between care teams during such hand-offs and settings may create conflict and hamper overall patient-centered care.[75,76] A structured process of hand-offs with an emphasis on clear communication with caregivers and among the health care teams during the transitions (for example, when a hospice sends a patient to the ED and vice versa) assists to streamline care and decrease conflict and assures that the patient goals of care are consistently met.[34,75,76]

PALLIATIVE EMERGENCIES IN THE ELDERLY

A palliative care emergency is an unexpected change in a patient's medical condition in the context of an underlying known advanced or serious illness, and this emergency often triggers an ED visit.[34,77,78] The recommended ED assessment and treatment plan should consider patients' overall goals of care as well as the following:

- What is the acute medical issue and is it potentially reversible?
- What would most likely be the patient's status after treatment?
- What is the person's recent performance level, the extent of the underlying disease, and overall prognosis?
- What are the burdens of any treatments that could be offered?
- What are the patient's/surrogate's wishes when informed of the potential benefits and burdens of treatment plan?

Some common emergencies seen in the elderly with known advanced underlying disease (especially malignancy) are presented in **Table 2**.

SYMPTOM MANAGEMENT

The challenge faced by ED physicians who are managing patients with life-limiting illness, specifically EOL patients, is to provide relief of symptoms. Whether a patient is admitted to the hospital or discharged to home should not interfere with this management initiative. A partial list of common symptoms and complaints that may need to be addressed at EOL includes

1. Agitation/confusion/delirium—see **Table 3**
2. Anxiety
3. Constipation—see **Table 4**
4. Diarrhea
5. Dyspnea
6. Nausea and vomiting—see **Table 5**
7. Pain—see **Table 6**
8. Pruritus
9. Stomatitis
10. Terminal oral secretions—see **Table 7**

Table 2
Palliative emergencies in the elderly patient

Emergency	Presentation	Cause	Therapeutic Plan
Cord compression[a,b]	Underlying malignant disease with • Worsening back/radicular pain • Progressive gait difficulties • Sphincter symptoms, such as urinary retention may occur late • Pain and temperature sensation are usually lost first	Vertebral metastasis Edema after radiation	• Dexamethasone when suspected (10 mg IV) • Urgent imaging (MRI scan) • Urgent referral for radiotherapy • Urgent surgical referral for decompression
Superior vena cava syndrome[c]	• Early: periorbital edema, facial swelling, cough, dyspnea • Late: engorged neck and chest veins, upper-extremity edema • Severe: headaches, seizures	Extrinsic pressure or invasion of tumor Intraluminal thrombus	• Raise head of bed and diuretics (temporary measures) • Radiation referral • Intravascular expandable metal stent • Lytic therapy if thrombosis • Dexamethasone
Hypercalcemia[d]	• Nausea, change in mentation, constipation, dehydration, cardiac arrhythmia	Multiple myeloma Malignancies	• Hydration • Loop diuretics (furosemide) • Bisphosphonates (pamidronate, zoledronic acid) • Steroids in lymphoid malignancies
Bowel obstruction[e,f]	Malignant bowel obstruction may present acutely or subacutely	Compression or intraluminal mass/tumors	• Antisecretory medications (eg, octreotide) to reduce the fluid load–associated vomiting and distress • Anticholinergic drugs (scopolamine, atropine, and glycopyrrolate) may decrease spasm • Avoid stimulants and prokinetic antiemetic (metoclopromide) in complete obstruction because they may worsen colicky pain (these may assist in partial obstructions) • Steroids help in decreasing edema and can relieve nausea • Initial decompression with nasogastric tube may be helpful • For intractable symptoms, consider a venting percutaneous gastrostomy • Surgery to relieve obstruction (if good functional status)

(continued on next page)

Table 2
(continued)

Emergency	Presentation	Cause	Therapeutic Plan
Dyspnea or respiratory failure[g,h,i]	Common at EOL	Reversible and nonreversible causes (pleural effusion, fluid overload, anemia, pneumonia, mucous plug, etc.)	• Suctioning and upright positioning • Supplemental oxygen may help • Morphine and lorazepam to decrease distress and anxiety • Noninvasive ventilation (BIPAP) as a bridge while decisions are being made • Treat reversible causes like anemia and pneumonia if they fit patient goals of care
Delirium[j,k,l]	Fluctuating mental state and disorganized thinking An abnormal state of arousal—either hyperactive/agitated or hypoactive	Medications Intracranial pressure rises Infections Underlying cognitive impairment	• Consider potentially reversible causes and screen early • Antipsychotic may be tried: haloperidol or newer atypical antipsychotics (olanzepine or risperidone)

[a] *Data from* George R, Jeba J, Ramkumar G, et al. Interventions for the treatment of metastatic extradural spinal cord compression in adults. Cochrane Database Syst Rev 2008;(4):CD006716. http://dx.doi.org/10.1002/14651858.CD006716.pub2.
[b] *Data from* Mehta R, Arnold R. Management of spinal cord compression. Fast facts and concepts 2011:238. Available at: http://www.eperc.mcw.edu/fastfact/ff_238.htm.
[c] *Data from* Wan JF, Bezjak A. Superior vena cava syndrome. Emerg Med Clin North Am 2009;27:243–55.
[d] *Data from* Siddiqui F, Weissman DE. Hypercalemia of malignancy. Fast Facts and Concepts 2006:151. Available at: http://www.eperc.mcw.edu/fastfact/ff_151.htm.
[e] *Data from* Von Gunten CF, Muir JC. Medical management of bowel obstructions, 2nd edition. Fast Facts and Concepts 2005. p. 45. Available at: http://www.eperc.mcw.edu/fastfact/ff_045.htm.
[f] *Data from* Ripamonti C, Mercadante S. How to use octreotide for malignant bowel obstruction. J Support Oncol 2004;2:357–64.
[g] *Data from* Navigante AH, Cerchietti LC, Castro MA, et al. Midazolam as adjunct therapy to morphine in the alleviation of severe dyspnea perception in patients with advanced cancer. J Pain Symptom Manage 2006;31:38–47.
[h] *Data from* LaDuke S. Terminal dyspnea and palliative care. Am J Nurs 2001;101:26–31.
[i] *Data from* Campbell ML. Terminal dyspnea and respiratory distress. Crit Care Clin 2004;20:403–17, viii–ix.
[j] *Data from* Carpenter CR, DesPain B, Keeling T, et al. The six item screener and AD8 for the detection of cognitive impairment in geriatric emergency department patients. Ann Emerg Med 2011;57:653–61.
[k] *Data from* Shuster JL. Delirium, confusion, and agitation at the end of life. J Palliat Med 1998;1:177–86.
[l] *Data from* Carpenter CR, Shah MN, Hustey FM, et al. High yield research opportunities in geriatric emergency medicine: Prehospital care, delirium, adverse drug events, and falls. J Gerontol A Biol Sci Med Sci 2011;66:775–83.

Table 3
Delirium: treatment

Generic Name (Common Brand Name)	Starting Dose	Dosing Interval	Max q24 h Dose	Formulations	EPS	Anticholinergic	Sedation	Comments
Risperidone (Risperdal)	0.25–1 mg	bid or up to q6 h prn	6 mg	0.25-, 0.5-, 1-, 2-, 3-, 4-mg tablets Available as ODT	++	+	+	Caution with renal failure
Olanzapine (Zyprexa)	2.5–10 mg Debilitated or elderly: 2.5 mg	Daily IM: q2 h (maximum: 3 doses daily)	20 mg	2.5-, 5-, 7.5-, 10-, 15-, 20-mg tablets Available as ODT and IM injection	+	++	++	Patients with hypoactive delirium, >70-y CNS malignancy may not respond well
Quetiapine (Seroquel)	12.5–50 mg	bid	800 mg	25-, 50-, 100-, 200-, 300-, 400-mg tablets	+	+	+++	Start daily at 4:00 PM for sundowning and then time subsequent, additional doses based on symptoms
Aripiprazole (Ability)	5–15 mg	qam	30 mg	2-, 5-, 10-, 15-, 20-, 30-mg Available as IM and oral solution	++	++	++	Useful for hyperactive delirium. Can cause insomnia if given at night

Abbreviations: CNS, Central nervous system; IM, Intramuscular; ODT, Oral dissolving tablet.
Data from UPMC supportive and palliative care pain card. University of Pittsburgh Medical Center, Pittsburgh, PA.

Table 4
Constipation and bowel protocol

Medication	Onset of Action	Usual Starting Dosage	Site and Mechanism of Action
Osmotic laxatives			
Lactulose	24–48 h	15–30 mL q12–24 h	Colon; osmotic effect
Polyethylene glycol	48–96 h	17 g (1tbsp) powder in 8 oz water q24 h	GI tract; osmotic effect
Sorbitol	24–48 h	15–30 mL q12–24 h, max 150 mL/d	Colon; delivers osmotically active molecules to the colon
Saline Laxatives			
Magnesium citrate	30 min–3 h	120–240 mL × 1; 10 oz q24 h	Small and large bowel; attracts and retains water in the bowel lumen
Magnesium hydroxide (MOM)	30 min–3 h	30 mL q12–24 h	Colon; osmotic effect and increased peristalsis
Stimulant laxatives			
Bisacodyl	6–10 h	5–15 mg × 1	Colon; stimulates peristalsis
Bisacodyl (PR)	15 min–1 h	10 mg × 1	Colon; stimulates peristalsis
Senna	6–10 h	2 tablets qhs	Colon; stimulate myenteric plexus, alters water and electrolyte secretion
Surface laxatives			
Docusate	24–72 h	100 mg q12–24 h	Small and large bowel; detergent activity; softens feces

Abbreviations: GI, gastrointestinal; MOM, Milk of Magnesia; PR, per rectum.
Data from UPMC supportive and palliative care pain card. University of Pittsburgh Medical Center, Pittsburgh, PA.

When patient and family agree to comfort measures rather than aggressive resuscitation, the goal of treatment is symptom management. EOL patient symptoms require appropriate assessment and intervention. For example, the management of an EOL patient who declines intubation but has dyspnea and respiratory failure is challenging. It is an ED physician's responsibility to keep that patient comfortable and permit the disease process to take its course. The treatment of dyspnea is not oxygen alone but a combination of therapies that includes opioids and benzodiazepines. Morphine works well in improving comfort, decreasing anxiety, and decreasing the feeling of breathlessness in the face of dyspnea.[79]

Knowledge and expertise in the management of these complaints is necessary to help patients meet their goals.[80] Remember to treat the patient as a person not as an EOL complaint.

ETHICAL ISSUES AT EOL IN THE EMERGENCY DEPARTMENT

"Palliative care at the EOL involves meeting the physical, psychological, social and practical needs of patients and caregivers."[81] Ethical issues arise from time to time in EDs when dealing with palliative care patients at the EOL. Ethical dilemmas in the ED setting are likely to include matters related to the use of artificial airways, artificial nutrition, and surrogate decision makers. If available, state-approved advanced directives in the form of do-not-resuscitate (DNR) orders, living wills, or durable powers of

Table 5
Nausea and vomiting: treatment

Drug (Generic Name)	Receptor Activity	Common Clinical Indications	Dosage/Route	Cost	Comments/Side Effects
Haloperidol	D2	Opioid-induced N/V	0.5–4 mg po or sq or IV q6 h	$	IV has less EPS compared with po
Metoclopramide	Peripheral D2	Impaired GI motility Opioid-induced N/V	5–20 mg po or sq or IV AC and HS	$	EPS, esophageal spasm, and colic in GI tract obstruction
Prochlorperazine	D2	Opioid-induced N/V N/V of unknown etiology	5–10 mg po or IV every 6 h or 25 mg pr q6 h	$	EPS and sedation
Scopolamine	Ach, H1	Motion-induced N/V	1.5-mg transdermal patch every 3 d	$	Dry mouth, blurred vision, ileus, urinary retention, and confusion
Ondansetron	5-HT 3	Chemotherapy or radiation induced N/V	4–8 mg po as a pill or dissolvable tablet or IV every 4–8 h	$$	Headache, fatigue, and constipation
Dexamethasone	Decrease ICP	N/V related to Increased ICP	4–8 mg qam or bid, po (as pill or liquid), and IV	$	Agitation, insomnia, hyperglycemia

Abbreviations: AC, Before meals; EPS, extrapyramidal symptoms; HS, hour of sleep; GI, gastrointestinal; ICP, intracranial pressure; N/V, nausea/vomiting.
    Data from UPMC supportive and palliative care pain card. University of Pittsburgh Medical Center, Pittsburgh, PA.

Table 6
Opioid conversions

Opioid Agonists	Parenteral mg[2]	Oral mg[3]	Duration of Effect
Morphine	10	30	3–4 h
Oxycodone		20–30	3–4 h
Hydromorphone	1.5	7.5	3–4 h
Meperidine[1] (not recommended)	75	300	3 h
Fentanyl[4]	0.1[a]		1–2 h
Codeine	130	200	3–4 h
Hydrocodone		25–30	
Oxymorphone	1	10	3–6 h

[a] Equivalency for a 1-time dose of IV fentanyl only.
    Data from UPMC supportive and palliative care pain card. University of Pittsburgh Medical Center, Pittsburgh, PA.

Table 7
Oral secretions at the end of life

Drug	(Trade Name)	Route	Starting Dose	Onset
Hyoscyamine hydrochloride	Scopolamine	Transdermal	1 (~1 mg/3 d)	12 h
Hyoscyamine sulfate	Levsin	Drops, tabs (oral)	0.125 mg	30 min
Glycopyrrolate	Robinul	Pills (oral)	1 mg	30 min
Glycopyrrolate	Robinul	Injection (SC IV)	0.2 mg	1 min
Atropine	Atropine	Injection	0.1 mg	1 min
Atropine	Multiple	Sublingual[a]	1 gtt (1%)	30 min

Tertiary amines which cross the blood-brain barrier (all but glycopyrrolate) cause CNS toxicity (sedation, delirium).

[a] Use atropine ophthalmic drops.

Data from Bickel K, Arnold R. Death Rattle and Oral Secretions, 2nd Edition. Fast Facts and Concepts. April 2008; 109. Available at: http://www.eperc.mcw.edu/fastfact/ff_109.htm.

attorney for health care[82] and/or physician orders for life-sustaining treatment[83] are valuable resources. In cases of advanced directives, ED physicians need to pay attention to the intent of the directive, not only the specific instructions.[84] Specifically, a DNR order does not equal "do not treat."[69] If time permits, gathering information from family, significant others, friends, and previous medical records can provide additional insight when making EOL decisions in an ED.[84] EDs must have specific procedures that address ethical issues as well as policies outlining how to request a consult with the ethics committee.

Physicians and their patients must evaluate the use of technology at their disposal, keeping in mind that the patient and/or surrogate has the right to decide on goals of care and treatment options. ED physicians need to confirm that the goals of care represent the patient's wishes.[84] If a treating physician cannot meet a patient's goals of care because of personal beliefs, it may be appropriate to transfer care to another physician. The American College of Emergency Physicians provides additional policies[85] and guidelines[86] for ED physicians and EOL care.

ED physicians have a responsibility to help EOL patients attain comfort by managing symptoms, such as anxiety or pain. Palliative care EOL patients should be kept as pain-free as possible so that they may die comfortably and with dignity.[87] In addition, every effort should be made to honor patients' wishes concerning the place in which they wish to die.[87] "Medicines capable of alleviating or suppressing pain may be given to a dying person, even if this therapy may indirectly shorten the person's life so long as the intent is not to hasten death."[87] It is a goal of care to make patients comfortable.

Futility

The term, *futility*, continues to be controversial because there are inconsistencies in definition and interpretation throughout the literature.[88–90] The American College of Emergency Physicians[88] suggests using terms, such as nonbeneficial, ineffectual, or having a low likelihood of success, when referring to medical interventions that may be unnecessary or unsuccessful.[89,90]

Disputes among family members, patients, and physicians regarding the medical plan of care for EOL ED patients should be resolved through increased communications, use of available institutional resources, and policies.[91] Another consideration for EDs physician is that of determining treatment goals when "defining an absence of benefit."[92] For example, it may be agreed to maintain ventilator support until family members can arrive at the bedside or maintain other medical interventions that support a patient's goal of seeing a granddaughter get married in a few days. Ultimately, treatment decisions should be based on standards of care, evidence-based data, and the patient and family wishes and goals of care as well as professional judgment.[88]

Palliative Sedation

Palliative sedation is often framed in ethical terms and is defined as "the use of specific sedative medications to relieve intolerable suffering from refractory symptoms by a reduction in patient consciousness, using appropriate drugs carefully titrated to the cessation of symptoms."[93] The primary ethical responsibility of physicians is to provide relief from suffering in a way that is consistent with the wishes, values, and norms of patients, their families, and medical professionals. The goal of palliative sedation is symptom relief.[94] Many palliative care patients reaching the EOL are unable to find relief from severe symptoms, such as pain or shortness of breath. The goals of care may shift from those of "prolonging life and optimizing function to maximizing the quality of remaining life."[94]

Palliative sedation requires continuous monitoring by physicians experienced with the medications and palliative sedation. The administration of palliative sedation needs to be guided by an institution's specific policies and procedures. The National Hospice and Palliative Care Organization[95] recommends that each institution's policies should address (1) criteria for administration of palliative sedation; (2) specific procedures for the administration of palliative sedation; (3) concomitant use of life-sustaining therapies, such as dialysis; (4) continuous education regarding clinical evidence and best practices; and (5) continuous quality improvement to monitor the use of palliative sedation in the institution.

MANAGING THE ELDERLY UNDER HOSPICE CARE IN THE EMERGENCY DEPARTMENT

Patients under hospice care often present to EDs for crisis events, and emergency clinicians who are familiar with the hospice model of care may be better able to guide EOL care for such patients.[34] Eligibility for hospice is primarily based on a prognosis of living 6 months or less if the disease were to run its natural course.[96] Patients may have any diagnosis to qualify for hospice care, and noncancer primary diagnoses now comprise more than half of all hospice admissions.[96,97]

Arrival of a patient under hospice care to an ED does not automatically equate to hospice care termination nor does it imply that patient seeks aggressive interventions.[34] Often, caregivers activate the 9-1-1 emergency response system as an automatic response to an inability to cope with patient deterioration.[34] Hospice providers may initiate patient transfers to an ED if they are unable to fully address a distressing symptom or imminent deterioration. It should not be assumed that a patient who embraced the comfort-based hospice philosophy would automatically choose a DNR directive (DNR is not a prerequisite for hospice). Such end-of-life conversations may take time and further discussions, even in patients under hospice care.[34] An initial assessment on ED arrival is needed to ascertain the underlying reasons (if any) for a shift in goals of care and the trigger for ED visit (**Box 2**).

A general management approach to ED management of patients under hospice care is listed in **Box 3**. It is important to highlight a multidisciplinary approach to optimizing care with early collaboration with hospice staff, social worker, and palliative team, if available.[3,34] Effective communication with all members of the team and caregivers is essential to emphasize ongoing commitment to patient. In general, it is best to avoid diagnostic/therapeutic modalities that do not match overall patient goals of care.[34,98–100]

Box 2
Common triggers for an emergency department visit by an elderly patient under hospice care

Triggers related to patient health care issues

- Poor control of symptoms especially pain, dyspnea, and delirium
- Loss or malfunction of a key support device, such as a tracheostomy or gastrostomy tube
- Inability to fill a new prescription (for example, pain medication on a weekend)
- New symptoms that require work-up (for example, fall and hip fracture in a patient with bone metastases)

Triggers related to other patient and caregiver issues

- Anxiety, fear, and inability to cope with impending loss of life
- Conflict about life-prolonging treatments (begun in past and discontinued or never started, for example, chemotherapy)
- Conflict with caregivers regarding approach to care (caregiver may want more aggressive interventions)
- Caregiver fatigue
- Dialing 9-1-1 as an automatic response to a perceived distress

Triggers related to hospice system

- Failure or inability to communicate with or address patient needs in a timely manner
- Equipment failure unable to be fixed in a timely manner (for example, home oxygen or nebulizer machine)
- Call initiated by hospice (unable to provide a particular aspect of care or patient is a full code)

Data from Lamba S, Quest TE. Hospice care and the emergency department: rules, regulations, and referrals. Ann Emerg Med 2010;53:282–90.

Patients under hospice care with imminent clinical deterioration present a major management challenge in EDs. Delineating patient wishes and underlying disease status in a life-threatening situation is difficult when a patient is unable to communicate and the family or primary provider is not readily accessible.[101–103] In such scenarios, the least-invasive modalities should be used first; however, imminent life-prolonging measures (ventilator) sometimes need to be instituted until it is determined that such measures are not desired and can then be withdrawn.[34]

Challenges to implementation of pre-existing advance planning documents exist, including an unanticipated change in health status, interfamily conflicts, and issues with institutional protocols.[14,34,69,70] Therefore, discussion of all relevant decisions ideally occurs in real time in EDs, with a rapid delineation of patient goals of care.[34,99,104] At minimum, EDs identify these needs and get a palliative consult or communicate the need in the transition of care the same as would be done with a bowel obstruction and surgical consult. Withdrawal of preinstituted life-prolonging interventions may sometimes be necessary in EDs if it is later determined that these measures are not desired or in conflict with patient goals.[105]

REFERRING AN ELIGIBLE EMERGENCY DEPARTMENT PATIENT TO HOSPICE CARE

Elderly patients with declining health and functional status and advanced disease have frequent ED visits, particularly in the last months of life, presenting a window of

Box 3
Approach to the management of a patient under hospice care in the emergency department

1. Notify hospice provider as soon as possible.

   a. Hospice providers have an ongoing understanding of patient-related issues.

   b. Hospice is legally/financially responsible for the patient's plan of care as well as medical costs related to the hospice-qualifying disease diagnosis.

2. Determine the main trigger for the emergency department visit.

   a. Pay attention not only to the distressing physical signs and symptoms but also to the underlying emotional and psychosocial issues.

   b. Involve social service/chaplaincy and palliative care team early, if needed.

3. Optimize management of distressing symptoms.

   a. Promptly address and optimize management of common distressing complaints related to pain, nausea, shortness of breath, altered mentation, and so forth.

4. Rapid goals of care discussions, especially if clinical deterioration is imminent.

   a. If imminent decisions are needed regarding the use of life-sustaining treatments (eg, intubation for respiratory failure), a rapid discussion of goals of care must occur.

      i. Determine the legal decision maker and review any completed advance directives.

      ii. Complete a rapid overall goals of care discussion (palliative team involvement early as needed).

      iii. Make clear recommendations, for example, "According to what you want for [the patient], I would/would not recommend...."

5. Care for the actively dying patient.

   a. Assess for cultural/spiritual needs and assure privacy.

   b. Identify family/patient preferences related to locations where patient could be safely transferred to for the dying process (eg, home, long-term care residence).

   c. Involve bereavement, chaplaincy, and palliative team support, as needed.

6. Carefully consider laboratory tests and diagnostics.

   a. May need to be limited or withheld until discussion with patient's hospice care team.

      i. Tests should be based on patient-defined goals of care.

      ii. Low burden, noninvasive means to reveal reversible pathology, or clarified prognosis should generally be used first.

7. Carefully consider therapeutic modalities.

   a. Management is based on patient-defined goals of care. Ensure that automatic algorithms (eg, antibiotics for pneumonia) are used only if they also meet patient goals of care.

8. Consider disposition based on patient goals and preferences.

   a. Determine after a discussion with hospice staff (and based on patient's goals).

   b. Return home with additional support or a direct admission to an inpatient hospice facility may be the best disposition rather than hospital admission (24-hour home support for those with difficult to manage symptoms is feasible).

9. Communicate plans of care clearly to patient or surrogate and hospice.

   a. The inpatient palliative care service (if available) and hospice should be notified if the patient is to be admitted to the hospital.

   b. Patient/caregiver should be made aware of next steps in plan of care (for example, a discharge home on adjusted pain medications or in-patient hospice).

Adapted from Lamba S, Quest TE, Weissman DE. Emergency Department management of hospice patients. Fast Facts and Concepts 2011:246. Available at: http://www.eperc.mew.edu/EPERC/FastFactsIndex/Documents/ff_246.htm. Accessed July 16, 2012; with permission.

Box 4
Approach to the management of a patient under hospice care in the emergency department

1. Assess patient eligibility for hospice care (Medicare Hospice Benefit guidelines).

   a. Does the patient have a prognosis that is 6 months or less if the disease runs its expected course?

   b. Ask the surprise question, "Would I be surprised if this patient died within the next 6 months?"

2. Discuss disposition to hospice care with the primary care provider for the patient.

   a. Discuss the current condition, prognosis, and prior goals of care conversations and proposed enrollment to hospice.

   b. Ask if the provider is willing to be the follow-up and continuing care physician of record for hospice.

3. Assess whether the patient goals of care are consistent with the hospice philosophy by asking clarifying questions:

   a. "What have you been told about the status of your illness and what to expect in the near future?"

   b. "Has anyone talked to you about your prognosis and how much time you likely have?"

   c. "Are there any plans for new treatments that will help you extend your life?"

   d. "What do you know about hospice?"

4. Introduce hospice as a care system to the patient and family.

   a. Discuss the core aspects of hospice and how some specific resources can help the patient (eg, 24/7 on-call assistance, home visits for symptom management, emotional, and chaplaincy support).

   b. Address concerns and clarify misconceptions.

   c. Phrase recommendations for hospice care in positive language, grounded in the patient's own goals: "I think the best way to help you stay at home, avoid the hospital, and stay as fit as possible for whatever time you have left is to receive hospice care at your home...."

5. Make a referral to hospice.

   a. When calling a hospice agency, anticipate commonly asked questions:

      i. What is the terminal illness or hospice qualifying diagnosis?

      ii. Who will be the following physician? (see Step 2)

      iii. What equipment will be needed immediately (eg, home oxygen)?

      iv. Is there a caregiver at home?

      v. What is the patient's code status?

   (A directive is not necessary for enrollment, but the hospice team needs to be aware of code status.)

6. Write orders.

   a. Sample ED-initiated hospice referral orders:

      i. Evaluate and admit/enroll Mr/Mrs_____ in hospice care.

      ii. Terminal diagnosis: _____.

      iii. Expected prognosis: terminal illness with a less than 6-month survival likely if the disease runs its normal expected course, or more specific as needed.

      iv. Dr _____ will follow the patient in hospice.

7. Ensure patient and surrogates understand the plan and next steps.

    a. Communicate the next steps after discharge from ED.

    b. Provide the name and contact number for hospice agency.

Adapted from Lamba S, Quest TE, Weissman DE. Initiating a hospice referral from the emergency department. Fast Facts and Concepts 2011:247. Available at: http://www.eperc.mcw.edu/EPERC/FastFactsIndex/Documents/ff_247.htm. Accessed July 16, 2012; with permission.

opportunity to assess patient needs/goals of care and initiate discussions about hospice in eligible patients.[35,96,100,103,106] Hospice may be considered in eligible patients when the pre-eminent care goal is relief of symptoms, such that they want therapy aimed at maintaining quality of life, without a major focus on life prolongation.[103]

Studies demonstrate that hospice enrollment may (1) provide optimal support for terminal disease-related physical and psychosocial symptoms, (2) provide assistance to family and caregivers with improved well-being as well as bereavement outcomes, (3) lead to increase in overall patient, family, and physician satisfaction with care at EOL, and (4) have an impact hospital outcomes, such as reduction in hospital length of stay, total health care expenditures, and repeat ED visits.[34,103,107] Hospice remains an underutilized resource, however.[34,35,97,103] Of the 2.4 million deaths in the United States in 2007, 38% of patients received hospice care. The median length of service under hospice is approximately 20 days with approximately one-third of patients receiving hospice care for 7 days or fewer.[97] Thus, many eligible patients if considered for hospice are enrolled too late in the course of disease to realize the full benefit of hospice.[34,97]

A stepwise approach to hospice referral is recommended, and assessing eligibility is the key initial step (**Box 4**). Effective communication about next steps with family and primary care provider is essential.[34,35,96,100] Hospice care is preferably set up at a location the patient calls home (a private residence or long-term care facility) and direct admissions to some hospice facilities can also occur. Patients can usually be enrolled in hospice care within 24 to 48 hours of referral. If a patient cannot be discharged home safely, observation versus short inpatient admission may be needed.[100]

MANAGING THE ACTIVELY DYING PATIENT IN THE EMERGENCY DEPARTMENT

Two distinct death trajectories have been recently discussed in ED literature: the so-called spectacular death—a resource-intensive event, for example, a traumatic, sudden event in a young person where multiple personnel are involved, and the so-called subtacular death, for example, ED death of an older person with a DNR directive who enters the final actively dying phase after a prolonged chronic illness.[106] Although it is important to give families a general idea of how long a patient might live, it is also necessary to advise them about the inherent unpredictability of the moment of death.[107–109]

It is important for clinicians to recognize the many physiologic changes related to the syndrome of imminent death.[107,109,110] An understanding of the underlying pathophysiology helps ED clinicians address each symptom effectively, support the family, and address concerns (**Table 8**). It may be helpful to reiterate that patient experiences may be different from what family perceives, for example, thirst issues may concern a family when oral intake declines but may not be distressing to the patient. Even though the loss of a loved one may have been expected for some time, family may

Table 8
Recognizing the signs and managing the actively dying patient in the emergency department

Changes as Death Approaches	Signs	Management
1. Fatigue	Inability to move or to lift head off pillow	Need not be treated (medications to manage fatigue may be discontinued)
2. Cutaneous ischemia	Erythema or skin breakdown (pressure ulcers)	• Turn frequently, cushioning and air mattress
3. Decreased oral intake of food	• Anorexia • Progressive weight loss (temporal wasting prominent)	• Dehydration/ketosis in the last hours may not cause distress, may stimulate endorphin release and promote sense of well-being[a] • Family support to explain the process
4. Decreased oral intake of fluids	• Dry mucous membranes	• Moisten oral mucosa often (artificial saliva, ice chips) • Lubricate lips/nose with petroleum jelly[a]
5. Cardiac and renal dysfunction	• Tachycardia • Decreased blood pressure • Cool, clammy, and pale skin • Cyanosis • Livedo reticularis • Dark urine and oliguria	Parenteral fluids not usually indicated if patient death is imminent because they may not reverse circulation shutdown
6. Neurologic dysfunction	• Decreasing level of consciousness (drowsy, nonresponsive to stimuli) • Decreased communication (monosyllabic responses, nonverbal) • Loss of swallowing ability • Incontinence • Loss of ability to close eyes • Death rattle (gurgling oropharyngeal and endobronchial secretions)	• Encourage family to talk to patient as if patient were conscious • Frequent artificial tears to avoid dry eyes • Encourage family to give the patient permission to let go ("We will miss you but we will be OK") • Oropharyngeal suction may not be helpful • Scopolamine or glycopyrrolate (0.2 mg SC every 4 h as needed) to decrease secretions[b]
7. Respiratory dysfunction	• Increased or decreased rates • Abnormal respiratory pattern (Cheyne-Stokes or agonal)	Reassurance to family
8. Pain	Facial grimacing	• Discontinue routine dosing or continuous infusions of morphine when renal clearance decreases and administer when needed • Recognize that grimacing/agitation may be signs of delirium and added opioid doses may worsen same

(continued on next page)

Table 8
(continued)

Changes as Death Approaches	Signs	Management
9. Terminal delirium	• Cognitive failure (eg, day-night reversal) • Agitation, restless, moaning	• Assess finality and irreversibility of situation and explain to family • Benzodiazepines (lorazepam elixir 1–2 mg every h as needed to settle patient) or sedating neuroleptics (haloperidol 0.5–2 mg SC, IV, or pr every 1 h as needed)[c]

[a] *Data from* McCann RM, Hall WJ, Groth-Juncker A. Comfort care for terminally ill patients: the appropriate use of nutrition and hydration. JAMA 1994;272:1263–6.
[b] *Data from* Hughes AC, Wilcock A, Corcoran R. Management of "death rattle." J Pain Symptom Management 1996;12:271–2.
[c] *Data from* Shuster JL. Delirium, confusion, and agitation at the end of life. J Palliat Med 1998;1:177–86.
  Data from Emanual L, von Gunten CF, Ferris FD, editors. The education for physicians on end-of-life care (EPEC) Curriculum. The EPEC Project. The Robert Wood Johnson, Foundation; 1999; and Ellershaw J, Ward C. Care of the dying patient: the last hours or days of life. BMJ 2003;326:30–4.

require intense support in these last hours; and allowing to be spent with the body may assist caregivers with acute grief.[107,111]

SUMMARY

It is impossible to put all aspects of palliative care into one article. The authors' objective is to give readers a broad overview of general principles. Geriatric care in EDs, by the nature of the specialty, must include an understanding of disease trajectory, prognostication, and symptom management in EOL as well as the psychosocial needs of dying patients and their families.

An understanding of palliative medicine is important for several reasons: palliative and hospice medicine is a subspecialty of EM; patients have the need for clinicians to have this expertise; and most people want to die in familiar surroundings. With knowledge of this subspecialty, physicians can help patients be symptom-free and transition care to a more appropriate venue, whether home with visiting nurses or in hospice care. Clinicians' knowledge of all aspects of palliative medicine helps patients better understand their disease and symptom and better meet their goal of care.

REFERENCES

1. World Health Organization. Definition of palliative care. Available at: http://www.who.int/cancer/palliative/definition/en/. Accessed August 15, 2011.
2. Recognition of subspecialty boards in emergency medicine. Available at: http://www.acep.org/content.aspx?id=34884. Accessed September 3, 2011.
3. Quest T, Marco C, Derse A. Hospice and palliative medicine: new subspecialty, new opportunities. Ann Emerg Med 2009;54:94–101.
4. Beemath A, Zalenski R. Palliative emergency medicine: resuscitating comfort care? Ann Emerg Med 2009;4:103–4.

5. Ciemins E, Blum L, Nunley M, et al. The economic and clinical impact of an inpatient palliative care consultation service: a multifaceted approach. J Palliat Med 2007;10:1347–55.
6. National Institutes of Health State-of-the-Science Conference Statement on Improving End-of-Life Care (2004). Available at: http://consensus.nih.gov/2004/2004EndOfLifeCareSOS024html. Accessed September 10, 2011.
7. Quest T, Asplin B, Cairns C, et al. Research priorities for palliative and end-of-life care in the emergency setting. Acad Emerg Med 2011;18:e70–6.
8. Penrod J, Deb P, Dellenbaugh C, et al. Hospital-based palliative care consultation: effects on hospital cost. J Palliat Med 2010;13:973–6.
9. Temel J, Greer J, Muzikansky A, et al. Early palliative care for patients with metastatic non-small-call lung cancer. N Engl J Med 2010;363:733–42.
10. Morrison RS, Penrod JD, Cassel B, et al. Cost savings associated with US hospital palliative care consultation programs. Arch Intern Med 2008;168:1783–90.
11. Smith TJ, Cassel JB. Cost and non-clinical outcomes of palliative care. J Pain Symptom Manage 2009;38:32–42.
12. Penrod J, Deb P, Luhrs C, et al. Cost and utilization outcomes of patients receiving hospital-based palliative care consultation. J Palliat Med 2006;9:855–60.
13. Meier D, Beresford L. Fast response is key to partnering with the emergency department. J Palliat Med 2007;10:641–5.
14. Stone S. Emergency department research in palliative care: challenges in recruitment. J Palliat Med 2009;12:867–8.
15. Grudzen C, Richardson L, Morrison M, et al. Palliative care needs of seriously ill, older adults presenting to the Emergency Department. Acad Emerg Med 2010; 17:1253–7.
16. Smith A, Fisher J, Schnoberg M, et al. Am I doing the right thing? Provider perspectives on improving palliative care in the Emergency Department. Ann Emerg Med 2009;54:86–94.
17. Ausband S, March J, Brown L. National prevalence of palliative care protocols in emergency medical services. Prehosp Emerg Care 2002;6:36–40.
18. Grudzen C, Stone S, Morrison R. The palliative care model for emergency department patients with advanced illness. J Palliat Med 2011;14:945–50.
19. The SUPPORT Principal Investigators. A controlled trial to improve care for seriously ill hospitalized patients: the study to understand prognoses and preferences for outcomes and risks of treatments (SUPPORT). JAMA 1995;274:1591–8.
20. Education in palliative and end-of-life care for emergency medicine. Available at: http://www.epec.net/epec.em.php. Accessed May 2, 2012.
21. Kuchn BM. Hospitals embrace palliative care. JAMA 2007;298(11):1263–5.
22. O'Mahony S, Blank A, Simpson J, et al. Preliminary report of a palliative care and case management project in an emergency department for chronically ill elderly patients. J Urban Health 2008;85:443–51.
23. Smith AK, McCarthy E, Weber E, et al. Half of older Americans seen in emergency department in last month of life; most admitted to hospital, and many die there. Health Aff (Millwood) 2012;31:1277–85.
24. Rosenwax LK, McNamara BA, Murrary K, et al. Hospital and emergency department use in the last year of life: a baseline for future modifications to end-of-life care. Med J Aust 2011;194:570–3.
25. Lamba S. Early goal-directed palliative therapy in the emergency department: a step to move palliative care upstream. J Palliat Med 2009;12:767.
26. Chan GK. End-of-life models and emergency department care. Acad Emerg Med 2004;11(1):79–86.

27. Lamba S, Nagurka R, Walther S, et al. Emergency-Department-initiated palliative care consults: a descriptive analysis. J Palliat Med 2012;15(6):633–6.
28. Lamba S, Mosenthal AC. Hospice and palliative medicine: a novel subspecialty of emergency medicine. J Emerg Med 2010, in press.
29. Goldstein NE, Morrison RS. The intersection between geriatrics and palliative care: a call for a new research agenda. J Am Geriatr Soc 2005;53:1593–8.
30. Hogan TM, Losman ED, Carpenter CR, et al. Development of geriatric competencies for emergency medicine residents using an expert consensus process. Acad Emerg Med 2010;17:316–24.
31. Chan G, Bryant EN, Lamba S, et al. Clinical practice guidelines: a technical assistance resource from the IPAL-EM Project. Center to Advance Palliative Care. Available at: http://ipal-live.capc.stackop.com/downlloads/ipal-em-clinical-practice-guidelineslpdf. Accessed July 20, 2012.
32. Glare PA, Sinclair CT. Palliative medicine review: prognostication. J Palliat Med 2008;11(1):84–103.
33. Head B, Ritchie CS, Smoot TM. Prognostication in hospice care: can the palliative performance scale help? J Palliat Med 2005;8:492–502.
34. Lamba S, Quest TE. Hospice care and the emergency department: rules, regulations, and referrals. Ann Emerg Med 2010;53:282–90.
35. Gazelle G. Understanding hospice—an underutilized option for life's final chapter. N Engl J Med 2007;357:321–4.
36. Grudzen CR, Hwang U, Cohen JA, et al. Characteristics of emergency department patients who receive a palliative care consultation. J Palliat Med 2012;15:396–9.
37. Lamba S, Nagurka R, Murano T, et al. Early identification of dying trajectories in emergency department patients: potential impact on hospital care. J Palliat Med 2012;15:392–5.
38. Glajchen M, Lawson R, Homel P, et al. A rapid two-stage screening protocol for palliative care in the emergency department: a quality improvement initiative. J Pain Symptom Manage 2011;42:657–62.
39. Weissman DE, Meier DE. Identifying patients in need of a palliative care assessment in the hospital setting: a consensus report from the Center to Advance Palliative Care. J Palliat Med 2011;14:1–5. http://dx.doi.org/10.1089/jpm.2010.0347.
40. Richards TC, Gisondi MA, Chang C, et al. Palliative care symptom assessment for patients with cancer in the emergency department: validation of the screen for palliative and end-of-life care needs in the emergency department instrument. J Palliat Med 2011;14:757–64.
41. Quest TE, Bryant EN, Waugh D. Palliative Care emergency department screening tool. A technical assistance resource from the IPAL-EM Project, Center to Advance Palliative Care. Available at: http://ipal-live.capc.stackop.com/downloads/ipal-em-palliative-care-ed-screening-tool.pdf. Accessed July 20, 2012.
42. Carpenter CR, DesPain B, Keeling T, et al. The six item screener and AD8 for the detection of cognitive impairment in geriatric emergency department patients. Ann Emerg Med 2011;57:653–61.
43. Carpenter CR, Bassett ER, Fischer GM, et al. Four sensitive screening tools to detect cognitive dysfunction in geriatric emergency department patients: brief Alzheimer's Screen, Short Blessed Test, Ottawa3DY, and the Caregiver Administered AD8. Acad Emerg Med 2011;18:374–84.
44. Carpenter CR, Griffey RT, Stark S, et al. Physician and nurse acceptance of geriatric technicians to screen for geriatric syndromes in the emergency department. West J Emerg Med 2011;12:489–95.

45. Smith AK, Schonberg MA, Fisher J, et al. Emergency department experiences of acutely symptomatic patients with terminal illness and their family caregivers. J Pain Symptom Manage 2010;39:972–81.
46. Curtis JR, Wenrich MD, Carline JD, et al. Understanding physicians' skills at providing end-of-life care perspectives of patients, families, and health care workers. J Gen Intern Med 2001;16:41–9.
47. Steinhauer KE, Clipp EC, McNeilly M. In search of a good death: observations of patients, families and providers. Ann Intern Med 2000;132:825–32.
48. Wenrich MD, Curtis JR, Shannon SE, et al. Communicating with dying patients within the spectrum of medicare care from terminal diagnosis to death. Arch Intern Med 2001;161:868–74.
49. Roberts CS, Cox CE, Reintgen DS, et al. Influence of physician communication on newly diagnosed breast patients' psychologic adjustment and decision-making. Cancer 1994;74:336–41.
50. Kaplan SH, Ware JE. The patients role in healthcare and quality assessment. In: Goldfield N, Nash DB, editors. Providing quality care: future challenges. Ann Arbor (MI): Health Administration Press; 1995. p. 26–7.
51. Fogarty LA, Curbow BA, Wingard JR. Can 40 seconds of compassion reduce patient anxiety? J Clin Oncol 1999;17:371–9.
52. Hofman JC, Wenger NS, Davis RB, et al. Patient preferences for communication with physicians about end-of-life decisions. SUPPORT Investigators. Study to understand prognoses and preference for outcomes and risks of treatment. Ann Intern Med 1997;127:1–12.
53. Clarke EB, Curtis JR, Luce JM, et al. Quality indicators for end-of-life care in the intensive care unit. Crit Care Med 2003;31:2255–62.
54. Abbott KH, Sago JG, Breen CM, et al. Families looking back: one year after discussion of withdrawal or withholding of life-sustaining support. Crit Care Med 2001;29:197–201.
55. Baker R, Wu AW, Teng JM, et al. Family satisfaction with end-of-life care in seriously ill hospitalized adults. J Am Geriatr Soc 2000;48:S61–9.
56. Azoulay E, Chevret S, LeLev G, et al. Half the families of intensive care unit patients experience inadequate communication with physicians. Crit Care Med 2000;28:3044–9.
57. Kaldjian LC, Curtis AE, Shinkunas LA, et al. Goals of care toward the end of life: a structured literature review. Am J Hosp Palliat Care 2009;25(6):501–11.
58. Arnold R, Nelson J, Prendergast T, et al. Critical Care communication (C3) Module III: Determining goals of care. Available at: www.capc.org/palliative-care-professional-development/Training/c3-module-ipal-icu.pdf.
59. Weissman DE, Quill TE, Arnold RM. The family meeting: end of life goal setting and future planning. Fast facts and concepts. 2010:227. Available at: http://www.eperc.mcw.edu/fastfact/ff_227.htm.
60. Kaldjian LC, Erekson ZD, Haberle TH, et al. Code status discussions and goals of care among hospitalized adults. J Med Ethics 2009;35:338–42.
61. Emanuel LL, Ferris FD, von Gunten CF. Education for Physicians on End-of-Life Care (EPEC). Am J Hosp Palliat Care 2002;19(1):17.
62. Sessums LL, Zembrzuska H, Jackson J. Does this patient have medical decision-making capacity. JAMA 2011;306:420–7.
63. Suhl J, Simons P, Reedy T, et al. Myth of substituted judgment. Surrogate decision making regarding life support is unreliable. Arch Intern Med 1994;154:90–6.
64. Singer PA, Robertson G, Roy DJ. Bioethics for clinicians: 6. Advance care planning. CMAJ 1996;155:1689–92.

65. Gillick MR. Advance care planning. N Engl J Med 2004;350:7–8.
66. Prendergast TJ. Advance care planning: pitfalls, progress, promise. Crit Care Med 2001;29:N34–9.
67. Tulsky JA. Beyond advance directives: importance of communication skills at the end of life. JAMA 2005;294:359–65.
68. Detering KM, Hancock AD, Reade MC, et al. The impact of a coordinated, systematic model of patient centered advance care planning in the ER in elderly patients: a randomized controlled trial. BMJ 2010;340:c1345.
69. Mirarchi F, Kalantzis S, McCracken E, et al. Triad II: do living wills have an impact on pre-hospital lifesaving care? J Emerg Med 2009;36:105–15.
70. Mirarchi F, Costello E, Puller J, et al. TRIAD III: Nationwide assessment of living wills and do not resuscitate orders. J Emerg Med 2012;42:511–20.
71. Adams DH, Snedden DP. How misconceptions among elderly patients regarding survival outcomes of inpatient cardiopulmonary resuscitation affect do-not-resuscitate orders. J Am Osteopath Assoc 2006;106:402–4.
72. Volandes AE, Paasche-Orlow MK, Barry MJ, et al. Video decision support tool for advance care planning in dementia: randomised controlled trial. BMJ 2009;338:b2159.
73. Marsella A. Exploring the literature surrounding the transition into palliative care: a scoping review. Int J Palliat Nurs 2009;15:186–9.
74. Gisondi MA. A case for education in palliative and end-of-life care in emergency medicine. Acad Emerg Med 2009;16:181–3.
75. Hauser JM. Lost in transition: the ethic of the palliative care handoff. J Pain Symptom Manage 2009;37:930–3.
76. Snow V, Beck D, Budnitz T, et al. Transitions of care consensus policy statement: American College of physicians-Society of general internal medicine-Society of hospital medicine-American geriatrics Society-American College of emergency physicians-Society of Academic medicine. J Hosp Med 2009;4: 364–70.
77. Barbera L, Paszat L, Chartier C. Indicators of poor quality end-of-life care in Ontario. J Palliat Care 2006;22:12–7.
78. Evans WG, Cutson TM, Steinhauser KE, et al. Is there no place like home? Caregivers recall reasons for and experience upon transfer from home hospice into inpatient facilities. J Palliat Med 2006;9:100–10.
79. Mosenthal AC, Francis Lee K. Management of dyspnea at the end of life: relief for patients and surgeons. J Am Coll Surg 2002;194:377–86.
80. Rosenberg M. Geriatric palliative care. 2012. Available at: http://www.acep.org/Clinical—Practice-Management/Geriatric-Videos.
81. Qaseem A, Snow V, Shekelle P, et al. Evidence-based interventions to improve the palliative care of pain, dyspnea and depression at the end of life: a clinical practice guidelines from the American College of Physicians. Ann Intern Med 2008;148:141–6.
82. ACEP. Ethical issues at the end of life. Clinical & Practice Management. 2008.
83. Center for ethics in health care. POLST. 2008. Available at: http://www.ohsu.edu/polst/programs/state+programs.htm.
84. Pauls M. Ethics in the trenches: preparing for ethical challenges in the emergency department. CJEM 2002;4:45–8.
85. ACEP. Ethical issues in emergency department care at the end-of-life. Ann Emerg Med 2008;52:592.
86. ACEP. Code of ethics for emergency physicians. 2012. Available at: http://www.acep.org.

87. United States Conference of Catholic Bishops. Ethical and religious directives for catholic health care services. 5th edition. Washington, DC; 2009. p. 32.

88. ACEP. The ethics of health care reform: issues in emergency-medicine – an information paper. 2012. Available at: http://www.acep.org.

89. Goold SD, Williams B, Arnold RM. Conflicts regarding decisions to limit treatment: a differential diagnosis. JAMA 2000;283:909–14.

90. Marco CA, Larkin GL, Moskop JC, et al. The determination of "futility" in emergency medicine. Ann Emerg Med 2000;35:604–12.

91. Parmley LC. Ethical consideration in end-of-life medicine. Internet J Emerg Intensive Care Med 1999;3(2). http://www.ispub.com/journals/IJEICM/Vol3N2/ethics.htm.

92. SAEM Ethics Committee. Guide to teaching ethics in emergency medicine residency programs. 2005:40–4. Available at: www.saem.org.

93. De Graeff A, Dean M. Palliative sedation therapy in the last weeks of life: a literature review and recommendations for standards. J Palliat Med 2007;10:67–85.

94. National Ethics Committee, Veterans Health Administration. The ethics of palliative sedation as a therapy of last resort. Am J Hosp Palliat Care 2007;23:483–91.

95. Kirk TW, Mahon MM. National hospice and palliative care organization position statement and commentary on the use of palliative sedation in imminently dying terminally ill patients. J Pain Symptom Manage 2010;39:914–23.

96. Centers for Medicare, Medicaid Services, Medicare Coverage Database. LCD (local coverage determination) for hospice: determining terminal status (L25678). Available at: http://www.cms.gov/mcd/viewlcd.asp?lcd_id_25678&;lcd_version_27&show_all#top. Accessed July 19, 2012.

97. National Hospice and Palliative Care Organization. NHPCO facts and figures: hospice care in America. Alexandria (VA); 2008. Available at: http://www.nhpco.org/files/public/Statistics_Research/NHPCO_facts-and-figures_Nov2007.pdf. Accessed January 14, 2012.

98. Lamba S, Quest TE, Weissman DE. Emergency Department management of hospice patients. Fast Facts and Concepts. 2011:246. Available at: http://www.eperc.mew.edu/EPERC/FastFactsIndex/Documents/ff_246.htm. Accessed July 16, 2012.

99. Reeves K. Hospice care in the emergency department. J Emerg Nurs 2008;34:350–1.

100. Lamba S, Quest TE, Weissman DE. Initiating a hospice referral from the emergency department. Fast Facts and Concepts. 2011:247. Available at: http://www.eperc.mcw.edu/EPERC/FastFactsIndex/Documents/ff_247.htm. Accessed July 16, 2012.

101. Chan GK. End-of-life and palliative care in the emergency department: a call for research, education, policy, and improved practice in this frontier area. J Emerg Nurs 2006;32:101–3.

102. Lamba S, Pound A, Rella JR, et al. Emergency medicine resident education in palliative care: a needs assessment. J Palliat Med 2012;15(5):516–20.

103. Meier DE. Increased access to palliative care and hospice services: opportunities to improve value in health care. Milbank Q 2011;89:343–80.

104. Von Gunten F, Weissman DE. Discussing DNR orders—part 1, 2nd edition. Fast facts and concepts. July 2005; fast fact 23. Available at: http://www.eperc.mcw.edu/fastfact/ff_023.htm. Accessed July 24, 2012.

105. Sedillot N, Holzapfel L, Jacquet-Francillon T, et al. A five-step protocol for withholding and withdrawing of life support in an emergency department: an observational study. Eur J Emerg Med 2008;15:145–9.

106. Bailey CJ, Murphy R, Porock D. Trajectories of end-of-life care in the Emergency Department. Ann Emerg Med 2011;57:362–9.
107. Emanual L, von Gunten CF, Ferris FD, editors. The education for physicians on end-of-life care (EPEC) curriculum. The EPEC project. The Robert Wood Johnson, Foundation; 1999.
108. Ellershaw J, Ward C. Care of the dying patient: the last hours or days of life. BMJ 2003;326:30–4.
109. Lichter I, Hunt E. The last 48 hours of life. J Palliat Care 1990;6:7–15.
110. Ellershaw JE, Sutcliffe JM, Saunders CM. Dehydration and the dying patient. J Pain Symptom Manage 1995;10:192–7.
111. Ferris FD, von Gunten CF, Emanuel LL. Competency in end of life care: the last hours of living. J Palliat Med 2003;6:605–13.

Evolving Prehospital, Emergency Department, and "Inpatient" Management Models for Geriatric Emergencies

Christopher R. Carpenter, MD, MSc[a,]*, Timothy F. Platts-Mills, MD[b]

KEYWORDS

- Geriatrics • Emergency medical services • Emergency service, hospital
- Case management/organization and administration • Models/organizational

KEY POINTS

- Ensuring high-quality and efficient emergency care for the growing number of older adults in the United States will require the development of alternative management strategies.
- Prehospital emergency care for older adults may be improved through the development of new methods for the early detection of acute severe illness and injury to guide timely condition-specific treatment.
- Prehospital providers may make an additional contribution to the health of older adults by conducting in-home assessments and referral of high-risk older adults.
- Emergency department care may be improved through a team approach and standardized screening procedures for important commonly overlooked conditions (eg, delirium, dementia, depression, drug-related adverse effects, neglect/abuse).
- For conditions with high mortality rates (eg, trauma, delirium), improved coordination of care during the transition from the emergency department to the inpatient setting may improve outcomes.

Dr Platts-Mills is supported by Award Number KL2 TR000084 and UL1 TR000083 from the National Center for Research Resources through the North Carolina Translational and Clinical Science Institute. The content is solely the responsibility of the authors and does not necessarily represent the official views of the National Center for Research Resources, the National Institutes of Health, or the North Carolina Translational and Clinical Science Institute.
No conflicts of interest to declare.

[a] Department of Emergency Medicine, Washington University in St. Louis, Campus Box 8072, 660 S. Euclid Avenue, St. Louis, MO 63011, USA; [b] Department of Emergency Medicine, University of North Carolina at Chapel Hill, 170 Manning Drive CB#7594, Chapel Hill, NC 27599-7594, USA
* Corresponding author.
E-mail address: carpenterc@wusm.wustl.edu

Clin Geriatr Med 29 (2013) 31–47
http://dx.doi.org/10.1016/j.cger.2012.09.003
0749-0690/13/$ – see front matter © 2013 Elsevier Inc. All rights reserved.

INTRODUCTION

A historically unprecedented increase in the world's geriatric population over the next 4 decades will challenge prehospital emergency medical services, health care providers, and hospital administrators to adapt the twentieth century infrastructure and management models to maintain reliable access to emergency medicine (EM) care.[1–5] EM nurses and physicians already identify geriatric patients as a significant source of clinical stress because of the higher burden of severe illness and injury and the greater complexity of medical decision making encountered in caring for this population.[6–10] The traditional emergency care model (**Fig. 1**A) focuses on purely diagnostic and therapeutic medical decision making, whereas the geriatric emergency care model incorporates essential elements of older adult well-being, including social isolation, transportation limitations, fixed incomes, cognitive status, and functional disability (see **Fig. 1**B).[11] Although the format and extent of change to existing organizations will depend on local resource availability and anticipated demand, almost

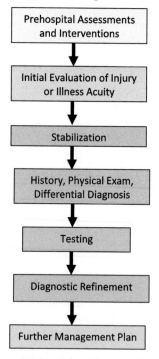

A   **Traditional EM Management Pathway***

Prehospital Assessments and Interventions

Initial Evaluation of Injury or Illness Acuity

Stabilization

History, Physical Exam, Differential Diagnosis

Testing

Diagnostic Refinement

Further Management Plan

Settings Where Processes Occur
Yellow = Home, Clinic, Accident-Scene or Nursing Home Environment
Blue = Waiting Room or Triage station
Red = ED patient room or hallway
Purple = Observation Unit, Inpatient or Outpatient Setting

Fig. 1. (*A*) Traditional EM management pathway. (*B*) Geriatric emergency care model. (*Adapted from* Sanders AB, Witzke DB, Jones JS, et al. Principles of care and application of the geriatric emergency care model. In: Sanders AB, editor. Emergency care of the elder person. St Louis (MO): Beverly-Cracom Publications; 1996. p. 59–93; with permission from the Society for Academic Emergency Medicine.)

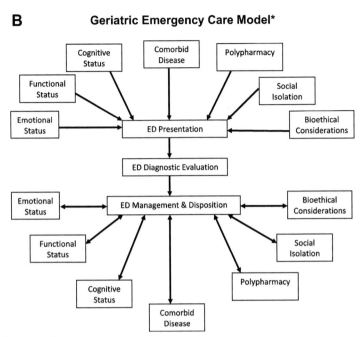

Fig. 1. (*continued*)

every health care system will need to adjust to some degree.[12] In addition, current policies that provide financial disincentives to short-term readmissions for common diagnoses have expanded the domain of EM to include the spectrum from proactive preventive care by prehospital providers to a paradigm-shifting concept of the "hospital at home." This article explores these evolving management models within the context of contemporary emergency care for geriatric adults.

The objective of EM care for the aging adult is to alleviate suffering while providing prompt diagnosis of life-threatening conditions to prolong quality of life, while respecting patient and family autonomy. Chronologic age is not always synonymous with physiologic age, and therefore neither a "one size fits all" nor an age-based approach to care exists. Instead, optimal care of the older adult requires attention to the psychosocial dynamic between the patient and the patient's family or care providers, thus distinguishing geriatric care from the traditional EM care model (see **Fig. 1**).[11] Emergency department (ED) management that neglects geriatric care principles produces suboptimal outcomes.[13] Therefore, these principles should be incorporated into prehospital provider and EM residency education. Unfortunately, EM graduate medical education has not emphasized geriatric principles in the past.[14]

Although the younger patient typically presents to the ED with a symptom-based chief complaint that is generally amenable to a focused diagnostic and therapeutic approach, geriatric adults more commonly report atypical or nonspecific symptoms that prompted the patient or their fatigued caregiver to seek medical care.[15] Although these symptoms can be the manifestation of an acute and reversible life-threatening illness, more often the symptoms are a result of a complex mix of chronic disease processes, some of which have not yet been diagnosed. In addition, the presenting complaint, whether life-threatening or not, may represent just one of the threats to the older patient's well-being, a situation that is far less likely in younger popula- tions.[16,17] These hidden threats are often viewed as outside the domain of traditional EM care and include physical or emotional isolation and neglect,[18,19] economic disparities, polypharmacy,[20–22] functional and cognitive decline,[23,24] malnutrition,[25,26] fall risk,[27,28] and inadequate access to transportation. To provide optimal evidence- based care incorporating geriatric principles, future EM management models will need to incorporate a sufficiently robust and adaptable organization that incorporates appropriately trained personnel; reliable streams of communication between preho- spital, ED, inpatient, and outpatient services; valid protocols; and a geriatric-friendly infrastructure.[3,8]

PREHOSPITAL GERIATRIC CARE OPPORTUNITIES

Because older adults often require assistance with transportation to the ED, prehospi- tal providers must and will likely continue to care for a disproportionate number of older patients. As of 2007, adults aged 65 years and older constituted 38% of all emer- gency medical services (EMS) transports in the United States.[29] In some regions, transports of older adults are anticipated to exceed 50% of total EMS transports in the next decade.[29,30] In 2003, the American Geriatrics Society and the National Council of State EMS Training Coordinators developed the Geriatric Education for Emergency Medicine Services (GEMS) curriculum.[31] Providers who have completed the GEMS course report improvement in communication, abuse assessments, and falls evaluation with elderly patients.[32] Internet-based learning for EMS providers is also possible.[33]

EMS providers are willing to promote geriatric health through proactive screening programs that extend beyond the traditional scoop-and-run approach, but simple screen-and-refer pathways are ineffective.[34,35] The burden of EMS care for older adults has generated 3 major areas of inquiry,[36] expressed here as questions:

1. For older adults with acute severe illness and injury, are there ways to improve the capacity of EMS providers to diagnose specific conditions to provide early treatment?
2. For older adults with nonsevere conditions, are alternatives methods of providing care available that are less costly than the traditional approach of EMS transport, ED evaluation, and EMS return transport?
3. Can prehospital providers serve as public health stewards by conducting rapid screening assessments to identify older adults in the community at high risk for adverse events?

Progress on each of these areas of inquiry is described.

Specific time-sensitive diseases that might benefit from rapid diagnostics include myocardial infarction, stroke, and trauma. Although electrocardiograms in the preho- spital setting are now broadly used, protocols that recognize that most older adults with ST-elevation myocardial infarction do not have chest pain have not been broadly implemented.[37] Prehospital stroke protocols have been developed and validated and have the potential to accelerate access to thrombolytic therapy.[38] However, the public health impact of these protocols is limited by the controversial benefit-to-risk ratio of thrombolytics for stroke in any age groups, and specifically in geriatric patients.[39–47] In prehospital trauma care, injury severity tends to be underrecognized in older adults,[48,49] a problem that also occurs when older patients reach the ED.[50] The incor- poration of age into trauma assessments may help prevent undertriage of older trauma patients.

Alternative methods of providing prehospital care for older adults who might otherwise seek care in the ED have the potential to reduce costs. Any such approach must also have the capacity to identify patients with time-sensitive illness and injury. One option is telemedicine, in which a patient assessment by a physician occurs verbally and visually via audio and video transmissions. Telemedicine is currently being studied as a method of reducing ED visits. Telemonitoring of older adults involves daily assessments using the same technology, but a randomized study did not find that this approach reduced ED visits or hospitalizations.[51] Increased access to primary care after an EMS evaluation has been shown to decrease ED use.[52,53] However, access to primary care for older adults in the United States continues to be a problem, reflecting both reimbursement problems and personnel shortages.[54,55]

The potential of prehospital providers to screen older adults for risk of falls, depression, or medication mismanagement has been demonstrated.[56] Prehospital screening for fall risk has yielded equivocal outcomes, but prospective referrals during the initial in-home evaluation are superior to retrospective EMS medical record review and refer models.[57–60] Ongoing research will assess the effectiveness of EMS fall screening in the near future.[61,62] The impact of EMS screening on ED use and other health outcomes has not been evaluated. Given the large number of at-risk older adults with limited access to primary care in the United States,[54] a large potential value exists in developing the capacity of EMS providers to identify older adults most likely to benefit from increased access to health care. Implementing this type of preventive care broadly will require additional research demonstrating an impact on important outcomes, and mechanisms to reimburse EMS systems.[63,64]

THE GERIATRIC ED

One method by which to classify ED clinical services for geriatric adults is to assess the availability of human resources, care processes, and community services linkages.[65] In general, specialized tertiary care EDs lack effective linkages to outpatient geriatric services, particularly when contrasted with the least-specialized community hospitals.[66] This article distinguishes 2 stylistic approaches to caring for geriatric emergencies: the geriatric-friendly ED versus the geriatric-specific ED. Although all general adult EDs should aspire to become geriatric-friendly, the geriatric-specific ED only manages older adults. Currently, very few geriatric-specific EDs exist, and most are within hospitals that also have a general adult ED, but they are geographically distinct, with separate staffing, protocols, and objectives. Most health care systems lack the resources to build a geriatric-specific ED. In contrast, geriatric-friendly EDs can be achieved in most settings and represent the baseline level of geriatric care to which all adult EDs should aspire. A quality assessment tool for the geriatric-friendly ED has been developed and incorporates 3 subscales: screening/assessment, discharge planning, and community services.[67] Although this instrument awaits validation, quality assessment tools for the geriatric-friendly ED will be essential for clinicians, managers, administrators, and payers to evaluate the merits of this concept.

The attributes of effective ED-based geriatric case management include an evidence-based practice model, nursing clinical involvement and leadership, high-risk screening protocols, focused geriatric assessments, the initiation of care and disposition planning in the ED, interprofessional and capacity-building work practices, post-ED discharge follow-up, and established quality improvement processes.[68] Clinical research in alternative ED management models that fails to demonstrate a clinically significant effect usually lack attention to more than one of these domains.[68,69] In particular, whether the hospital environment is rural or urban, academic or community, engaging nurses in protocol development and case management is essential, as demonstrated by the Regional Geriatric Programs of Ontario.[12]

Modification of the general adult ED toward a more geriatric-friendly ED that simultaneously yields optimal outcomes while minimizing resource consumption will need to incorporate focused staff education, pragmatic and evidence-based screening services, simple infrastructural considerations that accommodate the physiologic changes of aging, and readily available access to geriatricians (**Table 1**). Educational priorities for physicians and nurses to improve the care of older adults have been identified: recognition of atypical disease presentation; trauma assessment principles; recognition of cognitive decline; pain management alternatives; transition of care principles; and the contribution of comorbid illnesses to both disease presentation and effective management strategies.[14] In 2011, the American College of Emergency Physicians' (ACEP) and Society for Academic Emergency Medicine (SAEM) Geriatric Sections produced and disseminated contemporary educational modules for many of these core competencies (**Box 1**).[70]

Universal screening occurs when asymptomatic individuals are evaluated for a condition. Case finding refers to the screening of a subset of patients based on the presence of risk factors. EM leaders have long advocated for both universal screening and case finding programs for geriatric syndromes such as cognitive dysfunction, fall risk, and frailty.[24,71–73] At least 2 barriers obstruct the implementation of geriatric syndrome screening. First, very few appropriately brief, pragmatic ED screening instruments have been validated for these geriatric syndromes.[36,74] Research continues to identify screening instruments for dementia,[75–77] fall risk,[78,79] and functional decline,[80–82] but these instruments have yet to be validated in other settings, and important geriatric syndromes like frailty and delirium await instrument validation in the ED.[36,74] As a result, reviews and guidelines for ED management of geriatric syndromes such as dementia are often extrapolated from non-ED settings.[83]

The second barrier is daily ED crowding and ongoing nursing shortages, which limit the time available for providers to conduct screening. One alternative management strategy is to have a "geriatric technician" (GT), an individual who is neither a nurse nor a physician with the sole responsibility of assessing elderly patients in the ED

Table 1 Considerations for the geriatric-friendly ED	
Domain	**Examples**
Staff education	Recognition of atypical disease presentation Trauma resuscitation priorities Polypharmacy Transitions of care
Screening	Falls Cognitive dysfunction Frailty Functional decline Neglect
Infrastructure	Armchair Bedside commode Large-print instructions
Accessible consults	Mobile Acute Care for the Elderly unit Stay healthy clinics Palliative care Pain management

Box 1
Available geriatric EM educational modules
General assessment of the elder patient
Abdominal pain in the elderly
Altered mental status
Chest pain and dyspnea
The dizzy elder patient
End-of-life issues
Falls
Infectious diseases
Pharmacology and polypharmacy
Physiologic changes in aging
Data from American College of Emergency Physicians. Clinical & practice management: geriatric videos. Available at: http://www.acep.org/Clinical—Practice-Management/Geriatric-Videos/. Accessed October 9, 2012.

for geriatric syndromes using simple, reliable, and valid screening instruments. The GT workforce might consist of volunteers, students, or retirees. In one busy tertiary academic medical center, EM nurses and physicians recognized the potential for the GT model to promote patient safety and improve overall clinical care without reducing ED operational flow.[84]

Changes in infrastructure appropriate for a geriatric-friendly ED overlap with those described for geriatric-specific EDs, but are simpler to implement without a geographically distinct site of care or expensive reconstruction. Simple alterations to the structure of the ED that promote a geriatric-friendly milieu include an easy chair in addition to or in place of the traditional hospital bed. Wilber and colleagues[85] showed that in appropriate geriatric patients, the easy chair was preferred, with improved patient comfort and satisfaction scores and no adverse events noted. Another easy alteration that all EDs can implement is to increase the font of discharge instructions and prescriptions to accommodate the visually impaired.

Despite focused education of providers regarding geriatric care, ample screening mechanisms, and pragmatic infrastructural modifications, the diagnosis and short-term prognosis of some elderly patients remain poorly defined at the end of an ED evaluation. Because current inpatient funding models, which rely on diagnoses to request compensation, discourage admission of these individuals, alternative rapid access consult systems provide a means to increase the likelihood that patient outcomes do not suffer from payers' policies. One approach to this problem is the mobile Acute Care for the Elderly (ACE) team. Although the traditional ACE unit is solely an inpatient site, the mobile ACE team brings the medical expertise of the unit to the ED to conduct comprehensive geriatric assessment screening[86–88] and caregiver and patient psychosocial needs assessment, and ensure access to outpatient resources based on the results of their formal assessment.[36] Some settings have used hospitalists in the ED or hospital rather than geriatricians to staff the ACE unit.[89,90]

The geriatric-specific ED would incorporate all of the principles of the geriatric-friendly ED, but would staff a geographically distinct ED with nurses, physicians, social workers, and case coordinators specially trained to care for senior adults. This focus on geriatric adults permits an infrastructure that is completely modified for the older adult, including appropriate lighting to optimize visual acuity while minimizing nocturnal delirium or other confusional states; handrails in hallways and bathrooms; protocols for pain and agitation management and fall prevention; slip-proof flooring; palliative care resources; and multidisciplinary care services with geriatric expertise that maintain continuity of care for admitted patients.

GERIATRIC EMERGENCY CARE BEYOND THE ED

Acute care for older adults does not end in the ED. For older adults with severe illness and injury, coordination of ED and inpatient care can improve the transfer of patient information, ensure that key interventions are initiated early and are continued after the patient leaves the ED, and ensure that patient care preferences are communicated to all providers. In contrast, failure to coordinate ED and inpatient care has the potential to prolong ED lengths of stay and lead to frustration on the parts of patients, families, and providers. Trauma and delirium are 2 particular conditions in which coordination with inpatient specialists is likely to be of particular value.

In the case of trauma, care at a trauma center for adults aged 80 years and older and activation of a trauma team for patients aged 70 years and older with an Injury Severity Score of 15 or more have each been associated with improved outcomes compared with usual care.[91,92] Thus, for older adults with serious injuries, early care by the trauma team is appropriate. Aggressive treatment in elderly trauma patients has been examined in observational studies, with most studies indicating the value of intensive early treatment for older adults with life-threatening injuries.[93–95] These studies also show that, as with other conditions in older adults, functional status and comorbidities are stronger predictors of outcomes from a given injury than age.

Like trauma, delirium is also a common and potentially life-threatening condition in older adults and likely to benefit from early initiation of specific therapies.[96,97] Unfortunately, delirium is underdiagnosed in older patients in the ED.[98–102] As a result, any efforts to improve outcomes for patients with delirium in the ED must first ensure the early and accurate identification of delirious patients. Once identified, the goals of delirium care are to treat underlying causes while mitigating symptoms with a minimum of physical and chemical restraints. Compared with delayed management, early care of older adults with hyperactive delirium by geriatricians and psychogeriatricians has shown improved outcomes.[103] Specifically, early interventions for hyperactive delirium in patients admitted from the ED reduce the need for physical (44% vs 63%) or chemical (49% vs 76%) restraint, reduced hospital length of stay (17 days vs 25 days), reduced the duration of delirium (11 days vs 22 days), and lowered fall rates.[103]

Once delirium is recognized, emergency providers should initiate delirium treatment in the ED. Key components of a comprehensive approach to treating delirium have been described: orientation; nonpharmacologic sleep aids; early mobilization; visual aids; hearing aids; and the prevention of dehydration.[104] Furthermore, communicating this diagnosis to the inpatient team and developing methods for continuing delirium treatment in the hospital is likely to be beneficial. Inpatient care by a multidisciplinary team led by a geriatrician with an emphasis on avoiding potential harmful interventions (eg, Foley catheters, bed rest, some medications) has been associated with a greater improvement in physical function over usual care.[105,106] This inpatient model evolved from the traditional ACE unit to designate one area of the ACE unit as the "delirium room," which is situated to permit continuous nurse monitoring with the intent to minimize delirium-related morbidity. The delirium room concept has been replicated in other inpatient settings and is cost-effective, but opponents debate whether an ED-based observation unit for suspected delirium would be ethical, cost-effective, and used appropriately.[107,108] Trials continue exploring the effect of the delirium room on patient outcomes.[109,110]

THE HOSPITAL AT HOME MODEL

For admitted patients of all ages, ED boarding times continue to increase, a trend likely to increase as baby boomers become octogenarians.[111] Thought leaders, patient safety experts, and policy-makers urge proactive and creative solutions to the challenge of ED boarding.[112] In addition, hospital care itself can be a health risk for geriatric adults with commonly reported iatrogenic events, such as functional decline, pressure sores, falls, and delirium.[113] Alternatives to traditional inpatient management models exist and early trials have been promising. The "admission avoidance" Hospital at Home model carefully selects a subset of geriatric patients for whom ED personnel deem hospital admission appropriate and who meet explicit criteria (**Table 2**)[114] for a few diagnoses, including chronic obstructive pulmonary disease exacerbations, cellulitis, or pneumonia. The difference is that rather than being transferred to the hospital ward, these patients go home with an inpatient-like management plan.

Hospital at Home care includes telemetry, and at least 12 hours of nursing care and one physician home visit each day. One meta-analysis of 5 randomized trials including 844 patients showed improved 6-month mortality (adjusted hazards ratio, 0.62; 95% CI, 0.45–0.87) for the Hospital at Home model.[115] Additionally, family members report less stress with Hospital at Home management, and health care providers view it as viable and acceptable.[116,117] In Australia this model has been sustainable over 7 years, and fewer than 5% of patients fail the home care model by requiring transfer back to the hospital.[118] In the United States, the Hospital at Home model was developed by Johns Hopkins and has been slow to disseminate.[119] The barriers to wider-spread

Table 2	
Exclusion criteria for Hospital at Home model	
Diagnosis	**Exclusion Criteria**
Congestive heart failure	Associated arrhythmia
	Known or suspected severe valvular heart disease
	Unstable angina
	Myocardial infarction within previous 3 months
	Rales in more than half the lung field at completion ED treatment
Chronic obstructive pulmonary disease	Other significant pulmonary disease, such as lung cancer or pulmonary fibrosis
Community-acquired pneumonia	Suspected supportive infection (empyema, meningitis, endocarditis)
	Alternative explanation for abnormal chest radiograph
	Cavitating lesion on chest radiograph
	Other significant pulmonary disease, such as lung cancer or pulmonary fibrosis
	Pneumonia within previous 6 weeks
	Leukopenia with leukemia, HIV, lymphoma/myeloma, or cytotoxic medications

Data from Leff B, Burton L, Bynum JW, et al. Prospective evaluation of clinical criteria to select older persons with acute medical illness for care in a hypothetical home hospital. J Am Geriatr Soc 1997;45(9):1066–73.

implementation of this model in the United States include an insufficient understanding of health care system adoption and infrastructural alteration costs, and the contradictory fee-for-service payment system that provides little incentive for hospital to adopt less-expensive alternatives to admission.[120] However, in an era of increasingly constrained health care budgets, policy-makers are beginning to note that Hospital at Home care is consistently less costly than traditional hospital management and is preferred by patients.[121]

SUMMARY

Emergency care for an aging population represents a challenge and an opportunity for multidisciplinary management of acute health issues. Ample opportunity exists for the cross-disciplinary exchange of ideas through the American Geriatrics Society Section for Enhancing Geriatric Understanding and Expertise Among Surgical and Medical Specialists,[122] the SAEM Academy of Geriatric Emergency Medicine,[123] and the ACEP Geriatric Emergency Medicine Section.[124] A paradigm shift in the traditional ED management model and inpatient scenario will likely improve health care delivery for all age groups. However, the characteristics that define high-quality alternative management models for geriatric adults have yet to be delineated. In addition, the feasibility and financial sustainability of novel prehospital screening programs, geriatric friendly EDs, inpatient delirium rooms, and the Hospital at Home model remain largely untested.[36] Nonetheless, these alternative management strategies provide a template for heterogeneous emergency care environments around the world to begin exploring more efficient pathways of care for a rapidly aging society.

REFERENCES

1. Roberts DC, McKay MP, Shaffer A. Increasing rates of emergency department visits for elderly patients in the United States, 1993 to 2003. Ann Emerg Med 2008;51(6):769–74.
2. Banarjee J, Conroy S, O'Leary V, et al. Quality care for older people with urgent and emergency care needs. British Geriatrics Society; 2011. p. 102. Available at: http://www.bgs.org.uk/campaigns/silverb/silver_book_complete.pdf.
3. Fitzgerald RT. American College of Emergency Physicians White Paper. The future of geriatric care in our Nation's emergency departments: impact and implications. 2008. Available at: http://apps.acep.org/WorkArea/DownloadAsset.aspx?id=43376.
4. Fealy GM, Treacy M, Drennan J, et al. A profile of older emergency department attendees: findings from an Irish study. J Adv Nurs 2012;68(5):1003–13.
5. Gruneir A, Silver MJ, Rochon PA. Emergency department use by older adults: a literature review on trends, appropriateness, and consequences of unmet health care needs. Med Care Res Rev 2011;68(2):131–55.
6. Schumacher JG. Emergency medicine and older adults: continuing challenges and opportunities. Am J Emerg Med 2005;23:556–60.
7. Schumacher JG, Deimling GT, Meldon SW, et al. Older adults in the emergency department: predicting physicians' burden levels. J Emerg Med 2006;30(4):455–60.
8. Hwang U, Morrison RS. The geriatric emergency department. J Am Geriatr Soc 2007;55(11):1873–6.
9. Samaras N, Chevalley T, Samaras D, et al. Older patients in the emergency department: a review. Ann Emerg Med 2010;56(3):261–9.
10. Roethler C, Adelman T, Parsons V. Assessing emergency nurses' geriatric knowledge and perceptions of their geriatric care. J Emerg Nurs 2011;37(2):132–7.

11. Sanders AB, Witzke DB, Jones JS, et al. Principles of care and application of the geriatric emergency care model. In: Sanders AB, editor. Emergency care of the elder person. St Louis (MO): Beverly-Cracom Publications; 1996. p. 59–93.

12. Ryan D, Liu B, Awad M, et al. Improving older patients' experience in the emergency room: the senior-friendly emergency room. Aging Health 2011;7(6): 901–9.

13. Schnitker L, Martin-Khan M, Beattie E, et al. Negative health outcomes and adverse events in older people attending emergency departments: a systematic review. Australas Emerg Nurs J 2011;14:141–62.

14. Hogan TM, Losman ED, Carpenter CR, et al. Development of geriatric competencies for emergency medicine residents using an expert consensus process. Acad Emerg Med 2010;17(3):316–24.

15. Nemac M, Koller MT, Nickel CH, et al. Patients presenting to the emergency department with non-specific complaints: the Basel Non-specific Complaints (BANC) study. Acad Emerg Med 2010;17(3):284–92.

16. Keim SM, Sanders AB. Geriatric emergency department use and care. In: Meldon SW, Ma OJ, Woolard R, editors. Geriatric emergency medicine. New York: McGraw Hill; 2004. p. 1–3.

17. Birnbaumer DM. The elder patient. In: Marx JA, Hockberger RS, Walls RM, et al, editors. Rosen's emergency medicine: concepts and clinical practice. 7th edition. Philadelphia: Mosby Elsevier; 2010. p. 2348–52.

18. Hastings SN, George LK, Fillenbaum GG, et al. Does lack of social support lead to more ED visits for older adults? Am J Emerg Med 2008;26(4):454–61.

19. Papaioannou ES, Räihä I, Kivelä SL. Self-neglect of the elderly. An overview. Eur J Gen Pract 2012;18(3):187–90.

20. Hohl CM, Dankoff J, Colacone A, et al. Polypharmacy, adverse drug-related events, and potential adverse drug interactions in elderly patients presenting to an emergency department. Ann Emerg Med 2001;38(6):666–71.

21. Hohl CM, Zed PJ, Brubacher JR, et al. Do emergency physicians attribute drug-related emergency department visits to medication-related problems? Ann Emerg Med 2010;55(6):493–502.

22. Baena MI, Faus MJ, Fajardo PC, et al. Medicine-related problems resulting in emergency department visits. Eur J Clin Pharmacol 2006;62(5):387–93.

23. Gill TM, Gahbauer EA, Murphy TE, et al. Risk factors and precipitants of long-term disability in community mobility: a cohort study of older persons. Ann Intern Med 2012;156(2):131–40.

24. Sanders AB. Missed delirium in older emergency department patients: a quality-of-care problem. Ann Emerg Med 2002;39(3):338–41.

25. Dramé M, Novella JL, Lang PO, et al. Derivation and validation of a mortality-risk index from a cohort of frail elderly patients hospitalised in medical wards via emergencies: the SAFES study. Eur J Epidemiol 2008;23(12):783–91.

26. Gosch M, Joosten-Gstrein B, Heppner HJ, et al. Hyponatremia in geriatric inhospital patients: effects on results of a comprehensive geriatric assessment. Gerontology 2012;58(5):430–40.

27. Wiegand JV, Gerson LW. Preventive care in the emergency department: should emergency departments institute a falls prevention program for elder patients? A systematic review. Acad Emerg Med 2001;8:823–6.

28. Paniagua MA, Malphurs JE, Phelan EA. Older patients presenting to a county hospital ED after a fall: missed opportunities for prevention. Am J Emerg Med 2006;24(4):413–7.

29. Shah MN, Bazarian JJ, Lerner EB, et al. The epidemiology of emergency medical services use by older adults: an analysis of the National Hospital Ambulatory Medical Care Survey. Acad Emerg Med 2007;14(5):441–7.
30. Platts-Mills TF, Leacock B, Cabañas JG, et al. Emergency medical services use by the elderly: analysis of a statewide database. Prehosp Emerg Care 2010;14(3):329–33.
31. Geriatric education for emergency medical services. Available at: http://www.gemssite.com/. Accessed October 15, 2012.
32. Shah MN, Rajasekaran K, Sheahan WD, et al. The effect of the geriatrics education for emergency medical services training program in a rural community. J Am Geriatr Soc 2008;56(6):1134–9.
33. Shah MN, Swanson PA, Nobay F, et al. A novel internet-based geriatric education program for emergency medical services providers. J Am Geriatr Soc 2012; 60(9):1749–54.
34. Shah MN, Clarkson L, Lerner EB, et al. An emergency medical services program to promote the health of older adults. J Am Geriatr Soc 2006;54(6):956–62.
35. Lerner EB, Fernandez AR, Shah MN. Do emergency medical services professionals think they should participate in disease prevention? Prehosp Emerg Care 2009;13(1):64–70.
36. Carpenter CR, Shah MN, Hustey FM, et al. High yield research opportunities in geriatric emergency medicine research: prehospital care, delirium, adverse drug events, and falls. J Gerontol A Biol Sci Med Sci 2011;66(7):775–83.
37. Glickman SW, Shofer FS, Wu MC, et al. Development and validation of a prioritization rule for obtaining an immediate 12-lead electrocardiogram in the emergency department to identify ST-elevation myocardial infarction. Am Heart J 2012;163(3):372–82.
38. Kothari RU, Pancioli A, Liu T, et al. Cincinnati prehospital stroke scale: reproducibility and validity. Ann Emerg Med 1999;33(4):373–8.
39. Katzan IL, Furlan AJ, Lloyd LE, et al. Use of tissue-type plasminogen activator for acute ischemic stroke: the Cleveland area experience. JAMA 2000;283(9):1151–8.
40. Hoffman JR, Schriger DL. A graphic reanalysis of the NINDS trial. Ann Emerg Med 2009;54(3):329–36.
41. Gomez-Choco M, Obach V, Urra X, et al. The response to IV rt-PA in very old stroke patients. Eur J Neurol 2008;15(3):253–6.
42. Mishra NK, Ahmed N, Andersen G, et al. Thrombolysis in very elderly people: controlled comparison of SITS International Stroke Thrombolysis Registry and Virtual International Stroke Trials Archive. BMJ 2010;341:c6046.
43. Boulouis G, Dumont F, Cordonnier C, et al. Intravenous thrombolysis for acute cerebral ischaemia in old stroke patients >/= 80 years of age. J Neurol 2011; 259(7):1461–7.
44. Dirks M, Koudstaal PJ, Dippel DW, et al. Effectiveness of thrombolysis with intravenous alteplase for acute ischemic stroke in older adults. J Am Geriatr Soc 2011;59(11):2169–71.
45. Sung PS, Chen CH, Hsieh HC, et al. Outcome of acute ischemic stroke in very elderly patients: is intravenous thrombolysis beneficial? Eur Neurol 2011;66(2): 110–6.
46. Zacharatos H, Hassan AE, Vazquez G, et al. Comparison of acute nonthrombolytic and thrombolytic treatments in ischemic stroke patients 80 years or older. Am J Emerg Med 2012;30(1):158–64.
47. Wardlaw JM, Murray V, Berge E, et al. Recombinant tissue plasminogen activator for acute ischaemic stroke: an updated systematic review and meta-analysis. Lancet 2012;379(9834):2364–72.

48. Phillips S, Rond PC, Kelly SM, et al. The failure of triage criteria to identify geriatric patients with trauma: results from the Florida Trauma Triage Study. J Trauma 1996;40(2):278–83.
49. Chang DC, Bass RR, Cornwell EE, et al. Undertriage of elderly trauma patients to state-designated trauma centers. Arch Surg 2008;143(8):776–81.
50. Platts-Mills TF, Travers D, Biese K, et al. Accuracy of the Emergency Severity Index triage instrument for identifying elder emergency department patients receiving an immediate life-saving intervention. Acad Emerg Med 2010;17(3): 238–43.
51. Takahashi PY, Pecina JL, Upatising B, et al. A randomized controlled trial of telemonitoring in older adults with multiple health issues to prevent hospitalizations and emergency department visits. Arch Intern Med 2012;172(10):773–9.
52. McCusker CM, Verdon J. Do geriatric interventions reduce emergency department visits? A systematic review. J Gerontol A Biol Sci Med Sci 2006;61(1):53–62.
53. Coleman EA, Eilertsen TB, Kramer AM, et al. Reducing emergency visits in older adults with chronic illness. A randomized, controlled trial of group visits. Eff Clin Pract 2001;4(2):49–57.
54. Cohen RA, Bloom B, Simpson G, et al. Access to health care. Part 3: older adults. Vital Health Stat 10 1997;(198):1–32.
55. Kovner CT, Mezey M, Harrington C. Who cares for older adults? Workforce implications of an aging society. Health Aff 2002;21(5):78–89.
56. Shah MN, Caprio TV, Swanson P, et al. A novel emergency medical services-based program to identify and assist older adults in a rural community. J Am Geriatr Soc 2010;58(11):2205–11.
57. Gerson LW, Schelble DT, Wilson JE. Using paramedics to identify at-risk elderly. Ann Emerg Med 1992;21(6):688–91.
58. Weiss SJ, Chong R, Ong M, et al. Emergency medical services screening of elderly falls in the home. Prehosp Emerg Care 2003;7(1):79–84.
59. Kue R, Ramstrom E, Weisberg S, et al. Evaluation of an emergency medical services-based social services referral program for elderly patients. Prehosp Emerg Care 2009;13(3):273–9.
60. Comans TA, Currin ML, Quinn J, et al. Problems with a great idea: referral by prehospital emergency services to a community-based falls-prevention service. Inj Prev, in press.
61. Lowton K, Laybourne AH, Whiting DG, et al. Can Fire and Rescue Services and the National Health Service work together to improve the safety and wellbeing of vulnerable older people? Design of a proof of concept study. BMC Health Serv Res 2010;10:327.
62. Snooks H, Cheung WY, Close J, et al. Support and Assessment for Fall Emergency Referrals (SAFER 1) trial protocol. Computerised on-scene decision support for emergency ambulance staff to assess and plan care for older people who have fallen: evaluation of costs and benefits using a pragmatic cluster randomised trial. BMC Emerg Med 2010;10:2.
63. Halter M, Vernon S, Snooks H, et al. Complexity of the decision-making process of ambulance staff for assessment and referral of older people who have fallen: a qualitative study. Emerg Med J 2011;28(1):44–50.
64. Snooks H, Hutchings H, Russell I, et al. Bureaucracy stifles medical research in Britain: a tale of three trials. BMC Med Res Methodol 2012;12(1):122.
65. Borges-Da Silva R, McCusker J, Roberge D, et al. Classification of emergency departments according to their services for community-dwelling seniors. Acad Emerg Med 2012;19(5):552–61.

66. McCusker J, Roberge D, Ciampi A, et al. Outcomes of community-dwelling seniors vary by type of emergency department. Acad Emerg Med 2012;19(3):304–12.

67. McCusker J, Verdon J, Vadeboncoeur A, et al. The elder-friendly emergency department assessment tool: development of a quality assessment tool for emergency department-based geriatric care. J Am Geriatr Soc 2012;60(8):1534–9.

68. Sinha SK, Bessman ES, Flomenbaum N, et al. A systematic review and qualitative analysis to inform the development of a new emergency department-based geriatric case management model. Ann Emerg Med 2011;57(6):672–82.

69. Fealy GM, McCarron M, O'Neill D, et al. Effectiveness of gerontologically informed nursing assessment and referral interventions for older persons attending the emergency department: systematic review. J Adv Nurs 2009; 65(5):934–5.

70. Clinical, practice management: geriatric videos. Available at: http://www.acep.org/Clinical—Practice-Management/Geriatric-Videos/. Accessed October 15, 2012.

71. Gerson LW, Counsell SR, Fontanarosa PB, et al. Case finding for cognitive impairment in elderly emergency department patients. Ann Emerg Med 1994; 23(4):813–7.

72. Terrell KM, Hustey FM, Hwang U, et al. Quality indicators for geriatric emergency care. Acad Emerg Med 2009;16(5):441–9.

73. Carpenter CR, Heard K, Wilber ST, et al. Research priorities for high-quality geriatric emergency care: medication management, screening, and prevention and functional assessment. Acad Emerg Med 2011;18(6):644–54.

74. Carpenter CR, Gerson L. Geriatric emergency medicine. In: LoCicero J, Rosenthal RA, Katic M, et al, editors. A supplement to new frontiers in geriatrics research: an agenda for surgical and related medical specialties. 2nd edition. New York: The American Geriatrics Society; 2008. p. 45–71.

75. Wilber ST, Carpenter CR, Hustey FM. The six-item screener to detect cognitive impairment in older emergency department patients. Acad Emerg Med 2008; 15(7):613–6.

76. Carpenter CR, DesPain B, Keeling TK, et al. The Six-Item Screener and AD8 for the detection of cognitive impairment in geriatric emergency department patients. Ann Emerg Med 2011;57(6):653–61.

77. Carpenter CR, Bassett ER, Fischer GM, et al. Four sensitive screening tools to detect cognitive impairment in geriatric emergency department patients: brief Alzheimer's screen, short blessed test, Ottawa3DY, and the caregiver administered AD8. Acad Emerg Med 2011;18(4):374–84.

78. Close JC, Hooper R, Glucksman E, et al. Predictors of falls in a high risk population: results from the prevention of falls in the elderly trial (PROFET). Emerg Med J 2003;20(5):421–5.

79. Carpenter CR, Scheatzle MD, D'Antonio JA, et al. Identification of fall risk factors in older adult emergency department patients. Acad Emerg Med 2009;16(3):211–9.

80. McCusker J, Bellavance F, Cardin S, et al. Detection of older people at increased risk of adverse health outcomes after an emergency visit: the ISAR screening tool. J Am Geriatr Soc 1999;47(10):1229–37.

81. Meldon SW, Mion LC, Palmer RM, et al. A Brief risk-stratification tool to predict repeat emergency department visits and hospitalizations in older patients discharged from the emergency department. Acad Emerg Med 2003;10:224–32.

82. Boyd M, Koziol-McLain J, Yates K, et al. Emergency department case-finding for high-risk older adults: the Brief Risk Identification for Geriatric Health Tool (BRIGHT). Acad Emerg Med 2008;15(7):598–606.

83. Clevenger CK, Chu TA, Yang Z, et al. Clinical care of persons with dementia in the emergency department: a review of the literature and agenda for research. J Am Geriatr Soc 2012;60(9):1742–8.
84. Carpenter CR, Griffey RT, Stark S, et al. Physician and nurse acceptance of geriatric technicians to screen for geriatric syndromes in the emergency department. West J Emerg Med 2011;12(4):489–95.
85. Wilber ST, Burger B, Gerson LW, et al. Reclining chairs reduce pain from gurneys in older emergency department patients: a randomized controlled trial. Acad Emerg Med 2005;12:119–23.
86. Conroy SP, Stevens T, Parker SG, et al. A systematic review of comprehensive geriatric assessment to improve outcomes for frail older people being rapidly discharged from acute hospital: 'interface geriatrics'. Age Ageing 2011;40(4): 436–43.
87. Ellis G, Whitehead M, O'Neill D, et al. Comprehensive geriatric assessment for older adults admitted to hospital. Cochrane Database Syst Rev 2011;(7):CD006211.
88. Arendts G, Fitzhardinge S, Pronk K, et al. The impact of early emergency department allied health intervention on admission rates in older people: a non-randomized clinical study. BMC Geriatr 2012;12:8.
89. Chadaga SR, Shockley L, Keniston A, et al. Hospitalist-Led medicine emergency department team: associations with throughput, timeliness of patient care, and satisfaction. J Hosp Med 2012;7(7):562–6.
90. Wald HL, Glasheen JJ, Guerrasio J, et al. Evaluation of a hospitalist-run acute care for the elderly service. J Hosp Med 2011;6(6):313–21.
91. Demetriades D, Karaiskakis M, Velmahos GC, et al. Effect on outcome of early intensive management of geriatric trauma patients. Br J Surg 2002;89:1319–22.
92. Meldon SW, Reilly M, Drew BL, et al. Trauma in the very elderly: a community-based study of outcomes at trauma and nontrauma centers. J Trauma 2002; 52(1):79–84.
93. Shabot MM, Johnson CL. Outcome from critical care in the "oldest old" trauma patients. J Trauma 1995;39(2):254–9.
94. Battistella FD, Din AM, Perez L. Trauma patients 75 years and older: long-term follow-up results justify aggressive management. J Trauma 1998;44(4):618–23.
95. Richmond TS, Kauder D, Strumpf N, et al. Characteristics and outcomes of serious trauma injury in older adults. J Am Geriatr Soc 2002;50(2):215–22.
96. Kakuma R, Galbaud du Fort G, Arsenault L, et al. Delirium in older emergency department patients discharged home: effect on survival. J Am Geriatr Soc 2003;51(4):443–50.
97. Han JH, Shintani A, Eden S, et al. Delirium in the emergency department: an independent predictor of death within 6 months. Ann Emerg Med 2010;56(3): 244–52.
98. Lewis LM, Miller DK, Morley JE, et al. Unrecognized delirium in ED geriatric patients. Am J Emerg Med 1995;13(2):142–5.
99. Naughton BJ, Moran MB, Kadah H, et al. Delirium and other cognitive impairment in older adults in an emergency department. Ann Emerg Med 1995; 25(6):751–5.
100. Elie M, Rousseau F, Cole M, et al. Prevalence and detection of delirium in elderly emergency department patients. CMAJ 2000;163(8):977–81.
101. Hustey FM, Meldon SW. The prevalence and documentation of impaired mental status in elderly emergency department patients. Ann Emerg Med 2002;39(3): 248–53.

102. Han JH, Zimmerman EE, Cutler N, et al. Delirium in older emergency department patients: recognition, risk factors, and psychomotor subtypes. Acad Emerg Med 2009;16(3):193–200.
103. Lu JH, Chan DK, O'Rourke F, et al. Management and outcomes of delirious patients with hyperactive symptoms in a secured behavioral unit jointly used by geriatricians and pyschogeriatricians. Arch Gerontol Geriatr 2011;52(1):66–70.
104. Inouye SK, Bogardus ST, Charpentier PA, et al. A multicomponent intervention to prevent delirium in hospitalized older patients. N Engl J Med 1999;340(9):669–76.
105. Flaherty JH, Steele DK, Chibnall JT, et al. An ACE unit with a delirium room may improve function and equalize length of stay among older delirious medical inpatients. J Gerontol A Biol Sci Med Sci 2010;65(12):1387–92.
106. Flaherty JH, Little MO. Matching the environment to patients with delirium: lessons learned from the delirium room, a restraint-free environment for older hospitalized adults with delirium. J Am Geriatr Soc 2011;59(Suppl 2):S295–300.
107. Wong Tin Niam DM, Geddes JA, Inderjeeth CA. Delirium unit: our experience. Australas J Ageing 2009;28(4):206–10.
108. Modawal A. Model and systems of geriatric care: "delirium rooms"–but where and at what cost? J Am Geriatr Soc 2004;52(6):1023.
109. Chong MS, Chan MP, Kang J, et al. A new model of delirium care in the acute geriatric setting: geriatric monitoring unit. BMC Geriatr 2011;11:41.
110. Harwood RH, Goldberg SE, Whittamore KH, et al. Evaluation of a Medical and Mental Health Unit compared with standard care for older people whose emergency admission to an acute general hospital is complicated by concurrent 'confusion': a controlled clinical trial. Acronym: TEAM: trial of an elderly acute care medical and mental health unit. Trials 2011;12:123.
111. Pines JM, Hilton JA, Weber EJ, et al. International perspectives on emergency department crowding. Acad Emerg Med 2011;18(12):1358–70.
112. Rabin E, Kocher K, McClelland M, et al. Solutions to emergency department 'boarding' and crowding are underused and may need to be legislated. Health Aff 2012;31(8):1757–66.
113. Creditor MD. Hazards of hospitalization of the elderly. Ann Intern Med 1993;118(3):219–23.
114. Leff B, Burton L, Bynum JW, et al. Prospective evaluation of clinical criteria to select older persons with acute medical illness for care in a hypothetical home hospital. J Am Geriatr Soc 1997;45(9):1066–73.
115. Shepperd S, Doll H, Angus RM, et al. Avoiding hospital admission through provision of hospital care at home: a systematic review and meta-analysis of individual patient data. CMAJ 2009;180(2):175–82.
116. Leff B, Burton L, Mader SL, et al. Comparison of stress experienced by family members of patients treated in hospital at home with that of those receiving traditional acute hospital care. J Am Geriatr Soc 2008;56(1):117–23.
117. Marsteller JA, Burton L, Mader SL, et al. Health care provider evaluation of a substitutive model of hospital at home. Med Care 2009;47(9):979–85.
118. Montalto M, Lui B, Mullins A, et al. Medically-managed Hospital in the Home: 7 year study of mortality and unplanned interruption. Aust Health Rev 2010;34(3):269–75.
119. Leff B, Burton L, Mader SL, et al. Hospital at home: feasibility and outcomes of a program to provide hospital-level care at home for acutely Ill older patients. Ann Intern Med 2005;143:798–808.
120. Leff B. Defining and disseminating the hospital-at-home model. CMAJ 2009;180(2):156–7.

121. Cryer L, Shannon SB, Van Amsterdam M, et al. Costs for 'hospital at home' patients were 19 percent lower, with equal or better outcomes compared to similar inpatients. Health Aff 2012;31(6):1237–43.

122. Section for enhancing geriatric understanding and expertise among surgical and medical specialists. Available at: http://specialists.americangeriatrics.org/about.php. Accessed October 15, 2012.

123. Academy of geriatric emergency medicine. Available at: http://www.saem.org/academy-geriatric-emergency-medicine. Accessed October 15, 2012.

124. Geriatric Emergency Medicine Section. Available at: http://www.acep.org/geriatricsection/. Accessed October 15, 2012.

Transitions of Care for the Geriatric Patient in the Emergency Department

Chad Kessler, MD, MHPE[a,b,c,d],*, Meredith C. Williams, MD, MBA[e],
John N. Moustoukas, MD, MBA[f], Cleo Pappas, MLIS[g]

KEYWORDS

- Senior • Emergency department • Geriatric hand-off • Patient transfer
- Transfer of patients • Transitions

KEY POINTS

- Usage of the emergency department (ED) by elderly patients is distinct from that by non-elderly patients.
- The transfer of elderly patients to and from the ED has many challenges, because these patients have multiple providers, multiple comorbidities, and often cognitive impairments that limit their ability to participate in their care.
- Vital information such as the reason for transfer, vital signs, code status, medication lists, or baseline mental status is often missing in the documentation provided from a nursing home.
- Failed transitions are regularly implicated in major morbidity and mortality, caused by problems like medication errors, adverse drug events, lack of timely coordination follow-up care, and unnecessary rehospitalizations.
- Standardized communication has been evaluated as a solution to omissions, and may be helpful in reducing errors related to diagnostic uncertainty and care planning.
- There is a need to develop more robust metrics for the care provided to the geriatric patient in the ED and their transition from one provider to another.
- Federal economic quality incentives rewarding high-quality transitions could potentially improve the paradigm and improve behaviors of clinicians and institutions.

Funding Sources: Nil.
Conflict of Interest: Nil.
[a] Emergency Medicine, Jesse Brown VA Hospital, 820 South Damen Avenue, M/C 111, Chicago, IL 60612, USA; [b] Department of Emergency Medicine, Combined Internal Medicine/Emergency, Medicine Residency, University of Illinois-Chicago, 1700 West Taylor, Chicago, IL 60612, USA; [c] Department of Medical Education, Combined Internal Medicine/Emergency, Medicine Residency, University of Illinois-Chicago, 1700 West Taylor, Chicago, IL 60612, USA; [d] Department Internal Medicine, Combined Internal Medicine/Emergency, Medicine Residency, University of Illinois-Chicago, 1700 West Taylor, Chicago, IL 60612, USA; [e] Section of Emergency Medicine, Department of Medicine, University of Chicago, 5841 South Maryland Avenue, MC 5068, Chicago, IL 60637, USA; [f] Department of Emergency Medicine, University of Illinois-Chicago, 808 South Wood Street, M/C 724, Chicago, IL 60612, USA; [g] Library of Health Sciences - Information Services, University of Illinois at Chicago - Library of the Health Sciences, 1750 West Polk Avenue, Chicago, IL 60612, USA
* Corresponding author. Emergency Medicine, Jesse Brown VA Hospital, 820 South Damen Avenue, M/C 111, Chicago, IL 60612.
E-mail address: Chad.Kessler@va.gov

Clin Geriatr Med 29 (2013) 49–69
http://dx.doi.org/10.1016/j.cger.2012.10.005
0749-0690/13/$ – see front matter Published by Elsevier Inc.

INTRODUCTION

The graying of America is a phrase used to describe an anticipated change in America's demographics over the next decades. By 2030, more than 20% of US residents are expected to be 65 years or older, representing a 102% increase from the year 2000.[1] The phrase can also be used to describe the future of America's emergency departments (EDs). Elderly patients represent the fastest-growing segment of ED patients in the United States[2–5] and according to a study published in the *Annals of Emergency Medicine,* the annual number of patients aged 65 to 74 years visiting EDs is projected to increase from 6.4 million in 2003 to 11.7 million by 2013.[6]

Elderly patients are more likely than other groups to be transferred between facilities[6] and the ED has become a common touch point for elderly patients moving through our health care system. As elderly patients move from one health care setting to another, their medical information and history, which are often complicated and long, must follow with them and be successfully communicated to each new provider who is continuing care. This transition of care from one facility to another, from one provider to another, is wrought with challenges. Elderly patients represent not only a large percentage of ED visits each year, they are more likely to suffer from chronic illness, multiple medical comorbidities, cognitive and functional impairments that limit their ability to communicate, and preexisting social problems.[7–9] Elderly patients are also more likely than other groups to receive care from multiple providers, increasing the frequency that these transitions occur. A 2001 Harris poll found that patients with 1 or more chronic medical problems see, on average, 8 different physicians in a single year.[10] These factors make transferring the elderly patient a challenging process that is prone to errors.

The safe transfer of elderly patients from one health care setting to another has become an increasingly important area of research. The American Geriatrics Society (AGS) developed a research agenda for emergency medicine and the highest priority was given to identifying if alterations in the process of ED care can improve outcomes in older patients.[11] The goal of this article is to present a summary of the current literature surrounding the transitions of care for the geriatric patient in the ED. We review the transition of elderly patients to the ED, from the ED to inpatient, and from the ED back to the community, and provide an analysis of current proposals to improve care.

METHODS

A transparent search methodology ensures the reproducibility of results that characterize evidence-based research. The search strategy for this project was designed and conducted by a medical librarian (CP) with input from the clinical lead and coprincipal investigators. Medical subject headings unique to each database and relevant keywords were integrated. A comprehensive search of the following electronic databases was undertaken for primary studies:

a. Medline (1966–February 2012) was searched using the PubMed interface
b. EMBASE (1974–February 2012)
c. PscyInfo
d. CINAHL
e. Google Scholar
f. Web of Science (1993–February 2012)
g. ISI Web of Science was searched for articles that cite studies included in the review

Limits used in all databases were "10 years" and "English."

The following search strings show representative combinations of keywords and subject headings that were reconfigured to comply with indexing thesauri of each database.

PubMed: "Geriatrics"[Mesh] OR ("Aged"[Mesh] OR "Geriatric Assessment"[Mesh] OR "Geriatric Nursing"[Mesh] OR "Geriatric Psychiatry"[Mesh] OR "Geriatric Dentistry" [Mesh] OR "Health Services for the Aged"[Mesh]) AND "Patient Transfer"[Mesh.].

EMBASE: transition OR relocation OR transfer AND [2000–2012]/py AND 'aged'/ exp/mj OR 'geriatrics'/exp/mj AND [humans]/lim AND [english]/lim AND [2000– 2012]/py.

Google Scholar: ("client transfer" OR transfer OR relocation OR move) AND (aging OR aged OR "elder care" OR geriatrics OR geriatric OR gerontology).

Authors then reviewed titles and abstracts, and articles were sorted into 1 of 5 categories: "Presenting to the ED," "Transitions to Inpatient" "Discharge from the ED" "Systems and Costs," and "Irrelevant." Inclusion criteria were that the article had to discuss the ED and either elderly patients or transitions of care. Articles deemed irrelevant discussed neither. Articles were not limited to research published in the United States. Each remaining article was then read and analyzed. Bibliographies were also reviewed for further relevant articles not discovered through our initial search, and those were then added to their relevant category.

RESULTS

The initial search yielded 787 results citations. Sorting yielded 75 articles in the presenting category, 31 in the inpatient category, 59 in the discharge category, and 47 articles in the systems/costs category. A remaining 575 articles were determined to be irrelevant to the study. After bibliographic review, an additional 13 articles were added to the presenting category and 4 were added to the discharge category. The results are grouped into discussion threads for continuity (**Table 1**).

Use of the ED by Elderly Patients

ED use by older patients is well described, and the data suggest that elderly ED usage is distinct from that of nonelderly patients.[7,14–18] A 2002 literature review that compared older patients with younger ones found that older adults use emergency services at a higher rate, their visits are higher acuity, they have longer lengths of stay, have higher admission and recidivism rates, and suffer from higher rates of adverse health outcomes after discharge.[19]

The exposure to potential transition-associated errors is alarming, because elderly patients experience transitions often. The 1994 long-term care survey of postacute and skilled nursing facilities revealed that between 1992 and 1994, roughly 5 million patients older than 65 years made more than 15 million transitions.[20] Four key areas have been identified as reasons for elderly transfer: infections, falls, pain, or exacerbation of a chronic illness.[21] **Box 1** suggests symptoms most frequently endorsed at the time of transfer. In addition, elderly patients are more susceptible to the risks of transitional care because they are frail, often cognitively limited, and suffer from chronic illness, with multiple comorbidities.[22,23] Studies have shown that up to 40% are transferred to an ED within 30 days of their death[21] and as a population have been shown to have a higher medical acuity[24] in general. Transitions of care are generally believed to negatively affect quality of life for elderly patients as a result of medical errors, unnecessary treatments and hospitalizations, and additional stressors related to changing locations.[25,26]

Table 1
Search methodology and results

Database	Search Terms	Limits	Retrievals	Relevant Retrievals	Duplicates Removed	Total Added
PubMed	"Geriatrics"[Mesh] OR "Aged"[Mesh] OR "Geriatric Assessment"[Mesh] OR "Geriatric Nursing"[Mesh] OR "Geriatric Psychiatry"[Mesh] OR "Geriatric Dentistry"[Mesh] OR "Health Services for the Aged"[Mesh]) AND "Patient Transfer"[Mesh]	English, published in the last 10 y	581	320	0	320
EMBASE	transition OR relocation OR transfer AND 'aged'/exp/mj OR 'geriatrics'/exp/mj	[2000–2012]/py [humans]/lim AND [english]/lim	109	36	21	15
PsycInfo	transfer OR relocation OR move DE = "client transfer"	Earliest to current	135	20	7	13
Google Scholar	("client transfer" OR transfer OR relocation OR move) AND (aging OR aged OR "elder care" OR geriatrics OR geriatric OR gerontology) led to a previously undiscovered PubMed citation. A related articles search on this citation revealed 60 articles, which were uploaded to RefWorks		60	60	21	39
CINAHL	(((XX "transfer"¹² AND (XX "client"¹³)) OR (transfer) OR (relocation) OR (move)) AND ((aging) OR (aged) OR ("elder care") OR (geriatrics) OR (geriatric) OR (gerontology))) AND emergency department	2000–2012	99	72	30	42
Web of Science	Related records: Aaltonen, Mari. The impact of dementia on care transitions during the last two years of life. (References used: 30)	ENGLISH Publication Years = (2010 OR 2009 OR 2011 OR 2008 OR 2007)				10

Box 1
The most common chief complaints leading to transfer from nursing home (NH) to ED
Fever (77.5%)
Poor oral intake (70.4%)
Altered mental status (68.7%)
Respiratory symptoms (67.0%)
Electrolyte or other laboratory test abnormalities (62.2%)
Neurologic problems (61.9%)
Data from Ackermann RJ, Kemle KA, Vogel RL, et al. Emergency department use by nursing home residents. Ann Emerg Med 1998;31(6):749–57.

Transition to the ED: the Prevalence of Information Gaps

A large body of research has been conducted analyzing the transitional care experienced by elderly patients living in NHs and long-term care (LTC) facilities. Roughly 5% of elders live in NHs, and those who do are generally frail, with multiple medical problems and impairments,[27] and they are often subject to fragmented care with little continuity. The larger group of community-dwelling patients living in the community either alone or with a caregiver present to the ED from home rather than residential care setting. However, many of these patients are subject to similar risks of transition to elderly NH dwellers.[28,29] Multiple studies show that there is an information gap between the NH and the ED.[30–32] For example, elderly patients are often transferred to the ED with little documentation of their symptoms, recent treatments, or pertinent medical history.[23] Often, vital information such as the reason for transfer, vital signs, code status, medication lists, or baseline mental status is missing in the documentation provided from the NH.[9] Studies have suggested that information is missing for 74% to 90% of the patients presenting from NHs.[33] Cognitively impaired patients who are unable to provide health information are especially vulnerable to information gaps. Confusion related to living wills and code status negatively affects the care provided by emergency medical services (EMS) and ED providers.[34]

Several studies have indicated that deficiencies in communication in the care of the LTC patient increase the risk of potentially avoidable events.[35–40] Failed transitions are regularly implicated in major morbidity and mortality caused by prescription errors, adverse drug events, lack of timely coordination of follow-up care, and unnecessary rehospitalizations.[41–44] Several studies have described medication errors after transitions as potentially deadly in this patient segment.[28,43,44] Failed NH-ED transitions lead to unnecessary resource utilizations in emergency, inpatient, postacute, and ambulatory services.[20,45,46]

NH-ED relationships are often dysfunctional. The 2 institutions have different capabilities, scopes of practice, and goals of care. The transfers usually occur in urgent or emergent circumstances that do not permit adequate time spent on coordinating the transition. Another major factor identified as contributing to poor coordination of NH-ED transfers is the different financial and reimbursement structures in the NH and the ED, and subsequent lack of incentive for either provider to strive for superior communication.[47]

To address these shortcomings, various studies have looked at ways to improve NH-ED communication. In 1995, the Society for Academic Emergency Medicine (SAEM) Geriatric Task Force recommended the use of a 1-page transfer form, and various studies have analyzed the effect of transfer form use. The results have been mixed, with some finding that the gaps in information did decrease[31] but there was no change in case resolution time or disposition.[48] Staff members can believe that there is an improvement with the use of a standard envelop for care[49] but the effect is limited, because these forms are not used regularly and consistently.

Transitions to Inpatient: the Effect of Poor Communication on the Sickest Patients

More than 25% of NH residents receive ED care annually, and these patients are frequently admitted to acute-care hospitals.[50–52] Of those who do go to an ED, between one-third and one-half result in a hospital admission. These rates are between 2.5 and 4.6 times higher than the hospitalization rates for younger patients. Transfers of patient care between levels of care within the same institution (ie, from ED to inpatient) are known to be a source of communication errors resulting in adverse medical outcomes.[53–55] This topic has been thoroughly studied for general populations as a potential opportunity to improve quality of care. A Finnish study indicates that most elderly patients experience several transitions during their last 2 years of life, with an increasing frequency as they approach death.[56] It is now more common for older people in Europe and North America to die somewhere other than home.[57–60]

According to the 1997 National Institutes of Health National Nursing Home Survey adults aged 65 years and older averaged more than 300 visits to the ED and 200 hospital admissions per 1000 persons.[61] When admitted, older emergency patients are more likely to require a bed in an intensive care unit (ICU). Elderly patients in the ED with sepsis experience increased times to ICU admission, and slower dispositions to ICU are statistically related to increased in-hospital mortality.[62–67] Older adults undergo more diagnostic tests and procedures, their ED diagnoses tend to be less accurate, and ED stays are longer compared with younger patients in the ED.[68]

Although our literature search did not reveal any articles describing intrahospital transfers (ie, ED to floor) specifically for the elderly population, it is reasonable to assume that the challenges faced in any transfer of care apply to elderly patients admitted to the ED. The largest body of research on transfers has focused on hand-offs within a specialty[68,69] (ie, end-of-shift sign-outs between residents or nurses), with few studies examining the ED to floor transfer.[67,69–73] The hand-off that occurs between emergency physicians and internal medicine physicians is believed to be particularly high risk because of major cultural, social, and linguistic differences between the 2 practitioners.[74,75]

Certain factors were found to represent vulnerabilities in the hand-off process, creating an opportunity for error. Communication issues were most frequently identified in failed transfers. One survey of 264 internal medicine and emergency medicine physicians of a large academic hospital identified 40 examples of near misses in admitted patients that occurred after ED to floor transfers. The errors were categorized as diagnostic (N = 13), treatment (N = 14), and disposition (N = 13). Vital signs and other elements of the physical examination were most frequently not communicated to admitting teams, followed by test results, details of the medical history, and the ED course. The most cited content item absent in communication was the most recent set of vital signs, occurring in 28% of responses. In addition to absent diagnostic information and communication issues, there are also conflicting expectations of care responsibility, particularly for admitted patients boarded in the ED. Even although the patient may be physically in the ED, emergency physicians note few to no cases in which an internist notified the ED about problems or clinical updates.[76]

Environmental factors such as ED volume, time of day, and access to information technology were implicated in high-risk transfers. A hectic ED environment and pending diagnostic results cause hurried sign-outs and missed follow-up of ordered tests or procedures.[77] For example, patients requiring emergent advanced imaging or hemodialysis can be immediately transferred to an inpatient ward after the procedure, bypassing the ED and resulting in a missed opportunity for communication with the admitting service. Other risks of the ED to floor transfer include diagnostic uncertainty at the time of hand-off, cognitive biases, need to save face, or a need to prove that a patient meets admission criteria.[67,70,78] Thus, a seamless ED to floor transfer requires attention to the institutional social order, which varies by institution.[67,70,79–82]

Discharge from the ED: a Poorly Communicated Plan is the Same as No Plan At All

The lack of appropriate and timely follow-up care can quickly undermine the benefits achieved in the previous setting, resulting in further functional dependency and permanent institutionalization. Of all patients aged 65 years or older presenting to the ED, 23% are discharged with home care, 42% are discharged to another institution within 24 months, and 11.6% are discharged home.[83,84] When patients are discharged from the hospital, they may be uncertain about whether they should resume their previous medication regimen or take only the medications listed on their discharge instructions.[85–87] Because elderly patients are more likely to experience diagnostic errors or omissions, they can consequently be discharged with problems that are either overlooked or untreated.[18,84] This confusion causes many older patients to complain of the lack of complete resolution of their presenting symptoms after an ED visit. Many believe that their needs have not been met and often come back to the ER.[88]

When discharged, older patients are also more likely to experience higher rates of adverse health outcomes.[89] The risks are particularly high in the first 3 months after an emergency visit, with an average mortality of about 10%,[90–92] Although mortality and hospitalization rates tend to stabilize after the first 3 months, the cumulative rates of ED returns continue to increase in a slower fashion in the next 3 months[93] with a return rate of as high as 44% reported in a 6-month follow-up study. Those who have a higher base morbidity, an ED visit, or hospitalization within the past 6 months, or are triaged to the emergency unit over urgent care are particularly at risk for an adverse event.[94]

When adverse events occur or functional status declines, patients then return to the ED for more care. Recidivism (ie, bounce-back) within 14 days is known to occur more frequently in elderly patients.[7] In 1 study, 29% of patients older than 75 years returned to the ED within 14 days, 90% of them for the same medical condition.[7] Other studies show that 19% of patients return to the ED or another acute-care hospital within 30 days, and as many as 42% within 24 months.[95] Hospital readmissions are costly, disruptive to patients and families, and tend to interrupt the comprehensive care plan established between patients and their providers. Hospitalization also increases risks of acute delirium, iatrogenic illness, adverse drug reactions, and pressure ulcers.[90] However, the findings related to the changes in functional capacity are less conclusive because of the inconsistencies in the definitions and measures used across studies.

Several studies have looked for ways to reduce these high rates of recidivism. In 1 analysis, the incorporation of a standardized nursing assessment for people 65 years and older decreased functional decline. However, there was an associated increase in the rate of return visits to the ED as well as referrals to community resources and primary care providers.[89] Several studies have found that that a nurse who helped coordinate discharge care for elderly patients led to fewer ED return visits and fewer admission,[13,88,96] with improved mental status and decreased stress for caregivers,[97] but without change in overall health outcomes or mortality.[94,95] Many of these studies did not stratify patients according to risk factors, and when the trials selected for patients that were high risk, as opposed to just an age inclusion criterion, there was more consistent improvement in functional status. However, these trials are difficult to conduct, because they are difficult to blind and standardize.[96] The Comprehensive Geriatric Assessment is a validated tool that assists the prediction of the risk of readmission, but widespread ED adoption is limited by time required to perform analysis.[98] Numerous other more facile clinical decision-making tools for geriatrics exist.[12,99,100] A Swiss ED-based comparison of readmissions for 7440 patients aged 75 years or older found no statistical difference in unpredicted readmission rates between the Identification of Seniors at Risk Tool (ISAR) and the Triage Risk Stratification Tool.[101] EDs with dedicated care managers or geriatric teams may use these tools more effectively to assist with disposition decisions.

The Cost of Poor Transitional Care

The increase in transfers of elderly patients to the ED could exacerbate existing problems with overcrowding in many departments. Research has also shown that up to 40% of transfers of elderly patients to the ED may be inappropriate.[13] It has been estimated that as many as one-third of NH-ED transfers are potentially avoidable, placing an unnecessary strain on existing resources.[98] One study calculated a cost of $1.24 billion in avoidable transfers in New York State alone.[13] Many investigators have previously examined the multiple factors associated with unnecessary transfers.[12] NHs that provide expanded services, such as midlevel providers on staff and intravenous therapies, have shown lower relative admission rates for specific diagnosis categories.[99] Two successful examples of comprehensive health programs include Evercare and Program of All-Inclusive Care for the Elderly, both of which have shown a reduction health care use since the program implementation.[100,101] One example of comprehensive NH physician services involved daily visits to the NH by geriatric physicians, with specific attention paid toward advanced directives, in which patients could not be transferred before undergoing an evaluation by a physician.[102] Ideally, the potential for harm from an additional transition is weighed against the potential benefit in each case before any decision to transfer.[103–110] In any transfer, the patient's medical needs should justify any change in physical care setting. A comprehensive economic analysis of care transitions for this patient segment is outside the scope of this review, and is an area that necessitates further research and attention.

DISCUSSION
Barriers to Improvement

Several systemic obstacles exist that potentiate the problems associated with elderly transitional care. Coleman and colleagues[105] recognized barriers to effective transitions of care at the levels of the health care delivery system, the clinician, and the patient. The US health care delivery system has evolved into a system of separate silo facilities, which act independently and often impede successful transitional care. Because of the closed nature of the origin and receiving institutions, information is not adequately conveyed to the next provider.[45,111–115] As a consequence, vital components of the care plan such as advanced directives and results of laboratory and diagnostic tests are frequently lost in transition.[22,116–118] The patient is at a disadvantage because of this lack of collaboration.[119] Verbal communication between providers has been determined by the SAEM Geriatric Task Force as an essential element for high-quality transitions.[120] However, a 2010 survey of 155 NH and ED providers indicated that less than 50% of providers responded that verbal communication "should always occur" between transferring providers. In the same survey, only 2.6% and 16.1% of respondents "strongly agree" or "somewhat agree" that there is good communication between NHs and EDs, respectively.[103]

Clinician-level factors include behavioral biases and inadequate training in managing acute illness in elderly patients in the ED. In 1 survey of emergency physicians, 78% of respondents expressed "more difficulty" in managing elderly compared with nonelderly patients, and 53% believed that they were inadequately prepared for clinical geriatric care.[2] Of these providers, nearly 70% of surveyed physicians indicated that emergency geriatrics is inadequately represented in emergency medicine research and continuing education programs. An emerging concept in the behavioral practices of emergency health care workers treating elderly patients is that of ageism.[121] A survey of ED nurses indicated that many providers attach a negative association with age, creating a negative attitude that pervades the care of elderly patients in the ED.[121] Further research is necessary to determine the possible sequelae of ageism. These statistics could indicate a skills deficiency, which should be addressed by research and professional training in this increasingly important area.[120,122–126] Clinicians are also prone to behavioral biases, which can compromise transitional care.

Patient-level barriers to high-quality transitional cares are also multifactorial. First, elderly patients are frequently unable to provide history and often have no advocates to ensure that effective care is administered and the care plan is followed.[115,116,127,128] In many cases, those patients with high baseline cognitive function are not made aware of the reason for transfer nor allowed an active role in their care plan.[113,129,130] In these cases, neither the receiving provider nor the patient understands the reason for transfer, creating dissatisfaction for patients and providers alike.[114,127]

The Need for Transitional Care Metrics

Elderly patients represent a unique category of patients in the ED, as shown not only by the unique challenges that they pose to providers but also by the growing field of geriatrics and the increased recognition by many specialties for the need for more research regarding care for this population. The movement to improve quality care has been growing over the past decade since the publication of the Institute of Medicine's famous report *To Err is Human*. As Terrell and colleagues[123] recognized, "a prerequisite for assessing (and, where needed, improving) the quality of emergency medical care is ability to measure quality of care." Both the SAEM and the American College of Emergency Physicians have recognized that there is a paucity of measures for quality care specifically designed for the geriatric patient. This lack of data makes it not only difficult for researchers to have a strong database from which to conduct analyses but also prevents institutions and groups from having information about their own performance regarding the geriatric patient and how to improve it. To this end, the AGS's research agenda-setting process has identified as its highest priority determining if changes in the process of ED care improved outcomes in older patients.[11] What is clear is that increased focus on creating measures and processes that reflect the quality of care provided to the geriatric patient is necessary. One of the barriers that current practitioners face is a scarcity of information about their own performance and few guidelines or processes designed to facilitate the geriatric assessment.

Optimizing Patient Hand-Offs

Standardized communication has been evaluated as a solution to omissions, and may be helpful in reducing errors related to diagnostic uncertainty and care planning.[131] Standardization exists in many medical settings in the form of checklists, protocols, and sign-out templates.[132] Consistent communication styles has proved to be effective in error reduction in other high-risk, nonmedical sectors.[133–139] Emergency physicians rarely use protocolized hand-off tools that have been validated in other specialties.[67,93,140–143] A standard hand-off tool may also ameliorate the effect of interpersonal biases that can obscure communications across the cultures of the ED and admitting physicians.[144] Socialization issues are particularly problematic in communications within functionally diverse teams.[67,75,145] For example, 1 study showed that emergency physicians felt compelled by internist colleagues to name definitive diagnoses in cases that led to premature closure.[78] Differences in prioritization, coordination, and expectations of care result in dysfunctional relationships, with resulting increase in patient morbidity.[72,146] Designing a transfer tool for cross-specialty communication requires consistency as well as flexibility, which allows providers to collaborate. Multidisciplinary rounds, joint conferences, and real-time feedback cycles have been proposed as methods of maximizing institutional buy-in of a hand-off tool.[140,147] To reduce reliance on telephone conversations, institutions could benefit by investing in electronic record systems, which allow transparency in vital signs and clinical records.[141,142] Boarding patients and those with an intermediate destination before arrival to the floor have repeatedly been found to be at especially high risk for falling through the cracks as a result of ill-defined ownership of the patient.[70,72,73,93,143,144] Hospital-wide patient-tracking dashboard systems that tag boarding ED patients and open beds, lean, and 6 sigma methods also have the potential to reduce risks of transitional errors.[148,149]

Addressing the NH Transition

As has been shown, information gaps are a major dilemma and source of risk for patients transferred from NH to ED. The patient's medical history and the reason for transfer should be clearly documented and transferred with the patient to the receiving ED. Available documentation should include details about any new symptoms or problems, the patient's baseline cognitive function and ability to communicate, any changes from baseline, relevant past medical history, medication history, and advanced directives. Failure to transfer pertinent information that is easily accessible to NH staff results in performance of unnecessary tests and interventions, and increased risks of adverse outcomes.[9,150] The use of a standardized transfer form does provide benefit, assuming that it is completed accurately and is used. A suggestion is to discuss within communities if there is a way to create a standardized form that is common to the major institutions in an area, so that there is less confusion surrounding which elements are to be completed and where information should be located.

Improving Transitional Care

There is no currently accepted standard for transitional care. Transitions of care occur when patients are transferred between different levels of care. Transitions may occur across physical locations or within a single location, such as transferring from the ED to an ICU or subacute care unit.[151] Transitional care describes the set of actions that enables continuity of health care over the course of a transition.[152] In 2009, the National Quality Forum proposed that transitional care should be measured when assessing quality of care coordination.[153] Elements to be evaluated include the quality of communication between providers, the quality of information, and the coordination of care services after the patient's transfer. Literature describing the EMS perspective on geriatric transitional care is rare and is a potential area of high-yield research.[154] Methods of education of prehospital providers have shown promise in increasing EMS provider sensitivity and awareness.[155] Effective transitional care is wholly dependent on the quality of communication between sending and receiving providers. Components of an effective care transition are listed in **Box 2**. Additional research priorities in geriatric transitional care include improved provider education, cognitive screening, identifying at-risk patients, and medication management.[156]

Several studies have evaluated the effect of communications interventions in improving the transitional care of elderly patients between NHs and acute-care hospitals. Emphasis on emergency medicine resident training in geriatrics has not yet been adopted uniformly, although several models exist.[157,158] A 2010 SAEM expert consensus panel created 26 competencies in geriatrics care that could form the basis of a standardized resident evaluation.[159] Our review of these studies found benefit of these interventions in communicating current medications and advanced directives.[31,105,121,160–162] Previous studies have shown that when available, completed advanced directives can affect medical decision making.[22] In some cases, clear communication of advance directives might have prevented a transfer to the ED.[14]

Electronic communication tools have been proved to facilitate information transfer between physically separate institutions and improve transitional outcomes.[113,163] A uniform electronic instrument can provide varying amounts and richness of information, and can be used to arrange referrals and follow-up care. Paper communication tools are capable of providing adequate information about the transfer but they should be standardized and attentively completed. Switching to electronic records has the potential to achieve the effect of the 1-page transfer form recommended and reduce the risk that the form is left incomplete or ignored.

The ISAR is one of several screening interventions that targets high-risk elderly patients in the ED and has been validated for use in the ED.[164] Patients who screen positive can be referred to an in-house specialist (ie, nurse, discharge planner), with additional training in emergency geriatrics for further assessment and coordinating necessary follow-up.[19,55,92,165–168] Some trials have looked at using a midlevel provider who is accountable for following high-risk older patients longitudinally after discharge, and this has been effective in reducing readmissions, costs, and lengths of hospitalizations.[169–171] An extended care pathway is a protocolized method of planning for the various stages of a patient's care based on a multidisciplinary approach to a specific reason for transfer. These methods have proved effective in hip fractures, with improved outcomes for several systems.[172–174]

Effective transitional care for elderly patients therefore requires communication between transferring and receiving providers, sharing relevant information about the patient's preferences and clinical status, robust medication reconciliation, early discharge planning, and use of palliative care when appropriate.[55,91,93] Accurate communication of medical information is fundamental in maintaining continuity of care during transfers between settings in the health care system.[93] A care plan should

---

Box 2
Components of effective care transitions

Communication between the sending and receiving clinicians, including summary of care given, patient's goals of care, updated problem lists, and baseline mental and physical function

Preparation of the patient and caregiver for what to expect at the next site of care

Reconciliation of the patient's medications prescribed before the initial transfer with the current regimen

A follow-up plan for how outstanding tests and appointments are completed

An explicit discussion with the patient/caregiver regarding warning symptoms

Updated contact telephone numbers for all parties

Data from Jones JS. Geriatric emergency care: an annotated bibliography. Ann Emerg Med 1992;21:835–41.

contain accurate and thoughtful medication reconciliation, arrangement of follow-up for outstanding results and necessary appointments, and discussion of warning signs necessitating emergent medical evaluation.[112] The patient must not be neglected and should be adequately prepared for the transition.

Sustainable Sources of Funding

Although a full discussion of the financing, funding, and payment incentives for geriatric care is beyond the scope of this article, it is an area of great importance that is worth discussing. Several strategies to improve transitional care have been proposed, but robust quality evidence supporting effective methods in transitional care is lacking. Although there is a growing movement to improve the quality-of-care metrics and research agenda, it is limited, and there is no financial incentive or accountability for transitional care in the fee-for-service Medicare reimbursement system. Federal economic quality incentives rewarding high-quality transitions could improve the paradigm and improve behaviors of clinicians and institutions. Performance measures that assess the quality of transitional care would permit comparisons between health care systems. Quality measures can determine whether or not a certain process has occurred, as well as evaluate outcomes. Few items of existing performance measures are related to transitions of care; however, there are no validated methods of measuring the quality of transitional care. During our research many articles were originated as either British or Australian studies. Other countries are making significant investments in the improvement of care for their elderly populations, and there is much we can do to increase our own contribution to this area of research. The efforts of the AGS, American College of Emergency Physicians, and SAEM should continue to create a positive impact and help create new measures and processes of care.

SUMMARY

We completed a review of more than 200 articles related to geriatric transitions to EDs. Transitions analyzed included patients presenting to the ED to the time of disposition. Particular attention was paid to transitions from NHs to the ED. Patients aged 65 years and older represent a growing segment of patients treated in US EDs. This population poses specific challenges of transitional care related to complex medical comorbidities, dependence on others for daily living activities, polypharmacy, and a higher frequency of transitions. Elderly patients transferring through the ED are at a higher likelihood for adverse events and readmission. Communication issues were frequently identified as central to adverse outcomes and complications with transitions. Several recommendations and interventions are shown to be effective in improving communications and transitions. Improving transitional care for these patients will be an area of increasing focus because of increasing demands for elderly emergency care. We recommend that emergency providers and NHs consolidate transitional care planning by developing strategies that implement this evidence. We also support the further development of metrics for transitional care and sustained research and funding agendas supporting the needs of elderly patients in the ED.

REFERENCES

1. Kinsella K, Velkoff VA. An aging world: 2001 (US Census Bureau, Series P95 01-1). Washington, DC: US Government Printing Office; 2001.
2. McNamara R, Rousseau E, Sanders AB. Geriatric emergency medicine: a survey of practicing emergency physicians. Ann Emerg Med 1992;21:796–800.

3. Eliastam M. Elderly patients in the emergency department. Ann Emerg Med 1989;8:133–9.
4. Burt CW, McCaig LF. Trends in hospital emergency department utilization: United States 1992–99. Vital Health Stat 13 2002;(150):1–34.
5. Emergency department managers warned of 'catastrophic' crowding due to elderly. ED Manag 2008;20(2):13–5.
6. Roberts DC, McKay MP, Shaffer A. Increasing rates of emergency department visits for elderly patients in the United States, 1993 to 2003. Ann Emerg Med 2008;51(6):769–74.
7. Lowenstein SR, Crescenzi CA, Kern DC, et al. Care of the elderly in the emergency department. Ann Emerg Med 1986;15:528–35.
8. Dickinson ED, Verdile VP, Kostyun CT, et al. Geriatric use of emergency medical services. Ann Emerg Med 1996;27:199–203.
9. Stiell A, Forster AJ, Stiell IG, et al. Prevalence of information gaps in the emergency department and the effect on patient outcomes. CMAJ 2003;169:1023–8.
10. Partnership for Solutions. New poll reveals Americans' concerns about living with chronic conditions and desire for elected officials to take action to improve care. Available at: http://partnershipforsolutions.org/media/press-releases. Accessed October 22, 2012.
11. Wilber ST, Gerson LW. A research agenda for geriatric emergency medicine. Acad Emerg Med 2003;10:251–60.
12. Grabowski DC, O'Malley AJ, Barhydt NR. The costs and potential savings associated with nursing home hospitalizations. Health Aff 2007;26:1753–61.
13. Miller D, Lewis L, Nork M, et al. Controlled trial of a geriatric case-finding and liaison service in an emergency department. J Am Geriatr Soc 1996;44(5): 513–20.
14. Ackermann RJ, Kemle KA, Vogel RL, et al. Emergency department use by nursing home residents. Ann Emerg Med 1998;31(6):749–57.
15. Strange GR, Chen EH, Sanders AB. Use of emergency departments by elderly patients: projections from a multicenter database. Ann Emerg Med 1992;21: 819–24.
16. Ettinger WH, Casani JA, Coon PJ, et al. Patterns of use of the emergency department by elderly patients. J Gerontol 1987;42:638–42.
17. Singal BM, Hedges JR, Rousseau EW, et al. Geriatric patient emergency visits part I: comparison of visits by geriatric and younger patients. Ann Emerg Med 1992;21:802–7.
18. Baum SA, Rubenstein LZ. Old people in the emergency room: age-related differences in emergency department use and care. J Am Geriatr Soc 1987; 35:398–404.
19. Aminzadeh F, Dalziel WB. Older adults in the emergency department: a systematic review of patterns of use, adverse outcomes, and effectiveness of interventions. Ann Emerg Med 2002;39:238–47.
20. Murtaugh CM, Litke A. Transitions through postacute and long-term care settings: patterns of use and outcomes for a national cohort of elders. Med Care 2002;40(3):227–36.
21. Naylor MD, Kurtzman ET, Pauly MV. Transitions of elders between long-term care and hospitals. Policy Polit Nurs Pract 2009;10(3):187–94.
22. Morrison RS, Olson E, Mertz KR, et al. The inaccessibility of advance directives on transfer from ambulatory to acute care settings. JAMA 1995;274:478–82.
23. Coleman EA, Berenson RA. Lost in transition: challenges and opportunities for improving the quality of transitional care. Ann Intern Med 2004;141:533–6.

24. Wang HE, Shah MN, Allman RM, et al. Emergency department visits by nursing home residents in the United States. J Am Geriatr Soc 2011;59: 1864–72.

25. Naylor MD, Stephens C, Bowles KH, et al. Cognitively impaired older adults: from hospital to home. Am J Nurs 2005;105:52–61.

26. Meier DE, Beresford L. Palliative care's challenge: facilitating transitions of care. J Palliat Med 2008;11:416–21.

27. Vladeck BC, Miller NA, Clauser SB. The changing face of long-term care. Health Care Financ Rev 1993;14:5–23.

28. Coleman EA, Smith JD, Raha D, et al. Posthospital medication discrepancies: prevalence and contributing factors. Arch Intern Med 2005;165:1842–7.

29. Travers D, Kjervik D, Katz L. Insufficient access to elderly patients' advance directives in the emergency department. In: Funk SG, Tornquist EM, Leeman J, et al, editors. Key aspects of preventing and managing chronic illness. New York: Springer; 2001. p. 207.

30. Hwang U, Morrison RS. The geriatric emergency department. J Am Geriatr Soc 2007;55:1873–6.

31. Terrell KM, Brizendine EJ, Bean WF, et al. An extended care facility-to-emergency department transfer form improves communication. Acad Emerg Med 2005;12:114–8.

32. Terrell KM, Miller DK. Challenges in transitional care between nursing homes and emergency departments. J Am Med Dir Assoc 2006;7(8): 499–505.

33. Gaddis GM. Elder care transfer forms. Acad Emerg Med 2005;12:160–1.

34. Currie CT, Lawson PM, Robertson CE, et al. Elderly patients discharged from accident and emergency departments–their dependency and support. Arch Emerg Med 1984;1:205–13.

35. Hedges JR, Singal BM, Rousseau EW, et al. Geriatric patient emergency visits part II: perceptions of visits by geriatric and younger patients. Ann Emerg Med 1992;21:808–13.

36. Brookoff D, Minniti-Hill M. Emergency department-based home care. Ann Emerg Med 1994;23:1101–6.

37. McCusker J, Ardman O, Bellavance F, et al. Use of community services by seniors before and after an emergency visit. Can J Aging 2001;20:193–209.

38. Gerson LW, Rousseau EW, Hogna TM, et al. Multicenter study of case finding in elderly emergency department patients. Acad Emerg Med 1995;2(8): 729–34.

39. Brown-Williams H, Neuhauser L, Ivey S, et al. From hospital to home: improving transitional care for older adults. Berkeley (CA): University of California, Health Research for Action; 2006. p. 1–34. Available at: http://www.healthresearchforaction.org/hospital-home-improving-transitional-care-older-adults. Accessed October 22, 2012.

40. Coleman EA, Parry C, Chalmers S, et al. The care transitions intervention: results of a randomized controlled trial. Arch Intern Med 2006;166:1822–8.

41. Boockvar K, Fishman E, Kyriacou CK, et al. Adverse events due to discontinuations in drug use and dose changes in patients transferred between acute and long-term care facilities. Arch Intern Med 2004;164(5):545–50.

42. American Medical Director's Association. Improving care transitions from the nursing facility to a community based setting. Columbia (MD): 2010. Available at: http://www.amda.com/governance/whitepapers/transitions_of_care.cfm. Accessed October 22, 2012.

43. Foster AJ, Murff HJ, Peterson JF, et al. The incidence and severity of adverse drug events affecting patients after discharge from the hospital. Ann Intern Med 2003;138(3):161–7.
44. Page RL II, Ruscin JM. The risk of adverse drug events and hospital-related morbidity and mortality among older adults with potentially inappropriate medication use. Am J Geriatr Pharmacother 2006;4:297–305.
45. Clarfield A, Bergman H, Kane R. Fragmentation of care for frail older people–an international problem. Experience from three countries: Israel, Canada, and the United States. J Am Geriatr Soc 2001;49:1714–21.
46. McCloskey R. The 'mindless' relationship between nursing homes and emergency departments: what do Bourdieu and Freire have to offer? Nurs Inq 2011;18:154–64.
47. Dalawari P, Duggan J, Vangimalla V, et al. Patient transfer forms enhance key information between nursing homes and emergency department. Geriatr Nurs 2011;32(4):270–5.
48. Belfrage MK, Chiminello C, Cooper D, et al. Pushing the envelope: clinical handover from the aged-care home to the emergency department. Med J Aust 2009; 190(Suppl 11):S117–20.
49. Jones AL, Dwyer LL, Bercovitz AR, et al. National Center for Health Statistics. The National Nursing Home survey: 2004 overview. Vital Health Stat 13 2009; 13(167):1–155. Available at: http://www.cdc.gov/nchs/nnhs/nnhs_products. htm. Accessed October 22, 2012.
50. Bergman H, Clarfield AM. Appropriateness of patient transfer from a nursing home to an acute-care hospital: a study of emergency room visits and hospital admissions. J Am Geriatr Soc 1991;39(12):1164–8.
51. Nawar EW, Niska RW, Xu J. National hospital ambulatory medical care survey: 2005 emergency department summary. Adv Data 2007;386:1–32.
52. Jagsi R, Kitch BT, Weinstein DF, et al. Residents report on adverse events and their causes. Arch Intern Med 2005;165:2607–13.
53. Singh H, Thomas EJ, Petersen LA, et al. Medical errors involving trainees: a study of closed malpractice claims from 5 insurers. Arch Intern Med 2007;167:2030–6.
54. Kripalani S, LeFevre F, Phillips CO, et al. Deficits in communication and information transfer between hospital-based and primary care physicians: implications for patient safety and continuity of care. JAMA 2007;297:831–41.
55. LaMantia MA, Scheunemann LP, Viera AJ, et al. Interventions to improve transitional care between nursing homes and hospitals: a systematic review. J Am Geriatr Soc 2010;58:777–82.
56. Ahmad S, O'Mahony MS. Where older people die: a retrospective population based study. QJM 2005;98:865–70.
57. Jakobsson E, Johnsson T, Persson LO, et al. End-of-life in a Swedish population: demographics, social conditions and characteristics of places of death. Scand J Caring Sci 2006;20:10–7.
58. Klinkenberg M, Visser G, Broese van Groenou MI, et al. The last 3 months of life: care, transitions and the place of death of older people. Health Soc Care Community 2005;13:420–30.
59. Van den Block L, Deschepper R, Bilsen J, et al. Transitions between care settings at the end of life in Belgium. JAMA 2007;298:1638–9.
60. Wilson DM, Northcott HC, Truman CD, et al. Location of death in Canada. Eval Health Prof 2001;24:385–403.
61. Gabrel CS, Jones A. The National Nursing Home Survey: 1997 Summary. Vital Health Stat 13 2000;147:1–121.

62. Young MP, Gooder VJ, McBride K, et al. Inpatient transfers to the intensive care unit: delays are associated with increased mortality and morbidity. J Gen Intern Med 2003;2:77–83.
63. Chalfin DB, Trzeciak S, Likourezos A, et al. Impact of delayed transfer of critically ill patients from the emergency department to the intensive care unit. Crit Care Med 2007;35(6):1477–83.
64. Yurkova I, Wolf L. Under-triage as a significant factor affecting transfer time between the emergency department and the intensive care unit. J Emerg Nurs 2011;37(5):491–6.
65. Arora V, Johnson J, Lovinger D, et al. Communication failures in patient sign-out and suggestions for improvement: a critical incident analysis. Qual Saf Health Care 2005;14:401–7.
66. Horwitz LI, Krumholz HM, Green ML, et al. Transfers of patient care between house staff on internal medicine wards: a national survey. Arch Intern Med 2006;166:1173–7.
67. Beach C, Croskerry P, Shapiro M. Profiles in patient safety: emergency care transitions. Acad Emerg Med 2003;10:364–7.
68. Sinha M, Shriki J, Salness R, et al. Need for standardized signout in the emergency department: a survey of emergency medicine residency and pediatric emergency medicine fellowship program directors. Acad Emerg Med 2007; 14:192–6.
69. Behara R, Wears RL, Perry SJ, et al. A conceptual framework for studying the safety of transitions in emergency care. In: Henriksen K, Battles JB, Marks ES, editors. Advances in patient safety: from research to implementation, vol. 2. Rockville (MD): Agency for Healthcare Research and Quality; 2005. p. 309–21.
70. Eisenberg EM, Murphy AG, Sutcliffe KM, et al. Communication in emergency medicine: implications for patient safety. Comm Monogr 2005;72: 390–413.
71. Apker J, Mallak LA, Gibson SC. Communicating in the "gray zone": perceptions about emergency physician hospitalist handoffs and patient safety. Acad Emerg Med 2007;14:884–94.
72. Beach C. Lost in transition. AHRQ WebM&M [serial online]. Available at: http://webmm.ahrq.gov/case.aspx?caseID116. Accessed October 22, 2012.
73. Burke CS, Salas E, Wilson-Donnelly K, et al. How to turn a team of experts into an expert medical team: guidance from the aviation and military communities. Qual Saf Health Care 2004;13(Suppl 1):i96–104.
74. Bunderson JS, Sutcliffe KM. Comparing alternative conceptualizations of functional diversity in management teams: process and performance effects. Acad Manage J 2002;45:875–93.
75. Horwitz LI, Meredith T, Schuur JD, et al. Dropping the baton: a qualitative analysis of failures during the transition from emergency department to inpatient care. Ann Emerg Med 2009;53(6):701–10.
76. Coiera EW, Jayasuriya RA, Hardy J, et al. Communication loads on clinical staff in the emergency department. Med J Aust 2002;176:415–8.
77. Tversky A, Kahneman D. Judgment under uncertainty: heuristics and biases. Science 1974;185:1124–31.
78. Kelly R. Goings-on in a CCU: an ethnomethodological account of things that go on in a routine hand-over. Nurs Crit Care 1999;4:85–91.
79. Kerr MP. A qualitative study of shift handover practice and function from a sociotechnical perspective. J Adv Nurs 2002;37:125–34.

80. Lally S. An investigation into the functions of nurses' communication at the inter-shift handover. J Nurs Manag 1999;7:29–36.

81. Sherlock C. The patient handover: a study of its form, function and efficiency. Nurs Stand 1995;9:33–6.

82. Agency for Healthcare Research and Quality HCUPnet. Outcomes by patient and hospital characteristics for all discharges. 1999. Available at: http://hcup.ahrq.gov/HCUPnet.asp. Accessed October 22, 2012.

83. Barker WH, Zimmer JG, Hall WJ, et al. Rates, patterns, causes, and costs of hospitalization of nursing home residents: a population-based study. Am J Public Health 1994;84:1615–20.

84. Beers M, Sliwkowski J, Brooks J. Compliance with medication orders among the elderly after hospital discharge. Hosp Formul 1992;27:720–4.

85. Williams S, Moore C, Wisnevesky J, et al. Assessing medical errors related to the continuity of care from an inpatient to an outpatient setting [abstract]. J Gen Intern Med 2002;17(Suppl 1):218.

86. Kravitz R, Reuben D, Davis JW, et al. Geriatric home assessment after hospital discharge. J Am Geriatr Soc 1994;42:1229–34.

87. Meredith S, Feldman PH, Frey D, et al. Possible medication errors in home healthcare patients. J Am Geriatr Soc 2002;49:719–24.

88. Guttman A, Afilafo M, Guttman R, et al. An emergency department-based nurse discharge coordinator for elder patients: does it make a difference? Acad Emerg Med 2004;11(12):1318–27.

89. McCusker J, Dendukuri N, Tousignant P, et al. Rapid two-stage emergency department intervention for seniors: impact on continuity of care. Acad Emerg Med 2003;10(3):233–43.

90. Ouslander JG, Lamb G, Perloe M. Potentially avoidable hospitalizations of nursing home residents: frequency, causes, and costs. J Am Geriatr Soc 2010;58(4):627–35.

91. Parker SG, Fadayevatan R, Lee SD. Acute hospital care for frail older people. Age Ageing 2006;35(6):551–2.

92. National Transitions of Care Coalition. Improving transitions of care: the vision of the national transitions of care coalition. Little Rock (AR); 2008. Available at: http://www.ntocc.org/Portals/0/PolicyPaper.pdf. Accessed October 22, 2012.

93. Coleman EA, Boult C, The American Geriatrics Society Health Care Systems Committee. Improving the quality of transitional care for persons with complex care needs. J Am Geriatr Soc 2003;51:556–7.

94. Hastings N, Schmader K, Sloan R, et al. Adverse health outcomes after discharge from the emergency department–incidence and risk factors in a veteran population. J Gen Intern Med 2007;22(11):1527–31.

95. Kramer A, Eilertsen T, Lin M, et al. Effects of nurse staffing on hospital transfer quality measures for new admissions. In: Health Care Financing Administration, editor. Appropriateness of minimum nurse staffing ratios for nursing homes. Baltimore (MD): Health Care Financing Administration; 2000. p. 9.1–9.22.

96. Caplan G, Williams A, Daly B, et al. A randomized controlled trial of comprehensive geriatric assessment and multidisciplinary intervention after discharge of the elderly from the emergency department–the DEED II study. J Am Geriatr Soc 2004;52(9):1417–23.

97. Ballabio C, Bergamaschini L, Mauri S, et al. A comprehensive evaluation of elderly people discharged from an emergency department. Intern Emerg Med 2008;3(3):245–9.

98. Saliba D, Kington R, Buchanan J, et al. Appropriateness of the decision to transfer nursing facility residents to the hospital. J Am Geriatr Soc 2000;48(2):154–63.

99. Ouslander JG, Lamb G, Tappen R, et al. Interventions to reduce hospitalizations from nursing homes: evaluation of the INTERACT II collaborative quality improvement project. J Am Geriatr Soc 2011;59(4):745–53.

100. NCHS Data Brief Number 33, April 2010. Potentially preventable emergency department visits by nursing home residents: United States, 2004. Available at: http://www.cdc.gov/nchs/data/databriefs/db33.pdf. Accessed November 2, 2012.

101. Intrator O, Zinn J, Mor V. Nursing home characteristics and potentially preventable hospitalizations of long-stay residents. J Am Geriatr Soc 2004;52:1730–6.

102. Kane RL, Keckhafer G, Flood S, et al. The effect of Evercare on hospital use. J Am Geriatr Soc 2003;51:1427–34.

103. Bodenheimer T. Long-term care for frail elderly people–the On Lok model. N Engl J Med 1999;341:1324–8.

104. Tresch DD, Simpson WM Jr, Burton JR. Relationship of long-term and acute-care facilities: the problem of patient transfer and continuity of care. J Am Geriatr Soc 1985;33:819–26.

105. Coleman EA. Falling through the cracks: challenges and opportunities for improving transitional care for persons with continuous complex care needs. J Am Geriatr Soc 2003;51(4):549–55.

106. Gittell JH, Fairfield KM, Bierbaum B, et al. Impact of relational coordination on quality of care, postoperative pain and functioning, and length of stay. Med Care 2000;38:807–19.

107. Levine C. Rough crossings: family caregivers' odysseys through the healthcare system. New York: United Hospital Fund of New York; 1998.

108. Coleman E, Smith JD, Frank J, et al. Development and testing of a measure designed to assess the quality of care transitions. Int J Integrated Care 2002;2. Available at: http://www.ijic.org/. Accessed October 22, 2012.

109. Weaver FM, Perloff L, Waters T. Patients' and caregivers' transition from hospital to home. Needs and recommendations. Home Health Care Serv Q 1998;17:27–48.

110. Jones JS, Dwyer PR, White LJ, et al. Patient transfer from nursing home to emergency department. Outcomes and policy implications. Acad Emerg Med 2002; 4:908–15.

111. Ghusn HF, Teasdale TA, Jordan D. Continuity of do-not-resuscitate orders between hospital and nursing home settings. J Am Geriatr Soc 2002;445:465–9.

112. Grief CL. Patterns of ED use and perceptions of the elderly regarding their emergency care: a synthesis of recent research. J Emerg Nurs 2003;29(2):122–6.

113. Jones JS, Rousseau EW, Schropp MA, et al. Geriatric training in emergency medicine residency programs. Ann Emerg Med 1992;21:825–9.

114. Jones JS. Geriatric emergency care: an annotated bibliography. Ann Emerg Med 1992;21:835–41.

115. Sanders AB. Care of the elderly in emergency departments: conclusions and recommendations. Ann Emerg Med 1992;21:830–4.

116. Sanders AB. Care of the elderly in emergency departments: where do we stand? Ann Emerg Med 1992;21:792–5.

117. Sanders AB, Morley JE. The older person and the emergency department. J Am Geriatr Soc 1993;41:880–2.

118. Schwartz GR. Geriatric emergency medicine. In: Schwartz GR, Cayten CG, Mangelsen MA, et al, editors. Principles and practice of emergency medicine. 3rd edition. Philadelphia: Lea & Febiger; 1992. p. 2559–98.

119. Institute of Medicine. Crossing the quality chasm: a new health system of the 21st century. Washington, DC: National Academy Press; 2001.
120. Gerteis M, Edgman-Levitan S, Daley J, et al, editors. Through the patient's eyes. Understanding and promoting patient-centered care. San Francisco (CA): Jossey-Bass; 1993.
121. vom Eigen KA, Walker JD, Edgman-Levitan S, et al. Care partner experiences with hospital care. Med Care 1999;37:33–8.
122. Anderson M, Helms L. Communication between continuing care organizations. Res Nurs Health 1995;18:49–57.
123. Terrell K, Hustey F, Gerson L, et al. Quality indicators for geriatric emergency care. Acad Emerg Med 2009;16(5):441–9.
124. Horwitz LI, Moin T, Krumholz HM, et al. Consequences of inadequate sign-out for patient care. Arch Intern Med 2008;168(16):1755–60.
125. Pronovost P, Needham D, Berenholtz S, et al. An intervention to decrease catheter-related bloodstream infections in the ICU. N Engl J Med 2006;355: 2725–32.
126. Patterson ES. Structuring flexibility: the potential good, bad and ugly in standardization of handovers. Qual Saf Health Care 2008;17:4–5.
127. Horwitz LI, Moin T, Green ML. Development and implementation of an oral sign-out skills curriculum. J Gen Intern Med 2007;22:1470–4.
128. Lee LH, Levine JA, Schultz HJ. Utility of a standardized sign-out card for new medical interns. J Gen Intern Med 1996;11:753–5.
129. Petersen LA, Orav EJ, Teich JM, et al. Using a computerized signout program to improve continuity of inpatient care and prevent adverse events. Jt Comm J Qual Improv 1998;24:77–87.
130. Van Eaton EG, Horvath KD, Lober WB, et al. A randomized, controlled trial evaluating the impact of a computerized rounding and sign-out system on continuity of care and resident work hours. J Am Coll Surg 2005;200:538–45.
131. Vidyarthi AR, Arora V, Schnipper JL, et al. Managing discontinuity in academic medical centers: strategies for a safe and effective resident sign-out. J Hosp Med 2006;1:257–66.
132. Aydin CE, Rice RE. Bringing social worlds together: computers as catalysts for new interactions in health care organizations. J Health Soc Behav 1992;33:168–85.
133. Milliken FJ, Martins LL. Searching for common threads: understanding the multiple effects of diversity in organizational groups. Acad Manag Rev 1996; 21:402–33.
134. Davenport DL, Henderson WG, Mosca CL, et al. Risk-adjusted morbidity in teaching hospitals correlates with reported levels of communication and collaboration on surgical teams but not with scale measures of teamwork climate, safety climate, or working conditions. J Am Coll Surg 2007;205:778–84.
135. Rex JH, Turnbull JE, Allen SJ, et al. Systematic root cause analysis of adverse drug events in a tertiary referral hospital. Jt Comm J Qual Improv 2000;26: 563–75.
136. Ursprung R, Gray JE, Edwards WH, et al. Real time patient safety audits: improving safety every day. Qual Saf Health Care 2005;14:284–9.
137. Lardner R. Effective shift handover, etc., prepared for the United Kingdom, Health and Safety Executive, Offshore Safety Division. Available at: http://www.hse.gov.uk/research/otopdf/1996/ oto96003. Accessed October 22, 2012.
138. Patterson ES, Roth EM, Woods DD, et al. Handoff strategies in settings with high consequences for failure: lessons for health care operations. Int J Qual Health Care 2004;16:125–32.

139. Kuperman GJ, Boyle D, Jha A, et al. How promptly are inpatients treated for critical laboratory results? J Am Med Inform Assoc 1998;5:112–9.
140. Yen K, Gorelick MH. Strategies to improve flow in the pediatric emergency department. Pediatr Emerg Care 2007;23:745–9.
141. Smith PC, Araya-Guerra R, Bublitz C, et al. Missing clinical information during primary care visits. JAMA 2005;293:565–71.
142. Oakes SL, Gillespie SM, Ye Y, et al. Transitional care of the long-term care patient. Clin Geriatr Med 2011;27:2–32.
143. National Quality Forum. National voluntary consensus standards for hospital care: Additional priority areas–2005–2006. Available at: http://www.qualityforum.org. Accessed October 22, 2012.
144. Boockvar KS, Carlson LaCorte H, Giambanco V, et al. Medication reconciliation for reducing drug-discrepancy adverse events. Am J Geriatr Pharmacother 2006;4:236–43.
145. Spaite DW, Bartholomeaux F, Guisto J, et al. Rapid process redesign in a university-based emergency department: decreasing waiting time intervals and improving patient satisfaction. Ann Emerg Med 2002;39:168–77.
146. Moore C, Wisnivesky J, Williams S, et al. Medical errors related to discontinuity of care from an inpatient to an outpatient setting. J Gen Intern Med 2003;18: 646–51.
147. Kim CS, Spahlinger DA, Kin JM, et al. Lean health care: what can hospitals learn from a world-class automaker? J Hosp Med 2006;1:191–9.
148. Crotty M, Rowett D, Spurling L, et al. Does the addition of a pharmacist transition coordinator improve evidence-based medication management and health outcomes in older adults moving from the hospital to a long-term care facility? Results of a randomized, controlled trial. Am J Geriatr Pharmacother 2004;2: 257–64.
149. Tolle SW, Tilden VP, Nelson CA, et al. A prospective study of the efficacy of the physician order form for life-sustaining treatment. J Am Geriatr Soc 1998;46: 1097–102.
150. Madden C, Garrett J, Busby-Whitehead J. The interface between nursing homes and emergency departments: a community effort to improve transfer of information. Acad Emerg Med 1998;5:1123–6.
151. Katon W, Von Korf M, Lin E, et al. Collaborative management to achieve treatment guidelines. Impact on depression in primary care. JAMA 1995;273: 1026–31.
152. McCusker J, Bellavance F, Cardin S, et al. Detection of older people at increased risk of adverse health outcomes after an emergency visit: the ISAR screening tool. J Am Geriatr Soc 1999;47:1229–37.
153. McCusker J, Bellavance F, Cardin S, et al. Screening for geriatric problems in the emergency department: reliability and validity. Acad Emerg Med 1998;5: 883–93.
154. McCusker J, Bellavance F, Cardin S, et al. Prediction of hospital utilization among elderly patients during the 6 months after an emergency department visit. Acad Emerg Med 2000;36:438–45.
155. McCusker J, Cardin S, Bellavance F, et al. Return to the emergency department among elders: patterns and predictors. Acad Emerg Med 2000;7:249–59.
156. McCusker J, Healey E, Bellavance F, et al. Predictors of repeat emergency department visits by elders. Acad Emerg Med 1997;4:581–8.
157. Meldon SW, Mion LC, Palmer RM, et al. Implementation of a two-stage geriatric screen in the ED. Acad Emerg Med 1999;6:530–1.

158. Rubenstein LZ. The emergency department: a useful site for CGA? J Am Geriatr Soc 1996;44:601–2.
159. Naylor M, Brooten D, Campbell R, et al. Comprehensive discharge planning and home follow-up of hospitalized elders: a randomized clinical trial. JAMA 1999; 281:613–20.
160. Rich M, Beckham V, Wittenberg C, et al. A multidisciplinary intervention to prevent the readmission of elderly patients with congestive heart failure. N Engl J Med 1995;333:1190–5.
161. Stewart S, Pearson S, Horowitz J. Effects of a home-based intervention among patients with congestive heart failure discharged from acute hospital care. Arch Intern Med 2000;158:1067–72.
162. Zuckerman J, Sakales S, Fabian D, et al. Hip fractures in geriatric patients. Results of an interdisciplinary hospital care program. Clin Orthop 1992;274: 213–25.
163. Ogilvie-Harris D, Botsford D, Hawker R. Elderly patients with hip fractures. Improved outcome with the use of care maps with high-quality medical and nursing protocols. J Orthop Trauma 1993;7:428–37, 170.
164. Ethans K, MacKnight C. Hip fracture in the elderly: an interdisciplinary team approach to rehabilitation. Postgrad Med 1998;103:157–8.
165. Coleman E, Besdine R. Integrating quality assurance across sites of geriatric care. In: Calkins E, Wagner E, Boult C, et al, editors. New ways to care for older people. New York: Springer; 1998. p. 185–95.
166. National Chronic Care Consortium. Self-assessment for system integration tool. Bloomington (MN): SASI; 1998.
167. Joint Commission on Accreditation of Healthcare Organizations. Hospital accreditation standards. Oakbrook Terrace (IL): Joint Commission on Accreditation of Healthcare Organizations; 2002.
168. Wenger NS, Young RT. Quality indicators for continuity and coordination of care in vulnerable elders. J Am Geriatr Soc 2007;55:S285–92.
169. Naylor M, Brooten D, Campbell R, et al. Comprehensive discharge planning and home follow-up of hospitalized elders: A randomized clinical trial. JAMA 1999; 281:613–20.
170. Rich M, Beckham V, Wittenberg C, et al. A multidisciplinary intervention to prevent the readmission of elderly patients with congestive heart failure. N Engl J Med 1995;333:1190–5.
171. Stewart S, Pearson S, Horowitz J. Effects of a home-based intervention among patients with congestive heart failure discharged from acute hospital care. Arch Intern Med 2000;158:1067–72.
172. Zuckerman J, Sakales S, Fabian D, et al. Hip fractures in geriatric patients. Results of an interdisciplinary hospital care program. Clin Orthop 1992;274: 213–25.
173. Ogilvie-Harris D, Botsford D, Hawker R. Elderly patients with hip fractures. Improved outcome with the use of care maps with high-quality medical and nursing protocols. J Orthop Trauma 1993;7:428–37.
174. Ethans K, MacKnight C. Hip fracture in the elderly: An interdisciplinary team approach to rehabilitation. Postgrad Med 1998;103:157–8.

Emergency Department Observation Units and the Older Patient

Mark G. Moseley, MD, MHA, Miles P. Hawley, MD, MBA,
Jeffrey M. Caterino, MD, MPH*

KEYWORDS

- Geriatric • Observation • Emergency department • Elderly

KEY POINTS

- Older adults can successfully be cared for in emergency department observation units (EDOUs) with a variety of clinical protocols.
- EDOUs provide distinct advantages for the care of older adults, such as the ability to further assess functional status, response to therapy, home environment, and stability for discharge.
- There are specific EDOU inclusion and exclusion criteria that vary among individual EDOUs and by type of protocol patients are to be placed on.
- Protocols amenable to caring for older adults include chest pain, syncope, congestive heart failure, transient ischemic attack (TIA), vertigo, skin infection, urinary tract infection (UTI), trauma, and abdominal pain, among others.
- Placement in an EDOU is affected by both clinical and regulatory concerns.

INTRODUCTION

An increasing number of emergency departments (EDs) are providing extended care and monitoring for patients in EDOUs.[1] Reasons for the expansion of ED-based observation services are multifactorial and include both benefits to ED operational efficiency and a response to insurer policies regarding readmissions. These units provide a period of time (generally 24 hours) to complete diagnostic studies and initial therapeutic interventions for a large variety of conditions.[2] EDOUs can be particularly useful for older adults both as an alternative to hospitalization in appropriately selected patients and as a means of risk stratification for older adults with unclear presentations. They can

Funding sources: Jeffrey M. Caterino has funding from National Institute on Aging, Pfizer, and Mitsubishi and is a consultant for newMentor, Inc. Mark G. Moseley and Miles P. Hawley have no funding sources.
Conflict of interest: No conflicts to declare.
Department of Emergency Medicine, The Ohio State University, 376 West 10th Avenue, Columbus, OH 43035, USA
* Corresponding author.
E-mail address: jeffrey.caterino@osumc.edu

also provide a period of therapeutic intervention and reassessment for older patients in whom the appropriateness and safety of immediate outpatient care is unclear.[3,4] This article first discusses the general characteristics of EDOUs. Next, it discusses appropriate entry and exclusion criteria for older adults in EDOUs. Then, several of the most common observation unit protocols are reviewed, focusing on their relevance to older adults. Finally, regulatory implications of observation status for patients with Medicare are briefly reviewed.

DEVELOPMENT OF EMERGENCY DEPARTMENT OBSERVATION UNITS

EDOUs have been used for many years to extend and enhance the ability of ED clinicians to make more appropriate disposition and management decisions. The majority of such units began as efforts to more efficiently manage, risk stratify, and disposition patients with low-acuity chest pain.[5] Over time, interest developed in managing a larger number of conditions to help alleviate diagnostic or severity of illness uncertainty in clinical care for patients who were too sick for ED discharge but not sick enough to be admitted to the hospital. The literature surrounding EDOUs has consistently demonstrated their value to patient management and to both ED and hospital operations, including decreases in ED length of stay and admission rate from the ED.[6–8] Several studies have shown cost effectiveness and equivalent clinical outcomes of EDOUs in comparison with inpatient care.[8–12] Studies have demonstrated positive benefits to ED patient satisfaction,[13,14] low rates of ED recidivism, and improved continuity of care.[15,16]

As a result of these benefits, several organizations have advocated for the creation of more EDOUs. In June of 2006, the Institute of Medicine released its report, *Hospital-Based Emergency Care: At the Breaking Point*, which specifically cited the benefits of EDOUs.[17] In 2008, the American College of Emergency Physicians made similar recommendations for implementation of ED-based observation units.[18] The result has been a nationwide increase in the availability of observation services for ED patients, although adoption is still not universal, even for common conditions, such as chest pain.[2,19] Currently, more than 2.3 million ED patients each year are placed in observation units, approximately one-third of whom are over 65 years of age.[4,19]

CHARACTERISTICS OF EMERGENCY DEPARTMENT OBSERVATION UNITS

Currently, 34% of hospitals have an observation unit, 56% of which are classified as EDOUs and another 36% of which are housed within the hospital itself.[2,19] In a majority of cases, observation units are under the direction and clinical responsibility of the ED.[2] Most commonly, patients must be evaluated in an ED before placement in an observation unit.[2] Although the focus of this article is on EDOUs, they share many characteristics with the hospital-based units.[20] As a result, this article's conclusions can generally be applied to both types of units.

The specific characteristics of EDOUs vary by institution (outlined in **Box 1**). The sum total of these factors—admission procedures, staffing, protocols, and resources—dictates the inclusion or exclusion of individual patients from each EDOU. Some units only take low-risk to moderate-risk patients with specific, predefined pathways. Others are more aggressive, taking more ill or more complex patients or those with less well-defined conditions.

Admission Procedure

In most cases, patients eligible for EDOU care are initially seen and evaluated in an ED.[2] Although some units allow for patients to come directly from outpatient clinics

---

Box 1
Characteristics varying between individual emergency department observation units, which may affect patient selection

1. Admission procedure:

   a. Closed admission (only by ED physician after evaluation in the ED)

   b. Open admission (other physicians may place patients in unit; ED evaluation may or may not be required)

2. Staffing patterns:

   a. Physician coverage (type, availability, and other responsibilities)

   b. Midlevel provider coverage

   c. Nursing ratios

   d. Variation in coverage by time of day/day of the week

3. Protocol availability:

   a. Types of conditions cared for in the unit

   b. Important inclusion/exclusion criteria

   c. Variation by day of the week

4. Available resources:

   a. Ability to complete specific diagnostic tests, provide specific therapeutic interventions, and obtain specific specialty consultation

---

or doctors' offices, initial triage to determine appropriateness of care and screening for exclusion criteria is best accomplished in an ED under the auspices of the ED physician. For units with open admission policies, a referring physician should have a clear understanding of the capabilities and procedures of the unit. For example, it should be clear which physician is responsible for the care of a patient while in the unit.

Staffing Patterns

Staffing of an EDOU may include various combinations of coverage by emergency physicians concurrently working in the ED, physicians with sole responsibility for the EDOU, and/or midlevel providers. Staffing patterns have implications for the types of patients cared for in EDOUs. Units staffed by physicians also concurrently staffing an ED generally take specific patients only. In units staffed by a full complement of dedicated physicians and midlevel providers, there is greater ability to be aggressive in taking more complex and less well-defined patients. As a result, these units generally are more aggressive in their acceptance criteria. Nurse staffing ratios must also be considered in patient selection.

Available Protocols and Resources

Most EDOUs limit their patient populations to specific predefined treatment protocols and pathways (**Box 2**).[2] There are specific inclusion and exclusion criteria associated with each protocol that aid in the selection of appropriate patients. The goal is to choose patients who are likely to meet discharge criteria within 24 hours. In general, observation failure rates with subsequent admission from observation status of less than 30% are considered acceptable.[4,19,21]

For simplicity, EDOU patients can be classified into 2 groups: (1) diagnostic patients who have a chief complaint that requires monitoring and further diagnostic evaluation

---

Box 2
Potential emergency department observation unit protocols applicable to older adults

Cardiac

Chest pain

Syncope

Hypertensive urgency

Congestive heart failure

Neurologic

TIA

Vertigo

Headache

Infectious disease

Skin and soft tissue infection (SSTI)

UTI

Pneumonia

Other

Trauma

Allergic reaction

Abdominal pain

Dehydration

Nausea/vomiting

Low back pain

Adverse medication reaction

Nephrolithiasis

Asthma exacerbation

(eg, chest pain or abdominal pain) and (2) therapeutic patients in whom the diagnosis is known but whose severity of illness does not allow immediate safe discharge (for example, asthma or cellulitis). The breadth of protocols in a specific EDOU depends on the resources available to that unit, including those that have been arranged with other hospital services. Availability of resources may also vary by day of the week and time of day. For example, most EDOUs have protocols to rule out myocardial infarction, including stress testing while in the observation unit. This testing may be limited on weekends or holidays. The use of other protocols may depend on availability of imaging or consulting resources. **Box 3** presents a partial list of the types of services available in EDOUs.

THE ROLE OF EDOUS IN CARING FOR OLDER ADULTS

Older adults have been successfully cared for in EDOUs on a variety of protocols, generally demonstrating rates of admission equivalent to those of younger adults.[3,4,16,21–24] One study showed a slightly increased rate of admission for older adults (26% vs 18%), but their admission rate was still below a predetermined cutoff

---

Box 3
Sample of diagnostic modalities and therapies that may be available in an emergency department observation unit

Diagnostics

Serial clinical examinations

Telemetry monitoring

CT scan

MRI

Magnetic resonance angiography

Vascular ultrasound (eg, extremity and carotids)

Stress testing (multiple modalities)

Transthoracic echocardiogram

Ultrasound

Hepatobiliary iminodiacetic acid (HIDA) scan

Therapeutics

Intravenous (IV) hydration

Intravenous antibiotics

Antiemetics

Acute pain control

Specialty Consultations

Select medical and surgical subspecialties

Physical/occupational therapy

Social work/case management

Respiratory therapy

Pharmacy/medication review

---

of 30%.[4] Advanced age also has not been associated with increased revisit rates after EDOU stay compared with younger patients.[3,4,16] EDOUs can effectively care for older adults.

EDOUs provide an opportunity for further evaluation and management of older patients beyond what is possible in EDs. They provides time to obtain several services and assessments of particular concern to the older population, such as social work consultation, physical therapy assessment, and medication review and reconciliation. Some EDOUs have incorporated into their EDOU care some form of comprehensive geriatric assessment, which encompasses a multidisciplinary approach to patients, for example, by considering medical issues, functional status, and social issues, among other issues.[25,26] In one study from Singapore, this assessment included medical, social, and functional factors, such as fall history, timed up and go test, continence assessment, mental status evaluation, visual acuity testing, nutrition assessment, and questioning on behavior and mood. More than 70% of older EDOU patients had at least one need identified. The program resulted in decreased ED revisit (adjusted incident rate ratio of 0.59) and hospitalization rates (ratio of 0.64) over the succeeding year.[3]

CONTRAINDICATIONS TO OBSERVATION UNIT CARE FOR OLDER ADULTS

Prior to placing a patient in an EDOU, physicians must consider appropriateness both in light of specific inclusion/exclusion criteria and Centers for Medicare and Medicaid Services (CMS) rules regarding observation care (discussed later). Older adults may present unique challenges to an observation unit and several factors must be considered as potential contraindications to placement (**Box 4**). In addition to this list, there may be specific contraindications for individual protocols (discussed later). Specific inclusion and exclusion criteria are set by each EDOU.

Unstable Vital Signs

Patients with unstable vital signs are generally not appropriate for observation care due to their increased resource needs and severity of illness. One exception is a hypertensive urgency protocol, which accepts patients with severe elevation in blood pressure but without evidence of end-organ damage. One study found, however, that older adults with systolic blood pressures greater than or equal to 180 mm Hg were more likely to be admitted.[22]

Altered Mental Status

Altered mental status, including delirium and other alterations of consciousness, is often an exclusion criterion in EDOUs. Patients with altered mental status may have a greater likelihood of failing to improve within 24 hours. Also, EDOUs may not have nurse staffing ratios adequate to handle altered patients. In some cases, such as mild alterations in mental status in the setting of a UTI, placement in the EDOU may be considered.

Likely Need for Placement in a Skilled Facility

Patients who are expected to require placement in a skilled nursing or rehabilitation facility are also poor EDOU candidates. CMS rules require a 3-day hospital stay for before such placement.[27] Furthermore, the resources required to affect rapid placement in such facilities are generally not available in the EDOU. It is rare that such placement could be arranged within 24 hours.

Failure to Thrive

A diagnosis of "failure to thrive" covers a broad array of causes and symptoms.[28,29] Usually, these require substantial investigation and often require skilled nursing placement. Such evaluations are generally not easily accomplished in an EDOU. Patients with failure to thrive have often failed outpatient therapies for their conditions or could

---

Box 4
Factors excluding older adults from observation unit care

1. Unstable vital signs
2. Altered mental status
3. Likely need for placement
4. Failure to thrive
5. Exacerbations of chronic problems
6. Expected to take greater than 24 hours for significant improvement
7. Inability to ambulate

be considered unsafe discharges, both of which are considered indications for admission by CMS.

Exacerbations of Chronic Problems

Ongoing treatment of chronic problems is rarely appropriate for the EDOU. Patients with ongoing chronic conditions have usually failed adequate outpatient therapy and do not improve within 24 hours, requiring admission. In other cases, the problem is more appropriately treated in an outpatient setting. EDOUs are appropriate, however, for acute exacerbations of many chronic conditions, such as asthma or congestive heart failure. The general rule should be to place patients in an EDOU who require specific diagnostic or therapeutic interventions likely to change management or improve symptoms within 24 hours.

Expected to Require More Than 24 Hours of Care

Patients expected to require more than 24 hours to complete their care should be admitted rather than placed in an EDOU. Examples include patients with congestive heart failure severe enough likely to require more than 24 hours of diuresis or with severe SSTI likely to require more than 24 hours of IV antibiotics.

Inability to Ambulate

Inability to ambulate is a contraindication depending on the likelihood of improvement and ability for a safe discharge within 24 hours. Patients who obviously require placement or do not have the resources at home to aid in their care should be admitted. In some cases, EDOU placement is appropriate to obtain a physical therapy evaluation and/or arrange for additional home resources, such as family support, care providers, or outpatient physical therapy.

RELATIONSHIP OF SPECIFIC OBSERVATION UNIT PROTOCOLS TO THE CARE OF OLDER ADULTS

A summary of evidence for each of these protocols is available in **Table 1**.

Chest Pain

Chest pain is the most common EDOU admitting symptom.[5,30–32] Most EDOU chest pain patients, within a 24-hour period, receive telemetry monitoring, serial cardiac enzymes, serial ECGs, and noninvasive cardiac testing.[33] Cardiology consultation is also available if necessary. Chest pain is also the most common EDOU diagnosis for older patients.[4] Although older adults with chest pain are more likely to be admitted from the EDOU than younger patients, rates are within acceptable levels (<30%).[21,34] The increased rates are likely related to the increased prevalence of coronary artery disease in older adults, a known risk factor for positive stress testing and admission.[34] Older adults without known coronary artery disease are no more likely to be admitted then younger patients.[21]

An important component of patient selection for EDOU chest pain protocols is risk stratification. Patients with unstable angina or non–ST elevation myocardial infarction require admission for both severity of illness and intensity of service considerations. EDOUs are safe and cost effective for the evaluation of low-risk chest pain (for example, those with low-risk Thrombolysis in Myocardial Infarction [TIMI] risk scores [see **Box 5**]).[5,35] In addition, several recent studies have shown that intermediate-risk patients, including those with known coronary artery disease, can be safely evaluated in an EDOU setting.[34–36]

Table 1
Summary of selected evidence for specific EDOU protocols

Protocol	Study	Number of Patients	Mean/Median Age (if Reported)	Outcomes
Chest pain	Holly et al,[35] 2012	552		EDOU admission rate for intermediate risk chest pain patients was 16% No unanticipated adverse events at 30 d
	Miller et al,[12] 2012	120		Physician selected cardiac testing cost-effective vs prespecified testing ($1686 vs $2005)
	Miller et al,[10] 2011	109	56 y	EDOU-CMR decreased costs over 1 y compared with inpatient care ($3101 vs $742) Major cardiac events similar between groups (6% vs 9%)
	Jagminas and Partridge,[20] 2005	1413	Not reported	Compared EDOU to inpatient OU EDOU had decreased admission rates (7.9% vs 19.2%) and decreased cost ($889 vs $1039)
	Goodacre et al,[8] 2004	972	49 y	Decreased admissions from 54% to 37% Follow-up costs reduced
Syncope	Anderson et al,[29,41] 2012	323	66 y	In EDOU patients with syncope and normal ECG, 0/235 had structural cardiac abnormality identified
Congestive heart failure	Diercks et al,[52] 2006	538	61 y	27% of ED patients with heart failure meet criteria to be managed in an EDOU
	Storrow et al,[48] 2005	64	58 y	Decreased cost, length of stay and no difference in outcomes in EDOU vs admission
TIA	Ross et al,[9] 2007	149	68 y	Compared with inpatient, EDOU patients had • Lower median length of stay (25 vs 61 h) • Lower 90-d costs ($890 vs $1547) • Greater rates of imaging (97% vs 91% for carotids; 97% vs 73% for echocardiography)
	Nahab et al,[55] 2011	142	68 y	79% discharged Median length of stay decreased from 47 h (inpatients) to 26 h (EDOU patients) Lower median costs (cost difference $1643 vs inpatients)
SSTI	Schrock et al,[24] 2008	179	41 y	38% Failed EDOU care and required admission Advanced age was not associated with failure of EDOU care

(continued on next page)

Table 1
(continued)

Protocol	Study	Number of Patients	Mean/Median Age (if Reported)	Outcomes
UTI	Schrock et al,[63] 2010	633	32 y	29% of EDOU patients ultimately admitted
Trauma	Holly et al,[75] 2011	259	35 y	No deaths, intubations, or other adverse events One missed injury, which did not affect outcome Admission rate from EDOU 10%
	Kendall et al,[76] 2011	1169	31 y	6% of EDOU patients with blunt abdominal trauma admitted EDOU median length of stay 9.5 h Low-risk patients less likely to receive CT scans
	Menditto et al,[78] 2012	240	55 y	Decreased rates of ED revisit in patients with thoracic trauma from 12% without EDOU to 4% with EDOU Length of stay decreased from mean >94 h to 65 h after EDOU in place No change in per-patient cost
	Madsen et al,[38,79] 2009	364	35 y	No adverse events or significant missed injuries among selected trauma patients placed in an EDOU Average length of stay 12.75 h; 12% admission rate
	Menditto et al,[78,81] 2012	97	51 y	EDOU decreased ED revisit rates (4% vs 12% in patients with thoracic trauma Hospitalization rates also decreased from 49% to 24% with an EDOU

A variety of noninvasive cardiac testing modalities are available in EDOUs, including nuclear perfusion imaging, stress echocardiography, cardiac CT, and cardiac MRI.[5,10,36–39] Testing depends on provider preference, local availability, and patient characteristics. Choice of modality likely does not affect cost or outcomes in low-risk patients.[12,37] There is some suggestion that in intermediate-risk patients, cardiac MRI is safe and decreases long-term costs.[10] With the advent of radial artery access strategies for cardiac catheterization, select patients in certain EDOUs may also be able to receive cardiac catheterization, with patients not requiring an intervention recovered and discharged from the EDOU.[40] EDOUs have been shown successful in providing high-quality and efficient care for older adults through rapid testing and evidence-based care.

Syncope

Syncope is commonly managed in EDOUs, including in older adults. In the largest report of syncope care in an observation unit, the mean age of the 323 participants was 66 years, indicating that older adults with syncope can be successfully managed in an EDOU.[41] The evaluation usually involves cardiac monitoring, serial cardiac

---

Box 5
TIMI risk score for unstable angina and non–ST-elevation myocardial infarction with 14-day risk for cardiac events

TIMI Score	Points
Age ≥65 y?	1
Known coronary artery disease (stenosis ≥50%)?	1
Aspirin use in past 7 d?	1
Severe angina (≥2 episodes within 24 h)?	1
ST changes ≥0.5 mm?	1
+ Cardiac marker?	1

Fourteen-Day Risk of Cardiac Events (%)

Risk Score	Death/MI	Death/MI/Urgent Revascularization
0/1	3	5
2	3	8
3	5	13
4	7	20
5	12	26
6/7	19	41

Data from Antman EM, Cohen M, Bernink PJ, et al. The TIMI risk score for unstable angina/non-ST elevation MI: a method for prognostication and therapeutic decision making. JAMA 2000;284(7):835–42.

---

enzymes, and an evaluation for structural heart disease, most commonly with transthoracic echocardiogram. It may also include stress testing.

Older adults are more likely to have many of the factors associated with poor outcome in patients with syncope, including congestive heart failure, low hematocrit, abnormal ECG, or hypotension.[42–44] Because they have greater numbers of risk factors, these patients may require a more extensive work-up than younger adults.[41,42] The ability to accommodate the need for additional testing depends on the individual EDOU. When making disposition decisions, CMS guidelines based on the InterQual criteria suggest admission for patients with syncope and known coronary artery disease. Inpatient stays based on that criterion, however, have been one of the biggest targets for Recovery Audit Contractor audits and denials.[45]

Congestive Heart Failure

Acute decompensated heart failure causes more than 1 million hospital admissions annually, 75% of which originate in the ED.[46,47] Compared with inpatient admissions, observation unit heart failure patients have no difference in outcomes and may have cost savings and more efficiently delivered care.[48–50] As with other protocols, only those patients expected to complete their diagnostic and therapeutic evaluation within 24 hours are appropriate for care. This evaluation most commonly includes echocardiogram (if not recently completed), IV diuretics, appropriate adjustments to home medication regimens, and possible cardiology consultation to aid in management.[47,51] General factors that may make a patient inappropriate for EODU care for heart failure include need for large volume diuresis unlikely to be completed within 24 hours, presence of renal insufficiency or hypotension limiting volume or speed of diuresis, and presence of acute cardiac ischemia.

Older adults have been well represented in studies of heart failure protocols in EDOUs, and advanced age has not been associated with increased admission rates.

In a 2005 study in which mean age was 70 years, only a blood urea nitrogen value greater than 30 mg/dL was associated with admission.[46] A 2006 evaluation of similar patients with mean age 61 years suggested that patients with a normal troponin and a systolic blood pressure greater than 160 are most appropriate for an EDOU.[52] Prognosis may be particularly poor for older adults with heart failure in combination with other social and medical issues. The Multidimensional Prognostic Index identifies older adults at risk of mortality within 30 days after hospital admission based on activities of daily living, mental status, nutrition status, medications, and social support.[53] These additional factors should be taken into account when considering appropriateness for EDOU care.

Transient Ischemic Attack

Older adults with TIA are commonly cared for in EDOUs with an average age in published studies of 70 years.[54,55] EDOU TIA protocols have been shown to be safe and reduce length of stay compared with admissions.[9,54,55] When compared with patients discharged from the ED for outpatient follow-up, TIA protocols increase completion rates for recommended imaging studies.[9] A comprehensive EDOU TIA evaluation can generally be completed within 24 hours, faster and at less cost than in patients who are admitted.[9,54,55] Readmission and 30-day stroke rates were similar between those managed in the EDOU and as inpatients.[9,55]

Patients with persistent, severe neurologic deficits are not candidates for EDOU TIA protocols. Those whose deficits have resolved and, in some EDOUs, those with minor deficits (eg, paresthesias or subjective weakness) remain candidates. The primary advantage of the TIA protocol is that patients are able to rapidly complete the suggested diagnostic evaluation, which may include MRI of the brain, transthoracic echocardiogram with bubble study to rule out embolic sources, and assessment of neck and cerebral vasculature through carotid Doppler, magnetic resonance angiogram, or CT angiography.[9] In most units, a neurologist is available and either evaluates all TIA patients or is consulted as needed. With confirmation of the diagnosis of TIA, EDOU physicians can initiate guideline concordant secondary prevention therapies.[56] Patients with acute CVA or other identified pathology identified can be admitted for further care.

Vertigo

Vertigo is another condition amenable to care in EDOUs for older adults. Due to their higher incidence of central vertigo, the EDOU is an appropriate venue to obtain diagnostic imaging, including brain MRI and magnetic resonance angiography for evaluation of the posterior circulation to rule acute stroke.[57–59] Equally important, the EDOU stay provides a treating physician time to determine patient response to therapy and safety for discharge home.[60] The physician can gauge not only the control of symptoms but also the effect on gait and balance of the centrally acting medication regimens, such as meclizine and/or diazepam, used for treatment.[61] This can include bedside evaluation by physical therapy if necessary to ensure that patients can be safely discharged. Those who are unable to ambulate safely, because of vertigo symptoms or side effects of the treatment medications, can be appropriately admitted.

Skin and Soft Tissue Infection

Most EDOUs treat patients with SSTI.[4,19] Patients with infections of moderate severity who are expected to show improvement within 24 hours can be placed in the EDOU for a period of IV antibiotics and serial assessments. Older age has not been associated with increased observation failure rates.[24,62] Key elements in considering appropriateness of EDOU care for an older adult with SSTI include infection type, size, comorbid conditions, and effect on functional status. Those with deeper infections or with multiple comorbidities may benefit from more prolonged courses of IV antibiotics and may require admission. The EDOU also provides an opportunity to rule out certain complications of SSTI, such as osteomyelitis or septic arthritis, with appropriate imaging and diagnostic studies.

Urinary Tract Infection

Older adults with UTI, both cystitis and pyelonephritis, may also benefit from EDOU care.[63] The unique challenges surrounding diagnosis and presentation of UTI in older adults can make EDOUs particularly attractive. Older adults diagnosed with UTI are less likely than younger patients to have classic symptoms, such as dysuria or fever.[64] They are more likely to present with weakness, confusion, or other vague symptoms.[64–67] Accurate diagnosis is complicated by the frequent presence of asymptomatic bacteriuria, even in community-dwelling older adults.[68,69] As a result, the initial diagnosis of UTI in an older adult may be unclear and uncertain, particularly when cultures are pending.

The EDOU stay provides the ability to clarify a diagnosis both by awaiting results of a urine culture and by noting a patient's response to antibiotic therapy. For moderately ill patients, it allows a trial of antibiotics, usually given IV, then transitioned to oral, before discharge. This is particularly important given the prevalence of drug resistant organisms in older adults with UTI.[70–72] Patients who fail to respond to initial therapy can be admitted for further diagnostic studies or administration of alternative antibiotics. Finally, because UTIs can cause issues with mentation and balance in older adults, an EDOU stay allows sufficient time to confirm that patients can safely continue treatment in an outpatient home setting.[64,73,74]

Trauma and Minor Head Injury

Observation units have been shown to be appropriate for the care of patients after traumatic injury.[75–79] A majority of patients in these studies were younger adults with median age in the 30s.[75,76,79] In one study with mean age 60 years, however, patients with blunt thoracic trauma were safely managed in an EDOU.[78] It is likely that carefully selected older trauma patients can be managed in the EDOU but further study is needed.

EDOUs may be particularly appropriate for older adults with falls and minor closed head injury (Glasgow coma scale 14 or 15) who are receiving anticoagulation. The subset of older adults who are anticoagulated may be at risk of delayed intracranial hemorrhage after even minor head trauma, such as falls from standing.[80–82] As a result, current European guidelines recommend repeat head CT approximately 24 hours after a normal head CT in anticoagulated patients.[83,84] This approach is controversial because rates of delayed hemorrhage may be lower than previously believed.[77,85–87] Recent evidence from a multicenter US study of 1064 anticoagulated patients (warfarin or clopidogrel) with minor head injury and mean age 75 years showed very low rates of delayed hemorrhage (0.6%; 95% CI, 0.2%–1.5%).[85] As a result, the need for observation of these patients has been questioned. If observation is considered, recent EDOU studies have validated the safety of either observation alone or observation with repeat head CT scans in 24 hours in older adults receiving anticoagulation.[77,81]

Abdominal Pain

Abdominal pain is another common and high-risk clinical presentation in older adults due to high rates of surgical and medical emergencies.[88–90] Two types of older adults with abdominal pain may be appropriately managed in the EDOU. First, in patients with an initially negative or equivocal diagnostic workup, the EDOU can provide the benefit of serial examinations, repeat laboratory studies, and possibly further imaging studies to help clarify the clinical picture.[90,91] Importantly, the EDOU must not replace a thorough initial evaluation because delays in diagnosis of many conditions, such as mesenteric ischemia, can be catastrophic.[92] Second, older adults, in whom significant pathology is clearly ruled out or only minor pathology found, might be placed in the EDOU for a period of therapeutic intervention before discharge. For example, patients with mild diverticulitis, most importantly, those without evidence of perforation,[93,94] could receive initial doses of antibiotics and repeat examinations to ensure clinical improvement. Patients with gastroenteritis might receive IV fluids and antiemetics until adequate oral intake could be resumed. Patients with more severe pathology or with chronic symptoms unlikely to improve within 24 hours are more appropriately managed in the inpatient setting.

MEDICARE IMPLICATIONS OF OBSERVATION STATUS

An understanding of the definition of "observation status" is important and necessary for appropriate placement of patients in the EDOU. In the regulatory definition, observation status is a billing status of a patient, which may occur in an EDOU or on the floor in the hospital. The Health Care Financing Administration (the precursor organization to the CMS) published the rules for appropriate use of observation status in the September 1996 Medicare Hospital Manual, Publication 10:[95]

The purpose of observation is to determine the need for further treatment or for inpatient admission. Thus, a patient in observation may improve and be released, or be admitted as an inpatient…

Increasing attention to placing patients in the correct status of care after initial ED evaluation has created a paradox for many established EDOUs. Historically, patient selection was accomplished by inclusion and exclusion criteria based on a predetermined care pathway. This was independent of a patient's billing status and was a clinical decision made by an ED care provider. Increasingly, CMS beneficiary patients are screened based on standardized evidence-based clinical decision support criteria, such as InterQual or Milliman, to determine medical necessity of services and patient appropriateness for inpatient admission.[96] Other factors may also play into the determination of appropriate level of care, such as failure of outpatient management. Thus, otherwise appropriately selected patients for EDOU management may meet inpatient criteria. Conversely, patients selected for inpatient admission based on perception of not meeting EDOU inclusion criteria may only qualify for observation status. As a result of this paradox, hospitals have been forced to prospectively screen eligible beneficiaries in the ED to determine appropriate level of care. Seemingly in this system, the care setting becomes an afterthought and a patient's billing status supreme.

Acute care hospitals have a financial incentive to certify and place patients in the inpatient setting rather than in observation status due to the differential compensation for inpatient admission. In addition, for Medicare beneficiaries, copayments are significantly higher for outpatient services,[97] providing a patient preference for inpatient admission due to lower out of pocket costs, and currently are the basis of a class action lawsuit challenging the legality of observation status.[1] The CMS Recovery Audit Contractor program has commandeered many back payments and substantial penalties from hospitals based on their determination of inappropriate level of care determinations. One of their areas of closest scrutiny is that of 1-day and even 2-day hospital stays. From the CMS perspective, they advocate that such patients should have been in observation status. These complexities highlight the challenges inherent to the current system.

In summary, observation status is a level of care determination and billing status that is part of outpatient management. It is not a not a geographic location in the hospital. It is governed by complex regulatory rules that have made the landscape of patient selection for the EDOU more complex. This is particularly true for older adults; many of whom are Medicare beneficiaries. In general, older adults placed in an EDOU should meet both clinical criteria for the unit and regulatory requirements for observation status. Patients not meeting clinical criteria for the EDOU should be placed in an inpatient unit location under either observation or inpatient status, depending on billing rules.

SUMMARY

In conclusion, EDOUs can provide several benefits to appropriately selected older adults. They offer the opportunity for more comprehensive evaluation of many characteristics of particular importance to the care of older adults that cannot be accomplished during a short ED stay. EDOUs can provide both diagnostic and therapeutic services to ensure that older adults are safe for outpatient care. Older adults have been successfully managed with many EDOU protocols. Knowledge of local EDOU capabilities and polices will aid clinicians in appropriately managing their older adult patients.

REFERENCES

1. Feng Z, Wright B, Mor V. Sharp rise in medicare enrollees being held in hospitals for observation raises concerns about causes and consequences. Health Aff (Millwood) 2012;31(6):1251–9.
2. Mace SE, Graff L, Mikhail M, et al. A national survey of observation units in the United States. Am J Emerg Med 2003;21(7):529–33.
3. Foo CL, Siu VW, Tan TL, et al. Geriatric assessment and intervention in an emergency department observation unit reduced re-attendance and hospitalisation rates. Australas J Ageing 2012;31(1):40–6.
4. Ross MA, Compton S, Richardson D, et al. The use and effectiveness of an emergency department observation unit for elderly patients. Ann Emerg Med 2003; 41(5):668–77.
5. Amsterdam EA, Kirk JD, Bluemke DA, et al. Testing of low-risk patients presenting to the emergency department with chest pain: a scientific statement from the American Heart Association. Circulation 2010;122(17):1756–76.
6. Baugh CW, Venkatesh AK, Bohan JS. Emergency department observation units: a clinical and financial benefit for hospitals. Health Care Manage Rev 2011;36(1): 28–37.
7. Schull MJ, Vermeulen MJ, Stukel TA, et al. Evaluating the effect of clinical decision units on patient flow in seven canadian emergency departments. Acad Emerg Med 2012;19(7):828–36.
8. Goodacre S, Nicholl J, Dixon S, et al. Randomised controlled trial and economic evaluation of a chest pain observation unit compared with routine care. BMJ 2004;328(7434):254.
9. Ross MA, Compton S, Medado P, et al. An emergency department diagnostic protocol for patients with transient ischemic attack: a randomized controlled trial. Ann Emerg Med 2007;50(2):109–19.

10. Miller CD, Hwang W, Case D, et al. Stress CMR imaging observation unit in the emergency department reduces 1-year medical care costs in patients with acute chest pain: a randomized study for comparison with inpatient care. JACC Cardiovasc Imaging 2011;4(8):862–70.

11. Miller CD, Hwang W, Hoekstra JW, et al. Stress cardiac magnetic resonance imaging with observation unit care reduces cost for patients with emergent chest pain: a randomized trial. Ann Emerg Med 2010;56(3):209–19.

12. Miller CD, Hoekstra JW, Lefebvre C, et al. Provider-directed imaging stress testing reduces health care expenditures in lower-risk chest pain patients presenting to the emergency department. Circ Cardiovasc Imaging 2012;5(1): 111–8.

13. Rydman RJ, Roberts RR, Albrecht GL, et al. Patient satisfaction with an emergency department asthma observation unit. Acad Emerg Med 1999;6(3): 178–83.

14. Chandra A, Sieck S, Hocker M, et al. An observation unit may help improve an institution's press ganey satisfaction score. Crit Pathw Cardiol 2011;10(2):104–6.

15. Iannone P, Lenzi T. Effectiveness of a multipurpose observation unit: before and after study. Emerg Med J 2009;26(6):407–14.

16. Ross MA, Hemphill RR, Abramson J, et al. The recidivism characteristics of an emergency department observation unit. Ann Emerg Med 2010;56(1):34–41.

17. Committee on the Future of Emergency Care in the United States Health System. Hospital based emergency care: at the breaking point (future of emergency care). Washington, DC: National Academies Press; 2007.

18. American College of Emergency Physicians. Policy statement: emergency department observation services. American College of emergency Physicians 2008. Available at: http://www.acep.org/Content.aspx?id=29204. Accessed September 1, 2012.

19. Venkatesh AK, Geisler BP, Gibson Chambers JJ, et al. Use of observation care in US emergency departments, 2001 to 2008. PLoS One 2011;6(9):e24326.

20. Jagminas L, Partridge R. A comparison of emergency department versus inhospital chest pain observation units. Am J Emerg Med 2005;23(2):111–3.

21. Madsen TE, Bledsoe J, Bossart P. Appropriately screened geriatric chest pain patients in an observation unit are not admitted at a higher rate than nongeriatric patients. Crit Pathw Cardiol 2008;7(4):245–7.

22. Caterino JM, Hoover EM, Moseley MG. Effect of advanced age and vital signs on admission from an ED observation unit. Am J Emerg Med 2012. [Epub ahead of print].

23. Chan T, Arendts G, Stevens M. Variables that predict admission to hospital from an emergency department observation unit. Emerg Med Australas 2008;20(3): 216–20.

24. Schrock JW, Laskey S, Cydulka RK. Predicting observation unit treatment failures in patients with skin and soft tissue infections. Int J Emerg Med 2008;1(2):85–90.

25. Elsawy B, Higgins KE. The geriatric assessment. Am Fam Physician 2011;83(1): 48–56.

26. Stuck AE, Siu AL, Wieland GD, et al. Comprehensive geriatric assessment: a meta-analysis of controlled trials. Lancet 1993;342(8878):1032–6.

27. Centers for Medicare & Medicaid Services. Medicare benefit policy manual; chapter 8-coverage of extended care (SNF) services under hospital insurance. centers for medicare and medicaid services: medicare benefit policy manual 2012. Available at: http://www.cms.gov/Regulations-and-Guidance/Guidance/Manuals/downloads/bp102c08.pdf. Accessed September 1, 2012.

28. Rocchiccioli JT, Sanford JT. Revisiting geriatric failure to thrive: a complex and compelling clinical condition. J Gerontol Nurs 2009;35(1):18–24.

29. Anderson K, Baraldi C, Supiano M. Identifying failure to thrive in the long term care setting. J Am Med Dir Assoc 2012;13(7):665–9.

30. Diercks DB, Kirk JD, Amsterdam EA. Can we identify those at risk for a nondiagnostic treadmill test in a chest pain observation unit? Crit Pathw Cardiol 2008; 7(1):29–34.

31. Amsterdam EA, Kirk JD, Diercks DB, et al. Exercise testing in chest pain units: rationale, implementation, and results. Cardiol Clin 2005;23(4):503–16, vii.

32. Kirk JD, Diercks DB, Turnipseed SD, et al. Evaluation of chest pain suspicious for acute coronary syndrome: use of an accelerated diagnostic protocol in a chest pain evaluation unit. Am J Cardiol 2000;85(5A):40B–8B.

33. Chng YM, Kosowsky JM. A triage algorithm for the rapid clinical assessment and management of emergency department patients presenting with chest pain. Crit Pathw Cardiol 2004;3(3):154–7.

34. Madsen T, Bossart P, Bledsoe J, et al. Patients with coronary disease fail observation status at higher rates than patients without coronary disease. Am J Emerg Med 2010;28(1):19–22.

35. Holly J, Hamilton D, Bledsoe J, et al. Prospective evaluation of the treatment of intermediate-risk chest pain patients in an emergency department observation unit. Crit Pathw Cardiol 2012;11(1):10–3.

36. Hall ME, Miller CD, Hundley WG. Adenosine stress cardiovascular magnetic resonance-observation unit management of patients at intermediate risk for acute coronary syndrome: a possible strategy for reducing healthcare-related costs. Curr Treat Options Cardiovasc Med 2012;14(1):117–25.

37. Napoli AM, Arrighi JA, Siket MS, et al. Physician discretion is safe and may lower stress test utilization in emergency department chest pain unit patients. Crit Pathw Cardiol 2012;11(1):26–31.

38. Madsen T, Mallin M, Bledsoe J, et al. Utility of the emergency department observation unit in ensuring stress testing in low-risk chest pain patients. Crit Pathw Cardiol 2009;8(3):122–4.

39. Hoffmann U, Truong QA, Schoenfeld DA, et al. Coronary CT angiography versus standard evaluation in acute chest pain. N Engl J Med 2012;367(4):299–308.

40. Pristipino C, Trani C, Nazzaro MS, et al. Major improvement of percutaneous cardiovascular procedure outcomes with radial artery catheterisation: results from the PREVAIL study. Heart 2009;95(6):476–82.

41. Anderson KL, Limkakeng A, Damuth E, et al. Cardiac evaluation for structural abnormalities may not be required in patients presenting with syncope and a normal ECG result in an observation unit setting. Ann Emerg Med 2012; 60(4):478–84.e1.

42. Schladenhaufen R, Feilinger S, Pollack M, et al. Application of San Francisco syncope rule in elderly ED patients. Am J Emerg Med 2008;26(7):773–8.

43. Quinn J, McDermott D, Stiell I, et al. Prospective validation of the San Francisco Syncope Rule to predict patients with serious outcomes. Ann Emerg Med 2006; 47(5):448–54.

44. Serrano LA, Hess EP, Bellolio MF, et al. Accuracy and quality of clinical decision rules for syncope in the emergency department: a systematic review and meta-analysis. Ann Emerg Med 2010;56(4):362–73.

45. Report on Medicare Compliance: RAC medical necessity audits accelerate, but hospitals say some miss the boat. Available at: http://www ehrdocs com/pdf/news/RMC_09 05 11.pdf. Accessed September 5, 20, 31, 2011.

46. Burkhardt J, Peacock WF, Emerman CL. Predictors of emergency department observation unit outcomes. Acad Emerg Med 2005;12(9):869–74.

47. Peacock WF, Emerman CL. Emergency department management of patients with acute decompensated heart failure. Heart Fail Rev 2004;9(3):187–93.

48. Storrow AB, Collins SP, Lyons MS, et al. Emergency department observation of heart failure: preliminary analysis of safety and cost. Congest Heart Fail 2005; 11(2):68–72.

49. Peacock WF, Young J, Collins S, et al. Heart failure observation units: optimizing care. Ann Emerg Med 2006;47(1):22–33.

50. Peacock WF, Albert NM. Observation unit management of heart failure. Emerg Med Clin North Am 2001;19(1):209–32.

51. Peacock WF. Using the emergency department clinical decision unit for acute decompensated heart failure. Cardiol Clin 2005;23(4):569–88, viii.

52. Diercks DB, Peacock WF, Kirk JD, et al. ED patients with heart failure: identification of an observational unit-appropriate cohort. Am J Emerg Med 2006;24(3): 319–24.

53. Pilotto A, Addante F, Franceschi M, et al. Multidimensional Prognostic Index based on a comprehensive geriatric assessment predicts short-term mortality in older patients with heart failure. Circ Heart Fail 2010;3(1):14–20.

54. Stead LG, Bellolio MF, Suravaram S, et al. Evaluation of transient ischemic attack in an emergency department observation unit. Neurocrit Care 2009;10(2):204–8.

55. Nahab F, Leach G, Kingston C, et al. Impact of an emergency department observation unit transient ischemic attack protocol on length of stay and cost. J Stroke Cerebrovasc Dis 2011. [Epub ahead of print].

56. Furie KL, Kasner SE, Adams RJ, et al. Guidelines for the prevention of stroke in patients with stroke or transient ischemic attack: a guideline for healthcare professionals from the american heart association/american stroke association. Stroke 2011;42(1):227–76.

57. Karatas M. Central vertigo and dizziness: epidemiology, differential diagnosis, and common causes. Neurologist 2008;14(6):355–64.

58. Kerber KA, Brown DL, Lisabeth LD, et al. Stroke among patients with dizziness, vertigo, and imbalance in the emergency department: a population-based study. Stroke 2006;37(10):2484–7.

59. Delaney KA. Bedside diagnosis of vertigo: value of the history and neurological examination. Acad Emerg Med 2003;10(12):1388–95.

60. Jonsson R, Sixt E, Landahl S, et al. Prevalence of dizziness and vertigo in an urban elderly population. J Vestib Res 2004;14(1):47–52.

61. American Geriatrics Society 2012 Beers Criteria Update Expert Panel. American Geriatrics Society updated beers criteria for potentially inappropriate medication use in older adults. J Am Geriatr Soc 2012;60(4):616–31.

62. Sabbaj A, Jensen B, Browning MA, et al. Soft tissue infections and emergency department disposition: predicting the need for inpatient admission. Acad Emerg Med 2009;16(12):1290–7.

63. Schrock JW, Reznikova S, Weller S. The effect of an observation unit on the rate of ED admission and discharge for pyelonephritis. Am J Emerg Med 2010;28(6): 682–8.

64. Caterino JM, Ting SA, Sisbarro SG, et al. Age, nursing home residence, and presentation of urinary tract infection in U.S. Emergency departments, 2001–2008. Acad Emerg Med 2012;19(10):1173–80.

65. Ginde AA, Rhee SH, Katz ED. Predictors of outcome in geriatric patients with urinary tract infections. J Emerg Med 2004;27(2):101–8.

66. Juthani-Mehta M, Quagliarello V, Perrelli E, et al. Clinical features to identify urinary tract infection in nursing home residents: a cohort study. J Am Geriatr Soc 2009;57(6):963–70.

67. Nicolle LE. Urinary tract infection in long-term-care facility residents. Clin Infect Dis 2000;31(3):757–61.

68. Raz R. Asymptomatic bacteriuria—clinical significance and management. Nephrol Dial Transplant 2001;16(Suppl 6):135–6.

69. Aguirre-Avalos G, Zavala-Silva ML, az-Nava A, et al. Asymptomatic bacteriuria and inflammatory response to urinary tract infection of elderly ambulatory women in nursing homes. Arch Med Res 1999;30(1):29–32.

70. Nicolle LE. Resistant pathogens in urinary tract infections. J Am Geriatr Soc 2002; 50(Suppl 7):S230–5.

71. Wright SW, Wrenn KD, Haynes M, et al. Prevalence and risk factors for multidrug resistant uropathogens in ED patients. Am J Emerg Med 2000;18(2):143–6.

72. Nicolle LE. Urinary tract pathogens in complicated infection and in elderly individuals. J Infect Dis 2001;183(Suppl 1):S5–8.

73. Rhoads J, Clayman A, Nelson S. The relationship of urinary tract infections and falls in a nursing home. Director 2007;15(1):22–6.

74. Eriksson S, Strandberg S, Gustafson Y, et al. Circumstances surrounding falls in patients with dementia in a psychogeriatric ward. Arch Gerontol Geriatr 2009; 49(1):80–7.

75. Holly J, Bledsoe J, Black K, et al. Prospective evaluation of an ED observation unit protocol for trauma activation patients. Am J Emerg Med 2012;30(8):1402–6.

76. Kendall JL, Kestler AM, Whitaker KT, et al. Blunt abdominal trauma patients are at very low risk for intra-abdominal injury after emergency department observation. West J Emerg Med 2011;12(4):496–504.

77. Kaen A, Jimenez-Roldan L, Arrese I, et al. The value of sequential computed tomography scanning in anticoagulated patients suffering from minor head injury. J Trauma 2010;68(4):895–8.

78. Menditto VG, Gabrielli B, Marcosignori M, et al. A management of blunt thoracic trauma in an emergency department observation unit: pre-post observational study. J Trauma Acute Care Surg 2012;72(1):222–8.

79. Madsen TE, Bledsoe JR, Bossart PJ. Observation unit admission as an alternative to inpatient admission for trauma activation patients. Emerg Med J 2009;26(6): 421–3.

80. Itshayek E, Rosenthal G, Fraifeld S, et al. Delayed posttraumatic acute subdural hematoma in elderly patients on anticoagulation. Neurosurgery 2006;58(5): E851–6.

81. Menditto VG, Lucci M, Polonara S, et al. Management of minor head injury in patients receiving oral anticoagulant therapy: a prospective study of a 24-hour observation protocol. Ann Emerg Med 2012;59(6):451–5.

82. Peck KA, Sise CB, Shackford SR, et al. Delayed intracranial hemorrhage after blunt trauma: are patients on preinjury anticoagulants and prescription antiplatelet agents at risk? J Trauma 2011;71(6):1600–4.

83. Vos PE, Battistin L, Birbamer G, et al. EFNS guideline on mild traumatic brain injury: report of an EFNS task force. Eur J Neurol 2002;9(3):207–19.

84. Cohen DB, Rinker C, Wilberger JE. Traumatic brain injury in anticoagulated patients. J Trauma 2006;60(3):553–7.

85. Nishijima DK, Offerman SR, Ballard DW, et al. Immediate and delayed traumatic intracranial hemorrhage in patients with head trauma and preinjury warfarin or clopidogrel use. Ann Emerg Med 2012;59(6):460–8.

86. Li J. Admit all anticoagulated head-injured patients? A million dollars versus your dime. You make the call. Ann Emerg Med 2012;59(6):457–9.

87. Li J. Validation of the dime. Ann Emerg Med 2012;59(6):469–70.

88. Samaras N, Chevalley T, Samaras D, et al. Older patients in the emergency department: a review. Ann Emerg Med 2010;56(3):261–9.

89. Marco CA, Schoenfeld CN, Keyl PM, et al. Abdominal pain in geriatric emergency patients: variables associated with adverse outcomes. Acad Emerg Med 1998; 5(12):1163–8.

90. Lewis LM, Banet GA, Blanda M, et al. Etiology and clinical course of abdominal pain in senior patients: a prospective, multicenter study. J Gerontol A Biol Sci Med Sci 2005;60(8):1071–6.

91. Hustey FM, Meldon SW, Banet GA, et al. The use of abdominal computed tomography in older ED patients with acute abdominal pain. Am J Emerg Med 2005; 23(3):259–65.

92. Ragsdale L, Southerland L. Acute abdominal pain in the older adult. Emerg Med Clin North Am 2011;29(2):429–48, x.

93. Jacobs DO. Clinical practice. Diverticulitis. N Engl J Med 2007;357(20):2057–66.

94. Solomkin JS, Mazuski JE, Bradley JS, et al. Diagnosis and management of complicated intra-abdominal infection in adults and children: guidelines by the surgical infection society and the infectious diseases society of America. Clin Infect Dis 2010;50(2):133–64.

95. CMS Manual System: Medicare Benefit Policy Manual, Chapter 6 - Hospital Services Covered Under Part B, Revision 157. Department of Health and Human Services (DHHS), Centers for Medicare and Medicaid Services (CMS); 2012. Available at: http://www.cms.gov/Regulations-and-Guidance/Guidance/Manuals/downloads/bp102c06.pdf. Accessed October 18, 2012.

96. InterQual Evidence-based Clinical Content. McKesson Corporation 2012. Available at: http://www.mckesson.com/en_us/McKesson.com/Payers/Decision%2BManagement/InterQual%2BEvidence-Based%2BClinical%2BContent/InterQual%2BEvidence-based%2BClinical%2BContent.html. Accessed September 1, 2012.

97. Centers for Medicare and Medicaid Services. Are you a hospital inpatient or outpatient? Centers for medicare and medicaid services, CMS Product No 11435 2011. Available at: http://www.medicare.gov/Publications/Pubs/pdf/11435.pdf. Accessed September 1, 2012.

Generalized Weakness in the Geriatric Emergency Department Patient: An Approach to Initial Management

Robert S. Anderson Jr, MD[a],*, Sarah A.M. Hallen, MD[b]

KEYWORDS

• Geriatric • Weakness • Emergency department • Evaluation

KEY POINTS

• "Generalized weakness" as a nonspecific chief complaint in the emergency department is associated with poor outcomes.

• Infectious, metabolic, or oncologic processes are often discovered to be the etiology.

• In addition to history and physical, a reasonable workup includes an electrocardiogram, a complete blood count, a basic metabolic panel, and a chest radiograph. Urine testing, if ordered, should be interpreted in light of high prevalence of asymptomatic bacteriuria.

• If the weakness is acute or localized, neuroimaging with a head computed tomography scan should be considered.

INTRODUCTION

In 2008, there were 38.9 million persons aged 65 years or older in America. The United States Census bureau estimates that this number will nearly double by 2030 and come to encompass nearly 19.3% of the population.[1] This rapid increase in the elderly population has been referred to as the "Silver Tsunami." Current emergency physicians (EP) report feeling ill-prepared to care for older adults because of inadequate training, research, and continuing education in geriatric emergency medicine. EPs believe older patients require more time and resources than younger patients, even for common complaints such as abdominal pain, headache, chest pain, and dizziness.[2] Studies evaluating emergency department (ED) resource use support these views. Singal and colleagues[3] found that the elderly were more likely than younger patients to arrive by ambulance with conditions of either high or intermediate urgency and

[a] Department of Emergency Medicine, Maine Medical Center, Tufts University School of Medicine, 22 Bramhall Street, Portland, ME 04102, USA; [b] Geriatric Medicine, Maine Medical Center, Tufts University School of Medicine, 66 Bramhall Street, Portland, ME 04102, USA
* Corresponding author.
E-mail address: Robert.Anderson@tufts.edu

Clin Geriatr Med 29 (2013) 91–100
http://dx.doi.org/10.1016/j.cger.2012.10.002
0749-0690/13/$ – see front matter © 2013 Elsevier Inc. All rights reserved.

complicated by comorbid diseases. These patients had longer mean stays in the ED and higher rates of laboratory and radiology testing, with double the hospital admission rate. EPs will need to feel more comfortable in managing geriatric complaints despite the complexity of the workup and resource use.

A NEBULOUS COMPLAINT

One classic clinical scenario whereby geriatric inexperience intersects with the demands of a busy ED is the older adult presenting with "generalized weakness." It is estimated that 20% of geriatric patients present to the ED with a nonspecific complaint,[4] such as generalized weakness. These complaints need to be evaluated despite their ambiguity, because past studies have shown that these patients are at increased risk for a bad outcome. Nemec and colleagues[5] found that 58% of a sample of patients presenting to an urban ED with a nonspecific complaint developed a serious condition within 30 days. The majority of these conditions represented an acute new problem rather than a deterioration of an existing one. The 30-day mortality rate for these patients was 6%. Another study found that adding age over 65 and weakness or dizziness to a standardized triage scale significantly increased odds of hospital admission when compared with general patients with similar, urgent acuity.[6] Yet generalized weakness as a symptom is difficult to clinically conceptualize and even more difficult to define and treat.

One reason for this is that the term generalized weakness is poorly defined. Patients and physicians use it synonymously with other vague terms such as dizziness, fatigue, or malaise. Past comprehensive emergency medicine reviews on the topic avoid defining it[7,8] and focus instead on diseases that may cause it. Indeed many diseases may cause generalized weakness. Nickel and colleagues[9] studied ICD-10 codes used for patients presenting to the ED with generalized weakness and found that 14 different diagnostic categories represented 65% of the billing codes used.

The geriatric literature also struggles with weakness, using the term interchangeably with frailty or failure to thrive.[10–12] The term "weakness" is not indexed at all in one popular geriatrics text[13] and only as "weakness in [other disease states]..." in another.[14] Even so, weakness more closely resembles other prototypical geriatric syndromes like delirium or insomnia than a traditional medical diagnosis. Unlike a medical syndrome, whereby a single process can manifest with multiple signs and symptoms, a geriatric syndrome is defined when one symptom results from the complex interplay of multiple causes and mechanisms.[15] Although weakness is not listed as a traditional geriatric syndrome,[16] conceptualizing it as such may help with differential development and initial workup.

Patient History

Obtaining a thorough history is crucial to determining the cause of weakness in the elderly. To illustrate how generalized weakness is similar to a geriatric syndrome, consider this case: an elderly person is deconditioned owing to poor mobility from arthritis that causes her to be functionally incontinent and develop a urinary tract infection, which causes her to have nausea and vomiting. The nausea and vomiting cause dehydration and thus she develops hyponatremia, delirium, and falls. This patient's family, however, may only report confusion and weakness. In this case, one can argue that the weakness is due to the delirium or hyponatremia, but such a simple view does not take into account the complex chain reaction of compounding comorbidities and acute illnesses that led to her presentation. The multifactorial nature of weakness is what makes it similar to other geriatric syndromes and makes a thorough history particularly important.

Special attention to possible geriatric syndromes and other common conditions in the elderly is essential. The patient and/or family should be asked about falls and cognitive impairment. Depression is often underappreciated and underdiagnosed[17] in the elderly population, and can cause people to feel subjectively weak. Hypoactive delirium can also be mistaken for generalized weakness. Delirium is defined as the acute onset of mental status changes and inattention, often associated with disorganized thinking and/or altered level of awareness. Although most associate delirium with hyperactivity and agitation, it more commonly manifests as somnolence and weakness in the ED.[18–20] In addition, the literature is clear that delirium is often not diagnosed by emergency providers[19] and that inpatient services do not establish the diagnosis when it is missed in the ED,[20] which results in an increased risk of death and complications. Accepting the lack of a quick validated ED tool for diagnosing delirium, emergency providers are encouraged to consider any change from baseline, especially inattention, as potential delirium. Extra time may be required to obtain history from family, care providers, facilities, or friends.

Medications should be reviewed in detail. Polypharmacy can also complicate presentation. With a higher use of prescription medications and over-the-counter drugs, adverse drug reactions should be a consideration for every elder presenting to the ED. A large systematic review reported 10.7% of all elderly admissions were due to an adverse drug event.[21]

There are also social issues that potentially could be driving the presentation of illness. What is the patient's level of function at baseline? No other group of patients is as heterogeneous as the elderly population. A functional baseline is crucial in determining the expectations and prognosis of a patient, with increasing functional dependence being increasingly used a marker of poor outcome and mortality.[22] A family bringing in a patient for weakness may require respite or be attempting to tell care providers that the patient is unsafe at home and needs more assistance. Substance abuse[23] and elder abuse[24] may manifest as weakness as well.

"Weakness" History and Differential Diagnosis

As important as the history and physical is to defining the patient, it is equally important to attempt to define what the weakness is. Time course and focality are 2 important clues (**Fig. 1**).

Time course is important because of its ability to separate acute emergent causes from more indolent ones. Etiologies that can cause weakness acutely are often medical emergencies such as cardiac ischemia, electrolyte imbalances, delirium, sepsis, or rapid-onset anemia. Neurologic etiologies are often more indolent, but myasthenia crisis or Guillain-Barré can also come on rapidly. Medication interactions and intolerances can also present acutely. Etiologies that can cause subacute or chronic weakness often can go undiagnosed because of the gradual onset of symptoms. Vasculitis or inflammatory myopathies are often slower to develop, as are the sequelae of hypothyroidism or adrenal insufficiency. Neurologic etiologies such as amyotrophic lateral sclerosis can have a slower onset, as do paraneoplastic syndromes or general weakness caused by malignancy. Causes of weakness with geriatric specific history considerations are listed in **Table 1**.

Focality is also important to determine. In 2009 Nickel and colleagues[9] found that in a predominantly elderly population who presented for evaluation of generalized weakness, 35% of the weak patients actually had localized or focal weakness, and of those patients 76% had had a transient ischemic attack, stroke, or intracerebral hemorrhage.

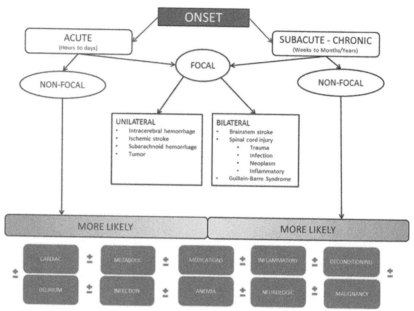

Fig. 1. Diagnostic network for weakness by onset and focality.

Unilateral or bilateral presentation is important because it can localize the lesion and direct imaging studies.

Physical and Laboratory Testing

Chew and Birnbaumer[7] last addressed nonfocal or generalized weakness in *The Clinics* in 1999. Similar to their recommendations, the authors recommend that the physical examination should be guided by what is known about a patient's medical history and medical comorbidities, with sensitivity to geriatric issues, including potentially causative social history. When performing the physical examination, the neurologic examination is particularly important to determine if symptoms are focal or nonfocal.

In terms of other testing, although strong evidence to guide testing choices is lacking, a small observational study found that 3 categories of illnesses were found in almost all patients presenting with nonspecific complaints such as weakness.[5] Those categories were infections (mostly pulmonary), followed by metabolic dysfunctions and then malignancies (**Table 2**).

Based on the available evidence, the authors recommend that initial testing should target these common and often coexisting etiologies. Geriatric considerations related to vital signs and other testing is outlined in **Table 3**.

The authors recommend obtaining a complete blood count, a basic metabolic panel, an electrocardiogram, and a chest radiograph.[7] Additional testing might include an erythrocyte sedimentation rate/C-reactive protein for inflammatory processes, and thyroid-stimulating hormone for hypothyroidism and urinalysis; however, the prevalence of asymptomatic bacteriuria must be considered when interpreting the results.

Up to 50% of women and 30% of men older than 65 have asymptomatic bacteriuria.[25] Asymptomatic bacteriuria does not warrant antimicrobial treatment. The presence of pyuria alone is not an indication for treatment either. Studies have shown that

Table 1
Differential diagnosis of weakness with geriatric history considerations

Category	Etiology	Geriatric History Considerations
Cardiac	Acute myocardial infarction (AMI) Valvular disease Heart failure	*AMI*: Atypical presentations common in geriatric populations; electrocardiograms are less likely to be diagnostic; outcomes can be much worse in acute coronary syndrome[27] *Heart failure*: Although dyspnea on exertion, fatigue, orthopnea are the most common symptoms associated with heart failure in older adults, it can also present atypically; symptoms can include: cognitive impairment, confusion, lethargy, and anorexia. Compared with younger patients, older patients are more likely to be women and to have a preserved left ventricular ejection fraction[30]
Delirium		More common in patients with underlying dementia and with functional impairment; patients in long-term care facilities may be especially at risk. Most likely coexisting with other common causes of weakness
Metabolic	Hypophosphatemia Hypo-/hyperkalemia Hypo-/hypercalcemia Hypo-/hypermagnesemia Hypo-/hypernatremia Hypo-/hyperglycemia Hypothyroidism Adrenal insufficiency	Consider electrolyte disturbances if patient has a recent history of poor intake, dehydration, or has started a new medication, especially diuretics *Hypothyroidism*: Because of insidious onset and nonspecific symptoms, the diagnosis can be missed; laboratory screening necessary Most common cause of *adrenal insufficiency* in older adults is chronic glucocorticoid therapy
Infectious	Urinary tract infection (UTI) Pneumonia Tick-borne illnesses	Patients with cognitive impairment and with functional impairment (especially in long-term care facilities) at higher risks of *UTI and pneumonia (aspiration)* *Tick-borne illnesses* (Lyme disease, ehrlichiosis, babesiosis) should be considered even in suburban areas
Medications	Diuretics Steroids Statins Antihypertensives Benzodiazepines Serotonin selective uptake inhibitors Hypnotics Narcotics Antipsychotics	If a new medication is started near the onset of symptoms, consider it potentially causative regardless of class

(continued on next page)

Table 1 (continued)		
Category	**Etiology**	**Geriatric History Considerations**
Anemia	Acute or chronic blood loss Pernicious anemia Myelodysplastic syndrome	*Anemia* is the most common age-related hematologic abnormality in older adults. Anemia of chronic disease and nutrient deficiencies (iron or vitamin B12/folate) are most common[31]
Neurologic	amyotrophic lateral sclerosis Myasthenia gravis Guillain-Barré Autonomic neuropathy Multiple sclerosis	
Inflammatory	Giant cell arteritis (GCA)/ polymyalgia rheumatica (PMR) Polymyositis/dermatomyositis	*GCA/PMR*: Prevalence increases with age and should be considered in all patients >50 y old who present with constitutional symptoms, including subjective weakness, and persistent pain or stiffness in upper arms, shoulders, hips, or thighs. Objective strength is often normal in these individuals. Predominant symptom is pain[32] *Polymyositis/dermatomyositis*: Unlike GCA/PMR, painless proximal muscle weakness is often the predominant symptom
Malignancy	Eaton-Lambert (paraneoplastic) Cachexia/catabolic effects in general	
Deconditioning		Consider with any chronic illness or comorbidity that may affect mobility

even in catheterized samples, pyuria is neither diagnostic of bacteriuria nor urinary tract infection. In addition, even though the presence of pyuria with bacteriuria when greater than 10 white blood cells per high-powered field are present has traditionally been considered evidence for infection, current guidelines currently recommend no treatment unless the patient is symptomatic.[26]

Table 2	
Top 3 diagnostic categories to explain generalized weakness in a small observational study	
Infections 60%	Respiratory tract, gastroenteritis, urinary tract, cholecystitis, pericarditis
Metabolic dysfunctions 18%	Acute renal failure, dehydration, hyponatremia, hypokalemia, acidosis, new-onset diabetes, Addison disease
Malignancy 10%	Previously known, new lung cancer, new myeloid leukemia

Data from Nemec M, Koller MT, Nickel CH, et al. Patients presenting to the emergency department with nonspecific complaints: the Basel Non-Specific Complaints (BANC) study. Acad Emerg Med 2010;17(3):284–92.

Table 3
Weakness evaluation with geriatric considerations

Testing	Geriatric Considerations
Vital signs	Geriatric physiology and medication effects reliably alter vital signs. Comparison trending of an *individual patient's* vital signs is critical and high yield[33] Fever can be absent or blunted in up to 30% of elders presenting with severe infection.[34] Fever in older adults has now been redefined as a consistent oral temperature of $\geq$37.2°C, a rectal temperature of $\geq$37.5°C, or a 1.1°C increase in temperature from baseline[35]
Labs: CBC, BMP, TSH UA, ESR/CRP	Older adults have a decrease in the reference range (lower normal): HCT, WBC, total protein, albumin[36] Interpret UA with caution: asymptomatic bacteriuria common in older adults (see text) >50 y, upper limit of normal for ESR increases to 20 mm/h in men and 30 mm/h in women[37]
Imaging: CXR Neuroimaging : head CT (noncontrast) or spine MRI	Clinician should consider lower threshold for neuroimaging after fall[38] Head CT with contrast: if suspected tumor or infection Brain MRI if suspected brainstem process
Other: ECG	Myocardial infarction can present as generalized weakness[27]

Abbreviations: BMP, basic metabolic panel; CBC, complete blood count; CRP, C-reactive protein; CT, computed tomography; CXR, chest radiograph; ECG, electrocardiogram; ESR, erythrocyte sedimentation rate; HCT, hematocrit; TSH, thyroid-stimulating hormone; UA, urinalysis.

In addition to the laboratory tests and imaging, the authors also advocate for a 12-lead electrocardiogram because myocardial infarction is known to present as general weakness in this population.[27] Lastly, consider neuroimaging if there are new focal findings on examination or concerns about intracranial bleeding or infection.

Disposition

Realistically most older adults who present to the ED with weakness will be admitted. Indeed, the admission rate for older adults presenting with nonspecific complaints in general is 80% to 90%.[5,28] Given the medical morbidity associated with generalized weakness and the often complex social factors that accompany it, careful consideration for admission is prudent. However, in the current financial climate, receiving payment for these admissions is increasingly difficult. The current Medicare reimbursement structure does not recognize common multifactorial geriatric problems such as "weakness."[15] In addition, if patients do not meet specified inpatient criteria, they may be admitted under observation or outpatient status, which can affect their ability to access postacute rehabilitation services. Such decisions can profoundly affect not only patients' out-of-pocket costs for the hospital bill but also shift financial responsibility for rehabilitation costs to the patient.[29] To combat this and anticipate the care needs of those individuals for whom social factors may be the predominant reason for presentation, more care managers and/or coordinators are needed.

SUMMARY

Ultimately the final evaluation of the older adult presenting to the ED with generalized weakness will be unique for each patient. This article is not meant to supplant clinical reasoning for this complex problem, but rather to share what little is known about it to inform clinical practice.

The authors advocate for basic testing in all patients with weakness or other nonspecific complaints because limited evidence suggests significant risks are associated with these chief complaints. Weakness should be differentiated into generalized or localized weakness, as well as chronic or acute weakness. Localized and/or acute weakness should warrant higher suspicion for an acute neurologic issue such as stroke or hemorrhage. An electrocardiogram, chest radiograph, and basic laboratory tests will identify some common causes of this nonspecific complaint in geriatric adults.

Generalized weakness, like many geriatric syndromes, exemplifies why geriatric care is so often difficult. Weakness may be due to multiple potential causes and mechanisms in this vulnerable, complex population. However, by focusing on history, presentation of the weakness, and reliance on high-yield testing and social intervention to aid with disposition issues, EPs can become more comfortable in managing geriatric complaints such as weakness and prepare for the "silver tsunami."

REFERENCES

1. Administration on Aging. A profile of older Americans: 2009. 2009.
2. McNamara RM, Rousseau E, Sanders AB. Geriatric emergency medicine: a survey of practicing emergency physicians. Ann Emerg Med 1992;21(7): 796–801.
3. Singal BM, Hedges JR, Rousseau EW, et al. Geriatric patient emergency visits. Part I: comparison of visits by geriatric and younger patients. Ann Emerg Med 1992;21(7):802–7.
4. Vanpee D, Swine C, Vandenbossche P, et al. Epidemiological profile of geriatric patients admitted to the emergency department of a university hospital localized in a rural area. Eur J Emerg Med 2001;8(4):301–4.
5. Nemec M, Koller MT, Nickel CH, et al. Patients presenting to the emergency department with non-specific complaints: the Basel Non-Specific Complaints (BANC) study. Acad Emerg Med 2010;17(3):284–92.
6. Ruger JP, Lewis LM, Richter CJ. Identifying high-risk patients for triage and resource allocation in the ED. Am J Emerg Med 2007;25(7):794–8.
7. Chew WM, Birnbaumer DM. Evaluation of the elderly patient with weakness: an evidence based approach. Emerg Med Clin North Am 1999;17(1):265–78, x.
8. LoVecchio F, Jacobson S. Approach to generalized weakness and peripheral neuromuscular disease. Emerg Med Clin North Am 1997;15(3):605–23.
9. Nickel CH, Nemec M, Bingisser R. Weakness as presenting symptom in the emergency department. Swiss Med Wkly 2009;139(17–18):271–2.
10. Clegg A, Young J. The frailty syndrome. Clin Med 2011;11(1):72–5.
11. Ko FC. The clinical care of frail, older adults. Clin Geriatr Med 2011;27(1):89–100.
12. Xue QL. The frailty syndrome: definition and natural history. Clin Geriatr Med 2011;27(1):1–15.
13. Hazzard's geriatric medicine and gerontology. 6th edition. New York: McGraw-Hill; 2003.
14. Brocklehurst's textbook of geriatric medicine and gerontology. 7th edition. Philadelphia: Saunders/Elsevier; 2010.

15. Inouye SK, Studenski S, Tinetti ME, et al. Geriatric syndromes: clinical, research, and policy implications of a core geriatric concept. J Am Geriatr Soc 2007;55(5): 780–91.
16. Pacala JT, Sullivan GM, editors. Geriatrics review syllabus: a core curriculum in geriatric medicine. 7th edition. New York: American Geriatrics Society; 2010. p. 179.
17. VanItallie TB. Subsyndromal depression in the elderly: underdiagnosed and undertreated. Metabolism 2005;54(5 Suppl 1):39–44.
18. Young J, Inouye SK. Delirium in older people. BMJ 2007;334(7598):842–6.
19. Han JH, Wilson A, Ely EW. Delirium in the older emergency department patient: a quiet epidemic. Emerg Med Clin North Am 2010;28(3):611–31.
20. Han JH, Zimmerman EE, Cutler N, et al. Delirium in older emergency department patients: recognition, risk factors, and psychomotor subtypes. Acad Emerg Med 2009;16(3):193–200.
21. Kongkaew C, Noyce PR, Ashcroft DM. Hospital admissions associated with adverse drug reactions: a systematic review of prospective observational studies. Ann Pharmacother 2008;42(7):1017–25.
22. Stineman MG, Xie D, Pan Q, et al. All-cause 1-, 5-, and 10-year mortality in elderly people according to activities of daily living stage. J Am Geriatr Soc 2012;60(3): 485–92.
23. Weintraub E, Weintraub D, Dixon L, et al. Geriatric patients on a substance abuse consultation service. Am J Geriatr Psychiatry 2002;10(3):337–42.
24. Thompson H, Priest R. Elder abuse and neglect: Considerations for mental health practitioners. Adultspan Journal 2005;4:116–28.
25. Fircanis S, McKay M. Recognition and management of extended spectrum beta lactamase producing organisms (ESBL). Med Health R I 2010;93(5):161–2.
26. Hooton TM, Bradley SF, Cardenas DD, et al. Diagnosis, prevention, and treatment of catheter-associated urinary tract infection in adults: 2009 international clinical practice guidelines from the infectious diseases society of America. Clin Infect Dis 2010;50(5):625–63.
27. Glickman SW, Shofer FS, Wu MC, et al. Development and validation of a prioritization rule for obtaining an immediate 12-lead electrocardiogram in the emergency department to identify ST-elevation myocardial infarction. Am Heart J 2012; 163(3):372–82.
28. Rutschmann OT, Chevalley T, Zumwald C, et al. Pitfalls in the emergency department triage of frail elderly patients without specific complaints. Swiss Med Wkly 2005;135(9–10):145–50.
29. ACEP. Utilization Review FAQs. Available at: http://www.acep.org/practres.aspx?id=36598. Accessed September 12, 2012.
30. Hunt SA, Abraham WT, Chin MH, et al. 2009 focused update incorporated into the ACC/AHA 2005 guidelines for the diagnosis and management of heart failure in adults: a report of the American College of Cardiology Foundation/American Heart Association Task Force on Practice Guidelines: developed in collaboration with the international society for heart and lung transplantation. Circulation 2009; 119(14):e391–479.
31. Eisenstaedt R, Penninx BW, Woodman RC. Anemia in the elderly: current understanding and emerging concepts. Blood Rev 2006;20(4):213–26.
32. Cantini F, Niccoli L, Nannini C, et al. Diagnosis and treatment of giant cell arteritis. Drugs Aging 2008;25(4):281–97.
33. Chester JG, Rudolph JL. Vital signs in older patients: age-related changes. J Am Med Dir Assoc 2011;12(5):337–43.

34. Gavazzi G, Krause KH. Ageing and infection. Lancet Infect Dis 2002;2(11): 659–66.
35. Norman DC. Fever in the elderly. Clin Infect Dis 2000;31(1):148–51.
36. Brigden ML, Heathcote JC. Problems in interpreting laboratory tests. What do unexpected results mean? Postgrad Med 2000;107(7):145–6, 151-2, 155-8 passim.
37. Desai SP, editor. Clinician's guide to laboratory medicine. 3rd edition. Hudson, OH: Lexi-Comp; 2004. p. 789.
38. Schrag SP, Toedter LJ, McQuay N Jr. Cervical spine fractures in geriatric blunt trauma patients with low-energy mechanism: are clinical predictors adequate? Am J Surg 2008;195(2):170–3.

Altered Mental Status in Older Patients in the Emergency Department

Jin H. Han, MD, MSc[a],*, Scott T. Wilber, MD, MPH[b]

KEYWORDS

- Delirium - Coma - Stupor - Emergency department - Epidemiology - Diagnosis
- Management

KEY POINTS

- Altered mental status is a common chief complaint among older patients in the emergency department (ED).
- Patients with acute changes in mental status are likely to have delirium, stupor, and coma, and these changes are commonly precipitated by an underlying medical illness that can be potentially life-threatening.
- Although stupor and coma are easily identifiable, the clinical presentation of delirium can be subtle and is often missed without actively screening for it.
- The ED management of patients with altered mental status should initially be focused on stabilizing the patient (airway, breathing, circulation) while searching for the underlying etiology.

INTRODUCTION

Altered mental status is a common chief complaint among older patients in the emergency department (ED). Despite the frequency of this complaint, the term "altered mental status" is vague and has several synonyms such as confusion, not acting right, altered behavior, generalized weakness, lethargy, agitation, psychosis, disorientation, inappropriate behavior, inattention, and hallucination.[1] Such lack of standardized terminology not only hinders the assessment and appropriate management of patients with altered mental status but also the advancement of knowledge through research.

Jin H. Han is supported by a grant from the National Institute on Aging, K23AG032355.
[a] Department of Emergency Medicine, Center for Quality Aging, Vanderbilt University School of Medicine, 703 Oxford House, Nashville, TN 37232-4700, USA; [b] Department of Emergency Medicine, Emergency Medicine Research Center, Summa Akron City Hospital, Northeastern Ohio Medical University, 525 East Market Street, Akron, OH 44309, USA
* Corresponding author.
E-mail address: jin.h.han@vanderbilt.edu

Altered mental status has varying time courses and degrees of severity. Acute changes in mental status are usually secondary to delirium, stupor, and coma, which are forms of acute brain dysfunction. These changes occur over a period of hours or days and are usually precipitated by an underlying medical illness that is potentially life-threatening. Chronic alterations in mental status (eg, dementia) occur over a period of months and years and are less likely to be precipitated by a life-threatening illness.[2] For these reasons, acute changes in mental status are the focus of this review. Altered mental status is rarely caused by psychiatric illnesses such as depression or schizophrenia, but in elder patients, these should be diagnoses of exclusion. Acute brain dysfunction (delirium, stupor, and coma) and their underlying etiology should be ruled out before considering any psychiatric diagnoses, especially in patients without a previous history of psychiatric illness.

The ED plays a critical role in the evaluation and management of older patients with altered mental status. The ED is often the initial point of entry for geriatric hospital admissions,[3] and it is tasked with rapidly identifying those who are critically ill while efficiently diagnosing the underlying etiology, and promptly initiating life-saving therapies. In the United States alone, the ED sees approximately 18 million patients who are 65 years and older each year.[4] Because of the projected exponential growth of the aging population in the United States over the next several decades, the number of elder ED patient visits will likely grow at a similar pace.[5] Hence, the emergency physician must be adept in evaluating and managing patients with acute alterations in mental status. This review discusses the epidemiology of delirium, stupor, and coma in the ED along with their effect on patients' outcomes. This article also reviews the mental status assessment of patients with acute brain dysfunction, as well as their diagnostic workup and treatment. Of all the forms of acute brain dysfunction, delirium is probably the most well studied and constitutes the focus of this review. However, the concepts pertinent to delirium can be generalized to stupor and coma, because there is significant overlap.

THE SPECTRUM OF ACUTE BRAIN DYSFUNCTION

Delirium, stupor, and coma represent a broad spectrum of acute brain dysfunction (**Fig. 1**) and are associated with an impairment of consciousness. There are 2 interrelated domains of neurologic function that are related to consciousness: content and level (also known as arousal) of consciousness.[6] The content of consciousness has many components such as orientation, perception, executive function, and memory, and is mediated at the cortical level. The level (or arousal) of consciousness signifies the patient's wakeful state and reactivity to surrounding stimuli, mediated at the ascending reticular activating system located in the brainstem.[6] Traditionally terms such as lethargic, drowsy, or somnolent have been used to describe level or arousal of consciousness. Because these descriptors can have different meanings for different clinicians, using a structured arousal scale such as the Richmond Agitation and Sedation Scale (RASS) may be a more reliable method to describe altered level of consciousness. This scale ranges from −5 (unresponsive to pain and voice) to +4 (extreme combativeness).[7,8] As the patient's level of consciousness becomes more disturbed, the concern for an underlying life-threatening acute medical illness should similarly increase. Patients with acute brain dysfunction not only can fluctuate between different RASS scores, but can also transition between delirium, stupor, and coma.

Stupor and Coma: Definitions and their Epidemiology in the Emergency Department

Stupor and coma occurs in 5% to 9% of older ED patients and when present, are considered to be medical emergencies that require immediate evaluation.[9,10] These

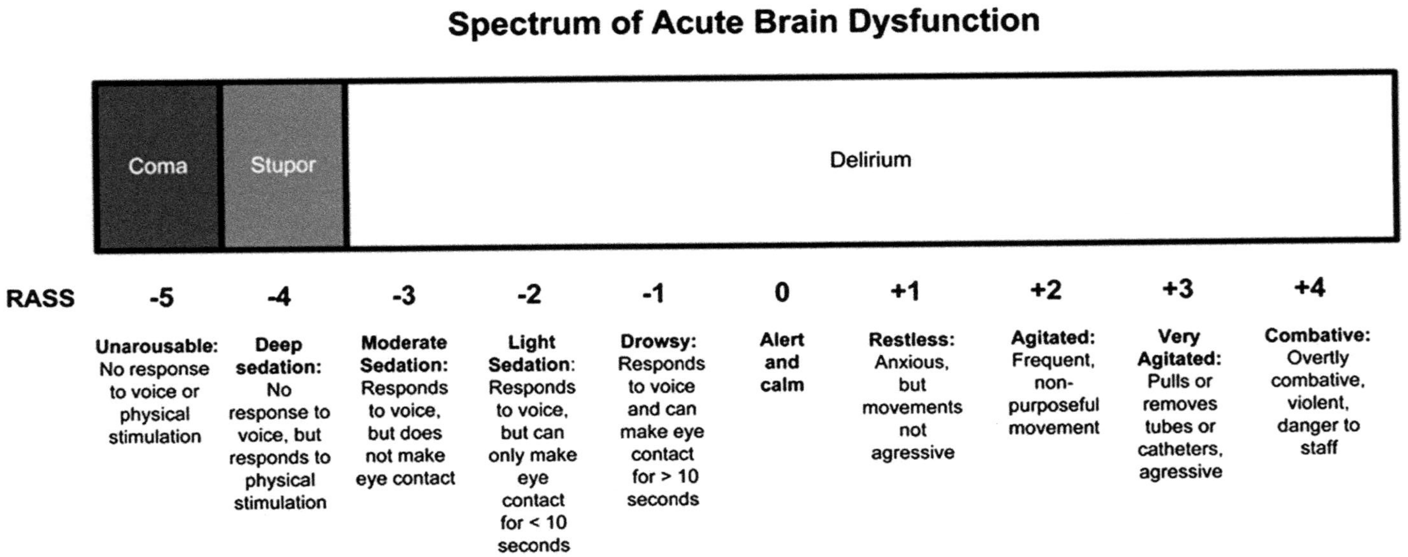

Spectrum of Acute Brain Dysfunction

RASS	-5	-4	-3	-2	-1	0	+1	+2	+3	+4
	Coma	Stupor				Delirium				
	Unarousable: No response to voice or physical stimulation	**Deep sedation:** No response to voice, but responds to physical stimulation	**Moderate Sedation:** Responds to voice, but does not make eye contact	**Light Sedation:** Responds to voice, but can only make eye contact for < 10 seconds	**Drowsy:** Responds to voice and can make eye contact for > 10 seconds	**Alert and calm**	**Restless:** Anxious, but movements not agressive	**Agitated:** Frequent, non-purposeful movement	**Very Agitated:** Pulls or removes tubes or catheters, agressive	**Combative:** Overtly combative, violent, danger to staff

Fig. 1. Spectrum of acute brain dysfunction based on the Richmond Agitation and Sedation Scale (RASS). (*Courtesy of* Vanderbilt University, Nashville, TN. Copyright © 2012; with permission.)

2 forms of acute brain dysfunction occur over a period of hours to days and represent the most severe disruptions in both the level and content of consciousness. Stupor (RASS −4) is a condition of deep sleep or similar behavioral unresponsiveness from which the patient can be aroused only with vigorous and continuous stimulation. Coma (RASS −5) is defined as a state of unresponsiveness from which the patient cannot be aroused with any stimuli.

Delirium: Definitions and its Epidemiology in the Emergency Department

Delirium is an acute disturbance of consciousness (ie, attention) accompanied by an acute loss in cognition that is not better explained by a preexisting dementia.[11] This form of acute brain dysfunction occurs in 8% to 10% of patients of older ED patients.[10,12–17] Similar to stupor and coma, delirium occurs over a period of hours and days, and its course tends to wax and wane throughout the day. In contrast to stupor and coma, however, some elements of the level and content of consciousness are maintained in patients with delirium. The degree of impairment in the level of consciousness can be variable, ranging from moderate sleepiness (RASS −3) to extreme combativeness (RASS +4). Patients with delirium also have inattention, which is considered a cardinal feature of delirium.[18,19] The impairment of content of consciousness is similarly variable and leads to an acute loss in cognition. Examples of such impairments observed in delirious patients are disorganized thought, perceptual disturbances, and disorientation (**Box 1**).[18]

The Psychomotor Subtypes of Delirium

Delirium can be further classified into 3 psychomotor subtypes: hypoactive, hyperactive, and mixed.[20] Hypoactive (RASS <0) delirium is described as "quiet" delirium and is characterized by psychomotor retardation; delirious patients with this subtype can appear drowsy, somnolent, or even lethargic. Because the clinical presentation can be very subtle, hypoactive delirium is frequently undetected by health care providers,[21] and is often attributed to other causes such as depression or fatigue.[22,23] To the contrary, patients with hyperactive delirium (RASS >0) have increased psychomotor

---

Box 1
Examples of impairments in the cognitive domains seen in patients with delirium

Disorganized thinking

The patient's thought process is disorganized and incoherent. The patient may ramble, make irrelevant statements, or have illogical flow of ideas. The following conversation is an example of disorganized thinking:

Physician: "Mr B, how are feeling today?"

Mr B: "I'm feeling horrible today. It reminds of the day I visited Italy when I was younger… those were the days of yesterday, today, and the future. The future is irrelevant to the past, and this makes me happy."

Perceptual disturbances

The patient may be seeing things that are not there (visual hallucinations) or hearing things that no one else can hear (auditory hallucinations). For example, a delirious patient with visual hallucinations is seen picking at her blanket thinking that she is picking up bugs, when in reality none are present.

Disorientation

The patient may not know where he is or what the date is.

activity and may appear restless, anxious, agitated, or combative. Hyperactive delirium is more easily recognized by health care providers. Mixed-type delirium exhibits fluctuating levels of psychomotor activity; the patient can exhibit hypoactive symptomatology at one moment and hyperactive symptomatology several hours or even seconds later. Hypoactive delirium and mixed-type delirium appear to be the predominant subtypes in older patients regardless of the clinical setting.[14,24–29] In the ED specifically, hyperactive delirium is the least common subtype.[14]

It is hypothesized that each psychomotor subtype has different underlying pathophysiologic mechanisms.[20,30] Although the mechanisms are unclear, it is hypothesized that each delirium subtype has differential neurotransmitter activity (cholinergic, dopamine, serotonin, and γ-aminobutyric acid).[20] Each psychomotor subtype may also be caused by differing etiology. Delirium caused by an infection or metabolic derangement is more likely to be the hypoactive subtype, whereas delirium caused by alcohol or benzodiazepine withdrawal is more likely to be the hyperactive subtype.[31] The psychomotor subtypes of delirium may also have a differential effect on clinical course and outcomes.[32] In 457 older patients admitted to a postacute care facility with delirium, Kiely and colleagues[33] observed that patients with hypoactive delirium had the highest 1-year mortality rate compared with the other subtypes.

Delirium Versus Dementia

Delirium is distinct from dementia (**Table 1**), yet many clinicians use these terms interchangeably. Of importance, however, is that dementia is an important predisposing factor to delirium, and patients can have both conditions concurrently. As previously mentioned, the loss of cognition observed in delirium tends to occur rapidly, and its course tends to fluctuate throughout the day. The loss of cognition observed in dementia is usually gradual (over months to years), and its course tends to be stable. Patients with delirium also have inattention, which is considered the cardinal feature of delirium, whereas attention is usually preserved in patients with dementia. Altered level of consciousness, disorganized thinking, sleep-wake cycle disturbances, and perceptual disturbances are also commonly observed in delirium, whereas these characteristics are typically absent in dementia.

There are instances when the clinical features of delirium and dementia overlap, making them difficult to distinguish from each other. This is especially the case in

Table 1
Key differences between delirium and dementia

Characteristic	Delirium	Dementia
Onset	Rapid over a period of hours or days	Gradual over months and years
Course	Waxing and waning	Stable
Inattention	Present	Absent[a]
Altered of level of consciousness	Usually present	Typically absent[a]
Disorganized thinking present	May be present	Typically absent[a]
Sleep-wake cycle disturbance	Present	Typically absent[a]
Perceptual disturbances and hallucinations	May be present	Typically absent[a]
Is cognitive decline reversible?	Usually reversible	Rarely reversible

[a] May be present in patients with severe dementia.

patients with end-stage dementia, whereby they can exhibit symptoms of inattention, altered level of consciousness, disorganized thinking, sleep-wake cycle disturbances, and perceptual disturbances in the absence of delirium.[34] When patients with end-stage dementia develop delirium, an acute change in mental status is still observed, and any preexisting abnormalities in cognition and level of consciousness will likely worsen. For this reason, diagnosing delirium can be extremely challenging in patients with end-stage dementia, and establishing their baseline mental status is critical to the diagnosis.

Delirium is classically thought of as reversible and is usually precipitated by an underlying medical illness. However, there is also a proportion of patients whose delirium is not transient and whose symptoms can persist for months or even years.[35,36] Dementia is thought of as irreversible and not secondary to an underlying medical illness. However, there are circumstances in which dementia may be reversible. Hypothyroidism, normal pressure hydrocephalus, vitamin B12 deficiency, and depression are examples of illnesses that can cause reversible dementia or a dementia-like illness (pseudodementia). One meta-analysis comprising 39 articles reported that 9% of dementia cases were potentially reversible, but only 0.6% showed any improvement in cognition after the reversible cause was addressed.[2]

Dementia with Lewy bodies is the second most common type of dementia (after Alzheimer) and deserves special mention because it can be very challenging to distinguish from delirium.[37] Similar to delirium, the loss of cognition observed in dementia with Lewy bodies can be rapid, and can fluctuate over several hours or days. Perceptual disturbances are also commonly observed in dementia with Lewy bodies. Patients with dementia with Lewy bodies, however, have Parkinsonian motor symptoms such as cog wheeling, shuffling gait, stiff movements, and reduced arm-swing during walking; such motor symptoms are usually absent in patients with delirium. Differentiating between dementia with Lewy bodies and delirium can be difficult in the ED, and may require a detailed evaluation by a neurologist or psychiatrist.

Other Illnesses that can Mimic Delirium, Stupor, and Coma

In patients with altered mental status, the emergency physician must also consider other medical neurologic diagnoses. In patients who appear unresponsive, locked-in syndrome, caused by focal injury to the ventral pons secondary to an infarct, hemorrhage, or trauma, should be considered. If secondary to an infarct, the distal basilar artery is usually occluded. Multiple sclerosis and central pontine myelinosis can also cause locked-in syndrome. Although the clinical presentation is variable, quadriplegia and anarthria are usually present, but vertical eye gaze and upper eyelid movement are usually retained.[38] Despite having the outward appearance of being unresponsive, patients with locked-in syndrome have normal levels of consciousness and are fully aware of their surroundings. If locked-in syndrome is suspected, prompt neuroimaging and neurology consultation are warranted. Patients with a suspected thromboembolic cause of locked-in syndrome should immediately be sent to interventional radiology for intra-arterial thrombolytic therapy, even if the symptoms have been ongoing for more than the traditional 3-hour window.[39] Without emergent intervention, survival and neurologic recovery for these patients can be poor.

Nonconvulsive status epilepticus (NCSE) should also be considered in patients who have altered mental status, especially if no obvious cause for their change in mental status is found. This diagnosis should strongly be considered if the patient has a seizure history or has had a seizure before arriving at the ED. One systematic review reported that NCSE occurred in 8% to 30% of patients with altered mental status (mean prevalence = 22%).[40] This systematic review consisted of 5 studies that predominantly enrolled patients in the hospital setting.[40] NCSE is underrecognized and is an important form of altered mental status that can only be diagnosed with electroencephalography (EEG). If this cause of altered mental status is considered, neurology consultation should be obtained promptly; the treatment for nonconvulsive status epilepticus (benzodiazepine and antiepileptic medications) is significantly different from that for other causes of altered mental status.

RISK FACTORS FOR DEVELOPING ACUTE BRAIN DYSFUNCTION

The etiology of delirium (and other forms of acute brain dysfunction) involves a complex interplay between patient vulnerability (or predisposing) factors and precipitating factors (**Fig. 2**).[41–43] Patients who are highly vulnerable (eg, a 92-year-old with severe dementia, poor functional status, and multiple comorbidities) will require a relatively benign insult to develop delirium. For these highly vulnerable patients, a simple urinary tract infection or small dose of narcotic medication can precipitate delirium. Because elderly patients are more likely to have multiple vulnerability factors, they are more susceptible to becoming delirious compared with their younger counterparts. Nursing home patients are particularly vulnerable.[44] For patients who are less vulnerable (eg, a 67-year-old with no dementia, little comorbidity burden, and who is still functionally independent), higher doses of noxious stimuli such as severe sepsis are required to develop delirium. Consequently, when a patient with little or no vulnerability factors presents to the ED with delirium, stupor, or coma, the clinician should have more concern for an underlying life-threatening illness. To develop stupor of coma, even higher doses of noxious stimuli are required.

Patient Vulnerability Factors for Acute Brain Dysfunction

A multitude of patient vulnerability factors for delirium have been identified in the hospital literature (**Box 2**) and can likely be extrapolated to stupor and coma.[45–48] Dementia is the most consistently observed vulnerability factor for delirium regardless of clinical setting.[41,45,49–55] A dose-response relationship seems to exist; as the

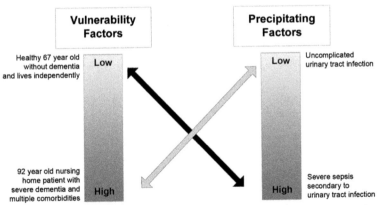

Fig. 2. Interrelationship between patient vulnerability and precipitating factors for developing acute brain dysfunction such as delirium. Patients who not vulnerable require significant noxious stimuli to develop acute brain dysfunction (*black arrow*). Patients who are highly vulnerable require only minor noxious stimuli to develop acute brain dysfunction (*gray arrow*). (*Adapted from* Inouye SK, Charpentier PA. Precipitating factors for delirium in hospitalized elderly persons. Predictive model and interrelationship with baseline vulnerability. JAMA 1996;275(11):852–7.)

Box 2
Patient vulnerability factors for delirium

Vulnerability Factors

Demographics

- Advanced age
- Male gender

Comorbidity

- Dementia
- Number of comorbid conditions
- Chronic kidney disease
- End-stage liver disease
- Terminal illness

Functional status

- Functional impairment
- Immobility

Medications and drugs

- Polypharmacy
- Baseline psychoactive medication use[a]
- History of alcohol or other substance abuse

Sensory impairment

- Hearing impairment
- Visual impairment

Decreased oral intake

- Dehydration
- Malnutrition

Psychiatric

- Depression

Increased severity of these vulnerability factors will increase the patient's susceptibility to delirium.

[a] Psychoactive medications include benzodiazepines, opioids, and medications with anticholinergic properties.
Modified from Refs.[46–48]

---

severity of dementia worsens, the risk of developing delirium increases.[56] Similarly, low education attainment also increases the patient's susceptibility to developing delirium.[57] Both dementia and education attainment may indicate poor cognitive reserve and reflect the inability of the brain to adequately compensate for any noxious or stressful physiologic insult. Other commonly observed vulnerability factors for delirium include poor functional status,[50,55] advanced age,[49,54] home psychoactive medication use such as narcotics, benzodiazepines,[49,58] and medications with anticholinergic properties,[51] history of alcohol abuse,[50,55] visual impairment,[41] high comorbidity burden,[55] and malnutrition.[42] There are limited data from the ED setting, but one study identified dementia, premorbid functional impairment, and hearing impairment as risk factors for delirium in the ED.[14] Another ED study also identified dementia as a risk factor for delirium,[59] and also observed that patients with advanced age, or a history of cerebrovascular disease and seizure disorder were more likely to be delirious in the ED.[59]

Precipitating Factors for Acute Brain Dysfunction

There are numerous precipitating factors of delirium that have been reported in the hospital literature (**Box 3**).[46–48] Generally speaking, patients with higher severities of illness are more likely to develop delirium,[41,58] and even higher doses are required to cause stupor and coma. Infections are probably the most common causes of delirium, occurring in 16% to 67% of cases[49,52–54,60–63]; urinary tract infection and pneumonia are common infectious causes. Other precipitants for delirium include electrolyte abnormalities such as hyponatremia, hypernatremia, hypercalcemia, and hypocalcemia[58,64]; organ failure[58,64]; Wernicke encephalopathy; thyroid dysfunction[65]; central nervous system insults such as cerebrovascular accidents, intracerebral hemorrhage, epidural and subdural hematomas, and subarachnoid hemorrhage[52,53,60,63]; ethanol and benzodiazepine withdrawal[66–68]; dehydration[41]; and cardiovascular illnesses such as congestive heart failure[53,54] and acute myocardial infarction.[69] Poorly controlled somatic pain (ie, extremity fracture patients) can also precipitate delirium.[70–72] Vital-sign abnormalities (hypertensive encephalopathy, hypotension, hyperthermia or hypothermia, or hypoxia), endocrine disorders (hyperglycemia, hypoglycemia, adrenal insufficiency), and hypercarbia can also precipitate delirium.[48,73] More often than not, multiple delirium precipitants will exist concurrently,[58] but in 13% of cases no obvious etiologic agent will be found.[63] Delirium can also be precipitated by iatrogenic events in the ED. Inouye and Charpentier[42] observed that the use of physical restraints or bladder catheters, or the addition of more than 3 medications were associated with delirium development.

Medication Risk Factors for Delirium

Medications are important vulnerability and precipitating risk factors for delirium, because polypharmacy is highly prevalent in the older patient population. Clegg and Young[74] performed a systematic review and observed that benzodiazepines, opioids, dihydropyridines (eg, nifedipine), and antihistamines may increase the risk for delirium. Of the opioids, meperidine is probably the most deliriogenic.[72,75–78] These medications, especially benzodiazepines and opioids, can also induce stupor and coma at higher doses.

Medications with anticholinergic properties are thought to be frequent causes of delirium. There are more than 600 medications with anticholinergic properties, and of these 11% are frequently prescribed to older patients.[79] Some examples of commonly prescribed medications with anticholinergic properties are diphenhydramine, promethazine, hydroxyzine, meclizine, lomotil, and heterocyclic antidepressants (eg, amitriptyline, nortriptyline, doxepin). In acute stroke patients, Caeiro and colleagues[80] found that patients on home medications with anticholinergic properties were more susceptible to developing delirium during hospitalization. In 278 older medical patients, Han and colleagues[81] observed that anticholinergic medications were associated with increased delirium severity. However, the evidence linking medications with anticholinergic properties and delirium is not consistently observed. Agostini and colleagues[82] observed a trend toward increase risk (relative risk = 2.1, 95% confidence interval: 0.9–4.7) of developing delirium in older hospitalized patients when diphenhydramine was used. Luukkanen and colleagues[83] found that older

Box 3
Precipitating factors for delirium

Precipitating Causes for Delirium

Systemic

- Infection/sepsis
- Inadequate pain control
- Trauma
- Dehydration
- Hypo- or hyperthermia

Central nervous system

- Meningitis/encephalitis
- Cerebrovascular accident
- Intracerebral hemorrhage
- Subarachnoid hemorrhage
- Subdural/epidural hematoma

Medications and drugs

- Medications and medication changes
- Recreational drug use or withdrawal

Metabolic

- Thiamine deficiency (Wernicke encephalopathy)
- Hepatic or renal failure
- Hypo- and hypernatremia
- Hypo- and hypercalcemia
- Hypo- and hyperglycemia
- Thyroid dysfunction

Cardiopulmonary

- Acute myocardial infarction
- Congestive heart failure
- Hypoxemia
- Hypercarbia
- Hypertensive encephalopathy
- Shock

Iatrogenic

- Procedures or surgeries
- Indwelling urinary catheters
- Physical restraints

Modified from Refs.[46–48]

patients who used more than 1 medication with anticholinergic properties were more likely to have delirium in the unadjusted analysis (27.0% vs 16.7%, $P = .05$). However, this relationship became nonsignificant after adjusting for age, gender, and comorbidity. In 147 hospitalized older patients, Campbell and colleagues[84] observed that anticholinergic medications were not associated with delirium that developed in the hospital. These discrepant observations may be a result of differing patient characteristics (stroke vs nonstroke, race, and so forth), or the method by which anticholinergic burden was measured. Despite these discrepant findings, the general consensus among geriatric and psychiatric experts is that medications with anticholinergic properties in older patients should be avoided, especially if safer alternatives exist.[85,86]

THE EFFECT OF ACUTE BRAIN DYSFUNCTION IN THE EMERGENCY DEPARTMENT ON OUTCOMES

There is a dearth of data with regard to acute brain dysfunction in the ED and its effect on patients' outcomes. Much of what is known is based on studies conducted in older hospitalized patients. Studies investigating the role of stupor and coma are mainly limited to the intensive care unit setting. It is clear that the development of stupor and coma portend adverse outcomes; multiple studies have observed that these patients are more likely to die and have poor functional outcomes regardless of underlying etiology.[87–91]

The link between delirium and patient outcomes is well established in older hospitalized patients. A recent meta-analysis that included 21 studies observed that hospitalized patients with delirium are twice as likely to die, have a 2-fold increased odds of being institutionalized, and have a 12-fold increased odds of developing dementia compared with patients without delirium.[92] Delirium also accelerates the rate of cognitive decline in patients with preexisting dementia, and it is hypothesized that delirium may cause irreversible brain injury.[93,94] In addition, delirium is associated with accelerated functional decline,[95] prolonged hospitalizations,[58] and higher health care expenditures.[96] The duration of delirium appears to be an important prognostic indicator, as every 48 hours of delirium increases the risk of 3-month death by 11%.[97] Furthermore, many patients with delirium can remember their delirious experience, and this can cause significant distress in 70% to 80% of patients.[98,99]

The consequences of acute brain dysfunction in the ED remain unclear. Although older patient cohorts are similar between the ED and hospital settings, caution must be taken when attempting to generalize the results of studies from one setting to another, especially with delirium. ED patients who are discharged home represent a significant proportion of older ED patients and are not represented in hospital-based studies. Up to 25% of delirious older ED patients are discharged home,[12,100] and likely represent a unique population. In addition, most hospital-based delirium studies enroll patients 24 to 48 hours after admission,[27,55,95,101,102] and this may not reflect what the patient's delirium status was in the ED. Delirium can rapidly fluctuate and can quickly resolve in less than 1 day in 20% to 51% of patients[103–105]; hospitalized patients who were classified as nondelirious in the hospital may have been delirious in the ED. Conversely, patients who were not delirious in the ED may have become delirious in the hospital at the time of enrollment. Such misclassification can also occur in stupor and coma studies that enrolled patients in the hospital; such patients may have been delirious or had normal mental status in the ED.

Although there are no studies investigating the role of stupor and coma in the ED on outcomes, there are limited data on the effect of ED delirium. Delirium in older ED patients appears to be a predictor of long-term mortality, and this relationship is independent of age, comorbidity burden, severity of illness, dementia, functional dependence, and nursing home residence.[106] Delirium is also a marker for death for those who are discharged from the ED. Kakuma and colleagues[17] observed that in older ED patients who were discharged from the ED, delirium was independently associated with 6-month mortality. Older ED patients with delirium are also more likely to have prolonged hospitalizations.[100] Only one ED study has investigated the relationship between delirium and long-term functional outcomes. Vida and colleagues[107] observed that delirium in the ED was associated with accelerated functional decline in patients without preexisting dementia in the unadjusted analysis only. However, this relationship disappeared after potential confounders were adjusted for in the multivariable model.[107] Even with the relatively small number of ED studies, it is likely that delirium in the ED is a marker for adverse patient outcomes.

UNDERRECOGNITION OF DELIRIUM IN THE EMERGENCY DEPARTMENT

Because of the severity of impairment observed, emergency physicians readily recognize stupor and coma with little difficulty. However, emergency physicians miss delirium in 57% to 83% of the cases,[10,12-17] because its clinical presentation can be subtle and can be missed if it is not actively sought. Missing delirium is considered by many to be a medical error and may have important downstream implications for clinical care.[108] Patients with delirium may be unable to provide an accurate reason of why they are in the ED,[109] and this may lead to inappropriate or inadequate diagnostic workups. Delirium may be ascribed to another psychiatric illness such as depression.[23] These patients may be erroneously admitted to a psychiatric ward and there may be delay in the diagnosis of their underlying medical illness.[110] Up to 25% of delirious older ED patients are discharged home,[12,100] but a significant proportion may not be able to comprehend their discharge instructions,[109] leading to noncompliance.[111] Older ED patients who are discharged home with unrecognized delirium are more likely to die at 6 months compared with those whose delirium was recognized.[17] Hustey and colleagues[12] observed that out of the 5 older ED patients who were discharged home with delirium, 1 patient fell and 2 patients returned to the ED within 3 days and were eventually hospitalized. Lastly, if the patient is admitted, more than 90% of delirium that is missed in the ED will also be missed in the hospital setting.[14]

ASSESSMENT OF THE DYSFUNCTIONAL BRAIN IN THE EMERGENCY DEPARTMENT

In any ED patient with acute alterations in mental status, the first step is to assess for the level of consciousness using a validated arousal scale such as the RASS. If the patient is in a sleeplike state, it is necessary to determine the intensity of stimulation that is needed to arouse the patient.[6] If a patient is unarousable to loud voice and vigorous shaking, a painful stimulus should be introduced, but every effort should be made to avoid causing tissue damage. Painful stimuli can be introduced by moderate compression of the nail beds, the supraorbital ridge, or the temporomandibular joint.[6] Patients with a RASS score of −4 and −5 are considered to be stuporous or comatose, respectively; these patients should then be assessed with a validated coma scale (see Assessment of Stupor and Coma). Patients with a RASS of −3 and above should be assessed for delirium (see Assessment of Delirium).

Assessment of Stupor and Coma

If the patient's RASS is −4 or −5, the patient is likely to be stuporous or comatose, for which several scoring assessments exist. The Glasgow Coma Scale (GCS) is probably the most widely used coma scale, and rates eye, verbal, and motor response to verbal and painful stimuli (**Table 2**).[112] Scores range from 3 (unresponsive) to 15 (normal). The GCS has prognostic significance as it predicts mortality,[113,114] but has several limitations because the verbal score is difficult to obtain in patients who are intubated or aphasic. The GCS can also have low interrater reliability because it is difficult to remember.[115] The Full Outline of Unresponsiveness (FOUR) is another coma score that assesses for eye response, motor response, pupillary reflexes, and breathing.[116] Because the FOUR Score does not evaluate verbal response, this scale can be performed in patients who are intubated or aphasic. However, the FOUR score is relatively complicated and is also difficult to remember. Hence, the FOUR score may have limited utility in the ED.

The AVPU is another commonly used scale to help describe impaired level of consciousness. AVPU stands for Alert, responsive to Verbal stimuli, responsive to Painful stimuli, and Unresponsive. The benefit of the AVPU scale is that it is easy to remember and allows for quick communication of the patient's global picture of level of responsiveness. However, it lacks granularity in detecting subtle impairments.[117]

Assessment of Delirium

For patients with altered mental status with a RASS score of −3 or greater (arousable to verbal stimuli), the patient should be assessed for delirium. It is important to remember that the minority of patients with delirium will have the chief complaint of "altered mental status" and the clinical manifestation of delirium can be subtle, especially if it is the hypoactive subtype. As a result, many cases of delirium will be missed unless it is actively screened for using validated delirium assessments. Recently, delirium screening has been proposed to be one of the key quality indicators for emergency geriatric care,[118] and a core competency for emergency medicine resident education.[119]

A psychiatrist evaluation using the *Diagnostic and Statistical Manual of Mental Disorders*, Fourth Edition, Text Revision (DSM-IV-TR) criteria is considered to be the

Table 2 Glasgow Coma Scale	
Points	**Scale Elements**
	Eyes
4	Opens eyes spontaneously
3	Opens eyes in response to voice
2	Opens eyes in response to painful stimuli
1	Does not open eyes
	Verbal
5	Oriented, converses normally
4	Confused, disoriented
3	Utters inappropriate words
2	Incomprehensible sounds
1	Makes no sounds
	Motor
6	Obeys commands
5	Localizes painful stimuli
4	Flexion/withdrawal to painful stimuli
3	Abnormal flexion to painful stimuli (decorticate response)
2	Extension to painful stimuli (decerebrate response)
1	Makes no movements

gold standard for delirium diagnosis.[11] To meet DSM-IV-TR criteria for delirium, a patient must have all of the following: (1) a disturbance of consciousness (ie, reduced clarity of awareness of the environment) with reduced ability to focus, sustain or shift attention; (2) a change in cognition or the development of a perceptual disturbance that is not better accounted for by a preexisting, established, or evolving dementia; (3) the disturbance develops over a short period of time (usually hours to days) and tends to fluctuate during the course of the day; and (4) there is evidence that the disturbance is caused by the direct physiologic consequences of a general medical condition or substance. Determining these criteria requires comprehensive neurocognitive testing and a detailed interview with a person who knows the patient well (ie, proxy or caregiver).

Obtaining routine psychiatric consultation to perform these DSM-IV-TR delirium evaluations may not be feasible for most hospitals, and these criteria are not routinely applied by nonpsychiatrists. The Confusion Assessment Method (CAM) was developed for nonpsychiatrists and is probably the most widely used delirium assessment in the medical setting,[120] and has undergone the most extensive validation.[121] The CAM operationalizes the DSM criteria for delirium and consists of 4 features: (1) altered mental status and fluctuating course, (2) inattention, (3) disorganized thinking, and (4) altered level of consciousness. Feature 1 (altered mental status and fluctuating course) is obtained from collateral history from one who knows the patient's baseline cognition (ie, family member, caregiver, nursing home, or primary care provider). Time of onset of the change in mental status should be established as well as the presence fluctuations ("Did the symptoms you noticed tend to come and go, or get worse and better over time"). In the ED, approximately 40% of older patients may not have a proxy available in the ED, and they may need to be contacted by telephone.[122] If the patient is grossly altered and a proxy is not readily available, information from the patient's medical record may be useful to help establish their mental status baseline. For example, if a patient is unable to follow simple commands and barely able to stay awake to verbal stimuli (RASS −3), but was able to provide a detailed history in a recent primary care provider clinic visit, this patient likely has an acute change in mental status. Feature 2 is inattention and considered to be a cardinal feature of delirium.[18,19,123] Patients with inattention are easily distractible to irrelevant stimuli and can have difficulty maintaining a conversation. Questions often have to be repeated to the patient when inattention is present. Patients who are inattentive may also fall asleep during the interview when disengaged. Inattention is also commonly assessed for by asking the patient to recite the months of year backward, recite the days of the week backward, or count backward from 20 to 1.[123,124] Patients with disorganized thinking (feature 3) exhibit incoherent thought processes; they may ramble or have irrelevant conversations. These patients may also display illogical flow of ideas, circumstantiality, or tangential thoughts. Feature 4 is altered level of consciousness whereby the patient is drowsy, lethargic, anxious, restless, or agitated (RASS other than 0).

For a patient to meet criteria for delirium, both features 1 and 2, and either 3 or 4 must be present. The original CAM validation study was conducted in hospitalized patients, and was found to have excellent sensitivity (94%–100%) and specificity (90%–95%) compared with a psychiatrist's assessment using DSM-III-R criteria.[120] The CAM is the only delirium assessment to be validated in the ED setting, albeit in patients from Brazil.[125] In 100 patients who were 60 years or older, the CAM's sensitivity was 94.1% and its specificity 97.4% when performed by a geriatrician.[125] The psychiatrist's DSM-IV assessment was the reference standard for this study. To assess all of the CAM's features, the training manual recommends performing the

Modified Mini-Cog and the Digit Span test, and can take approximately 5 minutes to complete.[126] If the patient is delirious or demented, the CAM may take even longer.[127] The CAM requires significant training and may be less sensitive when used by raters with less clinical experience.[128,129]

Detecting delirium in the ED can be challenging, because it is fast paced and the ED staff is usually under immense time constraints. As a result, spending 5 minutes performing a delirium assessment may not be feasible, and briefer (<2 minutes) delirium assessments may be needed in this difficult setting. The Confusion Assessment Method of the Intensive Care Unit (CAM-ICU) is based on the CAM and may be feasible to perform in the ED, because it takes less than 2 minutes to complete.[130] The CAM-ICU (**Fig. 3**) has been recently restructured and allows for early stoppage. For a patient to meet criteria for feature 1, a patient must have either altered mental status or fluctuating course; this is slightly different to the CAM, which requires both to be present. The CAM-ICU uses brief objective assessments to test for inattention and disorganized thinking. To test for inattention (feature 2), the CAM-ICU rater gives a series of 10 letters ("SAVEA-HAART") and asks the patient to squeeze the rater's hand whenever the letter "A" is heard. A picture recognition test, which tests the patient's short-term memory, is also

CAM-ICU

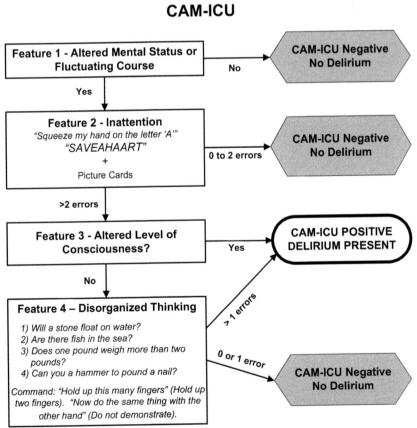

Fig. 3. Confusion Assessment Method for the Intensive Care Unit. (*Courtesy of* Dr Wes Ely and Vanderbilt University, Nashville, TN. Copyright © 2002; with permission. Available at: www.icudelirium.org.)

used to test for inattention. To test for disorganized thinking, 4 yes/no questions are asked as well as a simple command. The CAM-ICU incorporates the RASS to assess for altered level of consciousness (feature 3); a score other than 0 indicates altered level of consciousness. Additional details are available from www.icudelirium.org.

The CAM-ICU has excellent diagnostic performance in the critically ill patient population, but there are limited data evaluating the CAM-ICU's diagnostic performance in those who are noncritically ill. Neufeld and colleagues[131] evaluated the CAM-ICU performed by a layperson in 139 noncritically ill medical oncology patients whose median age was 57 years old. Its sensitivity was found to be 18% and its specificity 99% compared with a psychiatrist's DSM-IV assessment. In 129 patients with acute stroke and a median age of 72.5 years, the CAM-ICU's sensitivity and specificity was 76% and 98%, respectively.[132] It is unclear why the sensitivities are so discrepant, but it may be secondary to differences in median age, underlying disease, and severities of illness. Recently, the CAM-ICU was modified into the Brief Confusion Assessment Method (B-CAM) to improve its sensitivity. The B-CAM and CAM-ICU primarily differ on how they test for inattention. The B-CAM simply asks the patient to recite the months of the year backward from December to July. The CAM-ICU, B-CAM, and other brief delirium assessments specifically designed for the ED are currently being validated in the older ED patients.

Several very brief delirium assessments have been validated in other settings and may have promise for the ED. The Delirium Diagnostic Tool—Provisional (DDT-Pro) is brief delirium assessment that assesses for disorganized thinking, inattention, and sleep-wake cycle disturbances. In 36 patients with traumatic brain injury, the DDT-Pro was 100% sensitive and 94% specific when performed by a layperson in comparison with a psychiatrist's assessment.[133] However, the median age was 44 years, and patients were recruited from a rehabilitation hospital, indicating significant brain injury; the diagnostic performance may be different in older ED patients without head injury. The Single Question in Delirium (SQiD) is another promising delirium assessment that asks the patient's family or friend the following question: "Do you think [name of patient] has been more confused lately?" In 33 oncology inpatients, the SQiD was 80% sensitive and 71% specific compared with a psychiatrist's assessment.[134] Lastly, the modified Richmond Agitation and Sedation Scale (mRASS) may also have clinical utility in the ED; this assessment takes less than 30 seconds to complete and can easily be integrated into the ED clinical workflow.[134] The mRASS is based on the RASS but also incorporates the rater's observations of the patient's attentiveness. Using the psychiatrist's assessment as the reference standard, an mRASS other than 0 (altered level of consciousness or inattentive) is 64% sensitive and 93% specific for delirium in older hospitalized patients.[134] Performing serial mRASS assessments increases the sensitivity to 74% with a specificity of 92%.[134]

INITIAL MANAGEMENT OF PATIENTS WITH ALTERED MENTAL STATUS IN THE EMERGENCY DEPARTMENT

When a patient with altered mental status arrives to the ED, the first step is to determine whether this patient is critically ill or not. As the level of consciousness becomes more disturbed (ie, RASS −5 or RASS +4), the index of suspicion for a life-threatening illness that precipitated the acute change in mental status should similarly increase; this is particularly the case for patients who are stuporous and comatose. These patients should become the emergency physician's immediate priority, and the primary goal should be to promptly assess and stabilize the patient with as little delay as possible.

The initial evaluation and management for ED patients with altered mental status is summarized in **Table 3**. The patient's airway, breathing, circulation, and disability should be rapidly evaluated and addressed; the patient should be fully exposed to facilitate evaluation and treatment. Concomitantly, the patient should be placed on pulse oximeter and cardiac monitor, and an intravenous line should be established; if the patient is hemodynamically unstable, then 2 large-bore intravenous lines should be started in the antecubital fossa. Finger-stick blood glucose should be obtained immediately to rule out

Table 3		
Initial assessment and management of a patient with altered mental status		
	Assessment	**Intervention**
Airway	Is patient protecting his/her airway Look for airway obstruction including foreign bodies	Extend neck, provide chin lift or jaw thrust Suction oropharynx In cases of trauma, provide cervical spine immobilization Nasopharyngeal airway Oropharyngeal airway if no gag Endotracheal intubation patient is not able to protect airway
Breathing	Is there respiratory distress Is the patient hypoventilating Is the patient cyanotic or hypoxic Auscultate the chest	Provide high-flow oxygen[a] Provide bag-valve mask ventilation if hypoventilating
Circulation	Check for pulse while getting blood pressure measurement Look for other signs of hypoperfusion (ie, capillary refill, skin temperature) Place on electrocardiographic monitor to look for dysrhythmias Look for obvious bleeding If hypotensive or signs of hypoperfusion, consider bedside ultrasound[b]	Establish intravenous access Two large-bore intravenous lines are needed in patients who are hemodynamically unstable Fluid challenge with intravenous crystalloid if hypotensive or has other signs of hypoperfusion Stop hemorrhage if accessible
Disability	Examine pupils Assess responsiveness using a scale such as the GCS Check finger-stick blood glucose Consider toxicologic causes (ie, opioid overdose)	One ampoule (50 mL) of D50 in hypoglycemia Naloxone in suspected opioid overdose
Exposure	Expose the patient. Minimize heat loss in patients who are normothermic or hypothermic Look for transdermal drug patches (eg, fentanyl) that could cause mental status changes Look for signs of infection	Remove drug patches

Abbreviation: GCS, Glasgow Coma Scale.
 [a] In patients who have chronic obstructive pulmonary disease, high-flow oxygen may remove their respiratory drive especially in patients with chronic respiratory failure. Oxygen saturation should be titrated to the low 90s%.
 [b] Bedside ultrasonography is commonly used in emergency departments and intensive care units to rapidly rule out causes of hypotension such as cardiac tamponade and intra-abdominal blood. The inferior vena cava can also be assessed using the bedside ultrasound apparatus to assess whether a patient is hypovolemic (dehydration, hemorrhage) or hypervolemic (heart failure).

hypoglycemia. Vital signs should also be rapidly measured and if possible, a rectal temperature should be performed to accurately rule out hypothermia or hyperthermia.

If opioid overdose is suspected, intravenous naloxone should be given especially if the patient is comatose or stuporous. The initial dose of naloxone is not well established, but is generally considered to be 0.4 mg; this initial dose should be diluted in 10 mL of normal saline and be administered slowly over several minutes to avoid severe withdrawal symptoms. If there is no response, the dose can be escalated to 2 mg and up to 10 mg intravenously; higher doses may be needed if the patient is on a long-acting opioid medication such as methadone. Transdermal fentanyl patches should also be looked for while exposing the patient and, if present, should be removed immediately. Reversing benzodiazepine overdoses with flumazenil is not routinely recommended because it may elicit life-threatening withdrawal and seizures in patients who are chronic users. If the finger-stick blood sugar indicates hypoglycemia, one ampoule (50 mL) of D50 should be administered intravenously; if intravenous access is difficult to obtain, 2 mg glucagon can given intramuscularly. Thiamine, 100 mg given parenterally or intramuscularly, can also be considered if Wernicke encephalopathy is suspected; clinicians should have a high index of suspicion of this in patients who have a history of ethanol abuse or appear malnourished. Thiamine should be given before glucose administration. Based on animal models, there is a theoretical risk that glucose administration may worsen encephalopathy in those who are thiamine deficient.[135]

THE DIAGNOSTIC EVALUATION OF PATIENTS WITH ACUTE BRAIN DYSFUNCTION

In patients with delirium, stupor, or coma, the diagnostic evaluation should be focused on uncovering the underlying etiology. Although other causes of acute brain dysfunction are common, the emergency physician's first priority is to consider life-threatening causes. Life-threatening causes of acute brain dysfunction can be remembered using the mnemonic device "WHHHHIMPS" (**Box 4**).[73] Many of these life-threatening causes such as hypoglycemia or hypoxemia can be ruled out within the initial assessment mentioned in the previous section. Other diagnoses, such as meningitis, require a more extensive evaluation and should be considered if no other cause for the patient's acute brain dysfunction is found. Once these life-threatening causes have been considered, the ED evaluation can then focus on ruling out other less life-threatening causes of acute brain dysfunction as listed in **Box 3**.

Box 4
Life-threatening causes of delirium

Wernicke disease or ethanol withdrawal

Hypoxia or hypercarbia

Hypoglycemia

Hypertensive encephalopathy

Hyperthermia or hypothermia

Intracerebral hemorrhage

Meningitis/encephalitis

Poisoning (whether exogenous or iatrogenic)

Status epilepticus

Data from Caplan GA, Cassem NH, Murray GB. Delirium. In: Stern TA, editor. Massachusetts General Hospital comprehensive clinical psychiatry. 1st edition. Philadelphia, PA: Mosby/Elsevier; 2008.

History

Because a patient with acute brain dysfunction, including delirium, is unlikely to provide an accurate history,[109] obtaining a detailed history from a proxy is critical to uncovering the underlying etiology. This history may come from a family member, caregiver, or nursing home staff if the patient resides in one. Because so many medications can be deliriogenic, it is important to carefully review the patient's medication history. Medication histories obtained from triage or from electronic medical records are notoriously inaccurate and should be confirmed with the caregiver or their pharmacy.[136,137] A history of any recent changes or additions to the patient's home medication regimen should be elicited as well as increased dosages; the clinician should determine if these changes are temporally related to the development of symptoms. In addition to prescribed medications, a history of taking over-the-counter medications and alternative medications should also be obtained. A careful substance history should also be obtained, preferably from a proxy. A significant proportion of elderly patients are abusers of ethanol and sedative-hypnotics[138,139]; significant ingestion or withdrawal from these substances can precipitate delirium.

Physical Examination

The detailed physical examination (**Fig. 4**) is also crucial to uncovering the underlying etiology of delirium, especially if no collateral history is available. A head examination should look for any signs of recent trauma; the presence of trauma should increase one's suspicion for a subdural hematoma, subarachnoid hemorrhage, or other traumatic intracranial injury. A pupillary examination should also be performed looking for the presence of fixed or dilated pupils. The presence of miosis and mydriasis may also indicate opioid and anticholinergic medication toxicity, respectively. The pupillary examination may be difficult to assess in elderly patients with eye diseases, prior surgery, or in those who use ophthalmic eye drops. A fundoscopic examination can also be considered to look for papilledema suggestive of increased intracranial pressure or retinal subhyaloid hemorrhage suggestive of subarachnoid hemorrhage. If possible, an extraocular muscle examination should also be performed, especially in patients who appear to be unresponsive; the presence of vertical extraocular eye movements may suggest locked-in syndrome. Ophthalmoplegia can also be seen in patients with Wernicke encephalopathy or increased intracranial pressure. The presence of nystagmus may indicate intoxication with alcohol or other drugs.

A neck examination should look for thyromegaly and meningismus. Although the presence of meningismus greatly increases the likelihood of meningitis, its absence does not reliably rule it out. A lung examination should look for any signs of pulmonary edema or pneumonia. If febrile, the cardiac examination should be focused on looking for new murmurs that may suggest endocarditis. An abdominal examination is needed to rule out any acute surgical emergencies such as acute appendicitis, diverticulitis, or cholecystitis. The patient should also be completely exposed and the skin should be examined for medication patches (eg, fentanyl or scopolamine), signs of infection, petechiae, and sequelae of liver failure. A genitourinary examination should be performed to look for infected decubiti ulcers or perirectal or perianal abscesses. A rectal examination should be performed in patients with end-stage liver disease, as esophageal variceal bleeds can precipitate hepatic encephalopathy.

A focused neurologic examination should be also performed. The presence of focal, lateralizing neurologic symptoms is suggestive of a central nervous system insult (eg, cerebrovascular accident, intraparenchymal hemorrhage, or mass effect). In addition, the presence of repetitive movement of the eyelids, eyes, or extremities may be

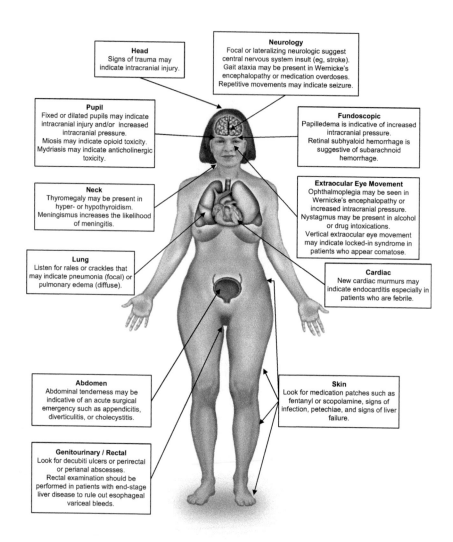

Head
Signs of trauma may indicate intracranial injury.

Neurology
Focal or lateralizing neurologic suggest central nervous system insult (eg, stroke). Gait ataxia may be present in Wernicke's encephalopathy or medication overdoses. Repetitive movements may indicate seizure.

Pupil
Fixed or dilated pupils may indicate intracranial injury and/or increased intracranial pressure.
Miosis may indicate opioid toxicity.
Mydriasis may indicate anticholinergic toxicity.

Fundoscopic
Papilledema is indicative of increased intracranial pressure.
Retinal subhyaloid hemorrhage is suggestive of subarachnoid hemorrhage.

Neck
Thyromegaly may be present in hyper- or hypothyroidism.
Meningismus increases the likelihood of meningitis.

Extraocular Eye Movement
Ophthalmoplegia may be seen in Wernicke's encephalopathy or increased intracranial pressure.
Nystagmus may be present in alcohol or drug intoxications.
Vertical extraocular eye movement may indicate locked-in syndrome in patients who appear comatose.

Lung
Listen for rales or crackles that may indicate pneumonia (focal) or pulmonary edema (diffuse).

Cardiac
New cardiac murmurs may indicate endocarditis especially in patients who are febrile.

Abdomen
Abdominal tenderness may be indicative of an acute surgical emergency such as appendicitis, diverticulitis, or cholecystitis.

Skin
Look for medication patches such as fentanyl or scopolamine, signs of infection, petechiae, and signs of liver failure.

Genitourinary / Rectal
Look for decubiti ulcers or perirectal or perianal abscesses.
Rectal examination should be performed in patients with end-stage liver disease to rule out esophageal variceal bleeds.

Fig. 4. The physical examination of the patient with delirium, stupor, or coma.

suggestive of seizure. The presence of gait ataxia may also be seen in patients with Wernicke encephalopathy or medication overdoses.

Laboratory Testing

Laboratory tests are routinely performed in patients with delirium, stupor, and coma. Because urinary tract infections are common delirium precipitants, a urinalysis should be performed in all patients. Serum electrolytes should also be routinely obtained to rule out electrolyte abnormalities such as hypernatremia, hyponatremia, hypercalcemia, or hypocalcemia. Because uremia can precipitate delirium, blood urea nitrogen and serum creatinine tests should be ordered. In patients with respiratory complaints or issues, an arterial or venous blood gas should be considered if hypercarbia is suspected. In patients with physical findings suggestive of end-stage liver disease, transaminases and ammonia levels can also be ordered. Thyroid-stimulating hormone and free T4 can also be considered to rule out hyperthyroidism and hypothyroidism. Serum drug levels should also be ordered if the patient is on medications that can be measured in the serum (ie, anticonvulsants, theophylline, and digoxin). Occasionally, patients with acute myocardial infarction can also present with delirium without chest pain[69,140]; hence, a 12-lead electrocardiogram and cardiac biomarkers should be considered, but their diagnostic yield in ED patients with delirium remains unknown. A lumbar puncture, though not routinely performed, should be strongly considered if there is a clinical suspicion for meningitis or encephalitis or if the patient has a fever or leukocytosis without an obvious source.[141,142] This diagnostic procedure can also be considered if no other causes of delirium, stupor, or coma are found. A urine drug screen can also be ordered but should be interpreted with caution, as it can mislead the clinician into thinking that the patient has a toxicologic cause for their acute brain dysfunction, when in fact another underlying illness, such as meningitis, exists. A patient who is on home opioids and benzodiazepines will likely have a positive urine drug screen for these substances. It also does not provide serum levels, and false-positive and false-negative results can occur.[143]

Radiographic and Other Testing

With regard to radiological testing, a chest radiograph can be considered to rule out pneumonia or pulmonary edema, especially in the setting of a history of cough and dyspnea, hypoxemia, or tachypnea. An abdominal ultrasonogram or abdomen and pelvis computed tomography (CT) should be considered if the patient has abdominal pain. For patients who are stuporous or comatose, they should promptly receive a head CT emergently to rule out any structural lesions. For delirious patients, however, there is little evidence-based guidance as to when a head CT is appropriate; their routine use is not recommended because its diagnostic yield may be low.[9] Based on 2 studies, a head CT's diagnostic yield is increased when performed in delirious patients with impaired level of consciousness, a recent history of a fall or head trauma, or a focal neurologic deficit.[9,144] It can also be considered when no other cause for delirium is found. Clinical judgment should be used when deciding whether a delirious patient requires a head CT.

Magnetic resonance imaging of the brain (brain MRI) and EEG are occasionally performed in patients with acute brain dysfunction including delirium, but their optimal role in the ED is yet to be determined. In addition, these diagnostic modalities may not be readily available in all settings, further limiting their use. Patients with cerebrovascular accidents involving the right parietal lobe can present with delirium as the sole manifestation and without any focal neurologic findings.[145] Early in the clinical course (several hours), the head CT may be nondiagnostic, and a brain MRI can help rule in this diagnosis. Nonconvulsive status epilepticus can also manifest as unusual mental status changes including delirium, but making this diagnosis can be challenging without an EEG. An early EEG should be considered in patients who had a reported seizure before ED arrival or have a seizure history. Although EEGs are difficult to obtain in the ED, the development of abbreviated (5-minute) EEG protocols[146] and portable EEG monitoring devices may improve the feasibility of obtaining this diagnostic modality quickly.[147] Early diagnosis of cerebrovascular accidents or nonconvulsive status epilepticus is important, because earlier intervention may improve patients' outcomes. If either of these diagnoses is being considered as a cause for altered mental status, prompt neurologic consultation in the ED is recommended to facilitate both diagnostic evaluation and therapeutic intervention.

EMERGENCY DEPARTMENT MANAGEMENT OF PATIENTS WITH DELIRIUM

The single most effective treatment for acute brain dysfunction is to diagnose and treat the underlying etiology. Beyond this, the clinical management of acute brain dysfunction is unclear, especially for delirium, and is secondary to the limited evidence available. Delirium care is slowly evolving, and nonpharmacologic and pharmacologic interventions currently exist, especially for those who are agitated. In general, non-pharmacologic interventions are favored as the initial management and pharmaco-logic means should be used as a last resort. The following sections can also be applied to patients in stupor or coma, as many of these patients will eventually transi-tion to delirium.

Nonpharmacologic Management

Although hyperactive delirium occurs less frequently in older ED patients, its manage-ment can be challenging if they are agitated or combative, and especially if patient, caregiver, and ED staff safety is a concern. Nonpharmacologic interventions should be attempted before considering pharmacologic interventions. Initial steps would be to modify the environment and may involve dimming or turning off the lights, mini-mizing auditory stimulation from beeping cardiac monitors or intravenous infusion pumps, and having family members and familiar objects from home at the patient's bedside.[47,148]

Flaherty and Little[149] recommend the "TADA" approach as a nonpharmacologic means to managing and preventing agitation. TADA stands for Tolerate, Anticipate, Don't Agitate. *Tolerating* behaviors that may appear to be potentially dangerous is the first step and is contrary to the nature of health care providers. For example, a delirious patient may attempt to get out of bed without assistance or pull on intra-venous lines, oxygen tubing, or cardiac monitoring devices. However, tolerating such behaviors allows patients to respond naturally to their circumstances and may provide them a sense of control while in their confused state. These behaviors may also be a cue that something is bothering them; they are so cognitively impaired that they are unable to communicate what is wrong. For example, a patient who is agitated and getting out of bed may really need to go to the bathroom. Tolerating behaviors require close supervision to maintain patient safety.[149] *Anticipating* behav-iors is where the health care provider prepares for what the patient might do and avoids inciting agents that may exacerbate agitation. Anticipation includes avoiding unnatural attachments or tethers that are not absolutely necessary for clinical care.[149] Examples of tethers are multiple intravenous lines, nasal cannula oxygen, and monitoring devices. Instead of giving intravenous normal saline continuously for maintenance fluids, intermittent boluses should be considered. Supplemental oxygen is not needed if the patient is not hypoxic or in respiratory compromise. Blood pres-sure cuffs, pulse oximeter, and cardiac monitoring devices should also be minimized if continuous monitoring is not necessary; intermittent vital-sign measurements should be used whenever possible.[149] Getting out of bed is also anticipated and encouraged by this approach as long as the patient's safety can be ensured. *Don't Agitate* is the final step and is considered the golden rule of this approach.[149] Some agitators are obvious (ie, urinary bladder catheters) and some are not. Reorientation can be unpre-dictable, as it can occasionally worsen agitation and should only be attempted if the patient is amenable to it.

Indwelling urinary bladder catheters deserve special mention because they are frequently placed in patients with acute brain dysfunction. These catheters should be avoided in delirious patients when there is no clear medical indication. Urinary bladder catheters cannot only agitate the patient further, but their use is also associated with increased in-hospital and 90-day mortality, longer stays in hospital, and a higher risk of developing delirium.[42,150] If the delirious patient has urinary incontinence and urine is needed for a urinalysis, straight catheterization should be used. Avoiding or removing urinary bladder catheters may not only help reduce agitation, but can also help minimize urethral trauma from forced self-removal and reduce the risk of catheter-associated infections.

Similarly, physical restraints should be avoided because they are associated with a 4-fold increase in delirium development during hospitalization and are associated with increasing delirium severity.[42] If placed for patient or provider safety, physical restraints should be a temporary measure and should be removed once nonpharmacologic or pharmacologic alternatives have taken effect. Having family members in the room or using sitters can help reduce the need for physical restraints; they can provide feedback to patients when they initiate dangerous behaviors such as climbing out of bed or attempting to go the bathroom without assistance.

Pharmacologic Management

Pharmacologic management is mainly focused on the agitated delirious patient (hyperactive), and can be considered if nonpharmacologic interventions fail. Benzodiazepines should be avoided as monotherapy in delirious patients whenever possible,[47,151] because they have high side-effect profiles and can exacerbate delirium. Breitbart and colleagues[152] performed a randomized controlled trial that compared antipsychotic medications with lorazepam, and observed a higher prevalence of treatment-limiting side effects such as oversedation and increased confusion in the lorazepam arm.

The National Institute of Health and Clinical Excellence (NICE) delirium guidelines recommend using antipsychotic medications in patients with agitation and who are at high risk for harming themselves and others.[151] However, these medications should be used only if verbal and nonverbal deescalation techniques have failed, and if used, the lowest dose possible should be given.[151] Antipsychotic medications are also used in delirious patients with behavioral disturbances and overt psychotic manifestations (ie, visual hallucinations and delusions). However, their routine use is controversial because most studies investigating the use of antipsychotics are limited by their nonblinded trial design, poor randomization, or inadequate power. Two systematic reviews investigated the role of antipsychotic medications in delirium management, and concluded that there was little evidence to support their routine use and that additional studies using more rigorous methodology were needed.[153,154]

Haloperidol is one of the most studied and widely used antipsychotic medications because its lacks anticholinergic properties and can be administered orally, intramuscularly, or intravenously.[47] Hu and colleagues[155] compared haloperidol with placebo, and observed that 70.4% of delirious patients who received haloperidol showed improvement in their delirium severity at the end of 1 week compared with 29.7% of the placebo group. For agitated elderly patients, 0.25 to 1.0 mg of haloperidol can be given every 30 to 60 minutes in the intravenous or intramuscular form. Special care must be taken when given in the intravenously, because torsades de pointes has been reported when given in this formulation.[156] If possible, a 12-lead electrocardiogram should be obtained before intravenous haloperidol administration to evaluate the patient's QTc interval, and should be avoided if the QTc interval is greater than 500 milliseconds. The benefit of the intravenous haloperidol is that it is the least likely to cause extrapyramidal symptoms, whereas the intramuscular formulation is associated with the highest incidence.

Atypical antipsychotic medications such as olanzapine, risperidone, and quetiapine are also commonly used by psychiatrists and geriatricians for the treatment of delirium. The advantage of these medications is the decreased incidence of extrapyramidal side effects compared with haloperidol.[157] Most atypical antipsychotics are given orally, but recently olanzapine, risperidone, ziprasidone, and aripiprazole have been made available in intramuscular formulations. Unfortunately, these forms may not be readily available in many EDs. Similar to haloperidol, there is limited evidence on the effectiveness of atypical antipsychotics, and few have been compared with placebo. Compared with placebo, olanzapine has been shown to improve delirium severity in one randomized controlled trial,[155] but its effectiveness may be attenuated in patients who are 70 years and older.[158] Tahir and colleagues[159] performed a double-blinded randomized controlled trial in 42 delirious patients, and observed that patients in the quetiapine arm recovered faster than those who received placebo.

In patients with diffuse Lewis body dementia or Parkinson disease, antipsychotic medications should be should be avoided or used with extreme caution.[160] These patients are highly sensitive to these medications and can easily develop extrapyramidal side effects.[151] If antipsychotic medications must be given to these patients, quetiapine is the least likely to have extrapyramidal side effects.[161] Regardless, if these patients are agitated and nonpharmacologic measures have failed, psychiatric and/or geriatric consultation may be warranted.

As previously mentioned, benzodiazepines should be avoided for the management of delirious patients. The exception to this recommendation is for patients who are withdrawing from ethanol (delirium tremens) or benzodiazepine.[47,162] Giving benzodiazepines to these patients will improve delirium severity and may also improve mortality and morbidity.[162] Because poorly controlled somatic pain can precipitate delirium,[70–72] using opioid medication in this subgroup may be beneficial and help reduce agitation.[71] Pain control can also be achieved by using regional anesthesia such as femoral nerve blocks in patients with lower extremity fractures.

Medications to Avoid in Patients with Delirium

Part of the management of patients with acute brain dysfunction is to avoid medications known to precipitate or worsen delirium. Recently, the Beers Criteria for Potentially Inappropriate Medication Use in Older Adults was updated. Based on "moderate quality evidence and strong strength of recommendation" from the panel, they recommend avoiding tricyclic antidepressants, medications with anticholinergic properties, benzodiazepines and other sedative-hypnotics, corticosteroids, and histamine-2 receptor antagonists in older patients because they may worsen or exacerbate delirium.[85] If the patient is on multiple medications with anticholinergic properties, reducing these medications may improve delirium severity; in a study of 34 delirious nursing home patients who were on at least 1 anticholinergic medication, subjects were randomly assigned to receive an intervention that reduced their anticholinergic load by 25%.[163] Those who received the intervention had significant improvements in delirium symptomatology.[163] There are several reports of histamine-2 blockers (cimetidine, ranitidine, and famotidine) precipitating delirium,[164] and they should be avoided in delirious patients because safer alternatives such as proton-pump inhibitors are available.

DISPOSITION

Patients who are stuporous or comatose need a hospital admission and likely require an intensive care unit. With delirium, however, there is little evidence-based guidance regarding the appropriate disposition of older ED patients. Most delirious patients will require hospitalization, especially if they have severe symptoms, have poor social support at home, or poor access to follow-up care. There is also evidence to suggest that older ED patients with delirium who are discharged home are more likely to die than their nondelirious counterparts; this relationship is further magnified when the delirium is missed by the ED.[17] However, for a small minority of delirious patients with reliable caregivers and accessible transportation, ED discharge can be considered if the etiology is unequivocally obvious and the delirium symptoms resolve (eg, accidental opioid overdose reversed with naloxone) or are mild, the patient can be closely supervised at home, and close outpatient follow-up can be arranged.

If admitted to the hospital, delirious patients should preferably be admitted to specialized geriatric unit such as an Acute Care for Elderly unit or a Delirium Room.[165,166] These units typically have multidisciplinary team of physicians, nurses, and social workers or case managers who specialize in geriatrics care and have expertise in managing delirious patients. The team also implements nonpharmacologic, multicomponent delirium interventions that (1) minimize the use of psychoactive medications such as benzodiazepines and medications with anticholinergic properties, (2) maximize mobility and limit the use of urinary bladder catheters and physical restraints, (3) implement the TADA approach as described earlier, (4) reduce sensory deprivation by offering eyeglasses or hearing devices, (5) provide cognitive stimulation and reorientation, and (6) encourage normal sleep-wake cycles (eg, minimize nighttime noise, use ear plugs at night).[148,166,167] However, the efficacy of these interventions is equivocal, especially for delirious medical inpatients.[168] Pitkala and colleagues[169,170] found that a multicomponent delirium intervention enhanced delirium resolution in the hospital and improved cognition and health-related quality of life at 6 months. However, they did not observe any differences in long-term mortality or institutionalization.[169,170] Regardless of which inpatient unit delirious patients are admitted to, their time spent in the ED should probably be minimized. Inouye and colleagues[42] observed that patients who were in the ED for longer than 12 hours were 2 times more likely to develop delirium in the hospital setting.

COMMUNICATION DURING TRANSITIONS OF CARE

Regardless of the patient's disposition, the patient's mental status in the ED should be communicated to the physician at the next level of care. The patient's delirium status and the delirium assessment used to make the diagnosis, the suspected underlying etiology, and treatments administered should be communicated. Communicating the patient's level of consciousness using an arousal scale such as the RASS may also be useful to provide information on the patient's psychomotor status (normal, hypoactive, or hyperactive). In addition, knowing a baseline RASS may be useful, as changes in RASS increase the likelihood that the patient has delirium.[134] If the delirious patient is being admitted, this information should be conveyed to the admitting physician. If the patient is being discharged home, his or her primary care provider should be notified. Similar communication should occur between ED physicians and nurses during shift change.

IMPROVING DELIRIUM RECOGNITION IN THE EMERGENCY DEPARTMENT: CHALLENGES AND FUTURE RESEARCH

Delirium is currently missed in the majority of older ED patients,[10,12–17] because EDs do not screen for this form of acute brain dysfunction. Improving delirium recognition in the ED will be challenging. Emergency physicians are usually under huge time constraints and have a limited amount of time to spend with the patient. These clinicians often take care of large numbers of patients at once, and their patient evaluations are also frequently interrupted (ie, radiologic testing or a higher-acuity patient arrives). Such a routine limits the feasibility of a prolonged mental status examination. Brief and efficient approaches to delirium monitoring that are specifically tailored for the ED setting are needed. Future research should focus developing these approaches. Such an approach may entail validating brief (<2 minutes) delirium assessments in older ED patients. These assessments should balance brevity with diagnostic accuracy, be easy to use, and be reliable when performed by nonphysicians such as nurses, paramedics, or patient care technicians. Nonphysicians may play a more instrumental role in ED delirium monitoring, because they may also have more time to spend with the patient at multiple time points in comparison with physicians.[171]

In addition, the utility serial measurements of global tests of cognition should be investigated. Decreasing scores in these cognitive assessments, such as the Mini-Mental State Examination, may be diagnostic of delirium.[172] However, the Mini-Mental State Examination can take 5 to 10 minutes to perform and may not be feasible to perform in the ED.[127] Brief cognitive assessments such as the Six-Item Screener,[173,174] Mini-Cog,[174] Ottawa 3DY,[175] and Brief Alzheimer's Screen exist,[175] but it is unclear as to how sensitive these assessments are in detecting changes in cognition observed in delirium. This approach would also require that routine cognitive screening be performed in the outpatient clinic and possibly the ED setting during non-delirious episodes to establish a baseline.

Delirium surveillance in the ED can further be optimized by performing assessments on patients who are at higher risk for having delirium. Ideally the process of identifying of high-risk patients should be automated and incorporated into the electronic medical record system to minimize ED staff workload. At present, there are few data to suggest what risk factors should be used to identify older ED patients at high risk for delirium. Future research should focus on developing and validating such clinical decision rules; these rules should use patient characteristics that are immediately and easily available to the clinician.

Perhaps the most significant obstacle to routine ED delirium monitoring is the absence of cost-effective interventions for delirious ED patients. Thus far, uncovering the underlying etiology remains the most effective treatment for delirium. Several non-pharmacologic multicomponent interventions have been developed (see Disposition) but, as previously mentioned, their efficacy is questionable in medical delirious patients. Perhaps initiating these interventions in the ED instead of the hospital setting would improve their efficacy. In addition, the role of antipsychotic medications in older ED patients with delirium remains unknown. It is also possible that there is a subgroup of delirious patients who may benefit more from these nonpharmacologic and pharmacologic interventions. Future studies using randomized controlled trial methodology are needed to test these hypotheses.

THE AMERICAN DELIRIUM SOCIETY

Delirium remains an underappreciated geriatric syndrome among clinicians outside of geriatrics and psychiatry. To increase delirium's awareness and recognition, and to advance its science, the American Delirium Society was recently created. The overall mission of this society is to "foster research, education, quality improvement, advocacy and implementation science to minimize the impact of delirium on short and long-term health and well being, and the effects of delirium on the health care system as a whole."[176] This organization consists of an interdisciplinary group of physicians, nurses, pharmacists, and social workers in psychiatry, geriatrics, emergency medicine, internal medicine, and critical care. Additional information can be found at www.americandeliriumsociety.org.

SUMMARY

Altered mental status is a common complaint in older ED patients. Acute changes are more concerning because they are usually caused by an underlying medical illness and can be life-threatening. Delirium, stupor, and coma are common causes of altered mental status, and these forms of acute brain dysfunction are associated with a multitude of adverse outcomes including higher death rates. Their etiology is multifactorial and is a result of a complex interplay between patient vulnerability and precipitating factors. Patients with acute brain dysfunction can fluctuate and transition from one state to another. A patient who is initially comatose in the ED frequently transitions to delirium. The initial evaluation of a patient with acute brain dysfunction should begin by assessing the level of consciousness using an arousal scale such as the RASS. If the patient is unresponsive (RASS −5) or responsive to painful stimuli (RASS −4) only, the patient is considered to be stuporous and comatose, respectively; a validated coma scale such as the GCS should be used. If the patient has a RASS of −3 and above, a delirium assessment such as the CAM should be used, but this takes 5 minutes to perform and may not be feasible for some EDs. Several briefer delirium assessments exist (CAM-ICU, B-CAM, SQiD, and mRASS) but require validation in older ED patients, and such studies are ongoing. Once acute brain dysfunction is detected in the ED, the primary goal is to find and treat the underlying cause. For agitated patients, nonpharmacologic interventions, such as the TADA approach, should be attempted initially. If nonpharmacologic interventions fail, antipsychotic medications such as haloperidol can be considered. Benzodiazepines should be avoided as monotherapy unless the patient is withdrawing from ethanol or benzodiazepines. Patients with delirium, stupor, or coma generally require admission. The optimal method for delirium monitoring and treatment in the ED remains unclear, and additional research is needed.

REFERENCES

1. Morandi A, Pandharipande P, Trabucchi M, et al. Understanding international differences in terminology for delirium and other types of acute brain dysfunction in critically ill patients. Intensive Care Med 2008;34(10):1907–15.
2. Clarfield AM. The decreasing prevalence of reversible dementias: an updated meta-analysis. Arch Intern Med 2003;163(18):2219–29.
3. Schuur JD, Venkatesh AK. The growing role of emergency departments in hospital admissions. N Engl J Med 2012;367(5):391–3.
4. Niska R, Bhuiya F, Xu J. National hospital ambulatory medical care survey: 2007 emergency department summary. Natl Health Stat Report 2010;26:1–31.
5. He W, Sengupta M, Velkoff VA, et al. U.S census bureau, current population reports, P23-209, 65+ in the United States: 2005. Washington, DC: U.S. Government Printing Office; 2005.
6. Posner JB, Plum F. Plum and Posner's diagnosis of stupor and coma. 4th edition. Oxford (United Kingdom), New York: Oxford University Press; 2007.
7. Sessler CN, Gosnell MS, Grap MJ, et al. The Richmond Agitation-Sedation Scale: validity and reliability in adult intensive care unit patients. Am J Respir Crit Care Med 2002;166(10):1338–44.

8. Ely EW, Truman B, Shintani A, et al. Monitoring sedation status over time in ICU patients: reliability and validity of the Richmond Agitation-Sedation Scale (RASS). JAMA 2003;289(22):2983–91.
9. Naughton BJ, Moran M, Ghaly Y, et al. Computed tomography scanning and delirium in elder patients. Acad Emerg Med 1997;4(12):1107–10.
10. Naughton BJ, Moran MB, Kadah H, et al. Delirium and other cognitive impairment in older adults in an emergency department. Ann Emerg Med 1995;25(6):751–5.
11. American Psychiatric Association. Task force on DSM-IV. Diagnostic and statistical manual of mental disorders: DSM-IV-TR. 4th edition. Washington, DC: American Psychiatric Association; 2000.
12. Hustey FM, Meldon SW, Smith MD, et al. The effect of mental status screening on the care of elderly emergency department patients. Ann Emerg Med 2003; 41(5):678–84.
13. Lewis LM, Miller DK, Morley JE, et al. Unrecognized delirium in ED geriatric patients. Am J Emerg Med 1995;13(2):142–5.
14. Han JH, Zimmerman EE, Cutler N, et al. Delirium in older emergency department patients: recognition, risk factors, and psychomotor subtypes. Acad Emerg Med 2009;16(3):193–200.
15. Elie M, Rousseau F, Cole M, et al. Prevalence and detection of delirium in elderly emergency department patients. CMAJ 2000;163(8):977–81.
16. Hustey FM, Meldon SW. The prevalence and documentation of impaired mental status in elderly emergency department patients. Ann Emerg Med 2002;39(3): 248–53.
17. Kakuma R, du Fort GG, Arsenault L, et al. Delirium in older emergency department patients discharged home: effect on survival. J Am Geriatr Soc 2003;51(4): 443–50.
18. Meagher DJ, Moran M, Raju B, et al. Phenomenology of delirium. Assessment of 100 adult cases using standardised measures. Br J Psychiatry 2007;190:135–41.
19. Meagher DJ, Maclullich AM, Laurila JV. Defining delirium for the International Classification of Diseases, 11th revision. J Psychosom Res 2008;65(3):207–14.
20. Meagher DJ, Trzepacz PT. Motoric subtypes of delirium. Semin Clin Neuropsychiatry 2000;5(2):75–85.
21. Inouye SK, Foreman MD, Mion LC, et al. Nurses' recognition of delirium and its symptoms: comparison of nurse and researcher ratings. Arch Intern Med 2001; 161(20):2467–73.
22. Nicholas LM, Lindsey BA. Delirium presenting with symptoms of depression. Psychosomatics 1995;36(5):471–9.
23. Farrell KR, Ganzini L. Misdiagnosing delirium as depression in medically ill elderly patients. Arch Intern Med 1995;155(22):2459–64.
24. Peterson JF, Pun BT, Dittus RS, et al. Delirium and its motoric subtypes: a study of 614 critically ill patients. J Am Geriatr Soc 2006;54(3):479–84.
25. Liptzin B, Levkoff SE. An empirical study of delirium subtypes. Br J Psychiatry 1992;161:843–5.
26. O'Keeffe ST. Clinical subtypes of delirium in the elderly. Dement Geriatr Cogn Disord 1999;10(5):380–5.
27. Kelly KG, Zisselman M, Cutillo-Schmitter T, et al. Severity and course of delirium in medically hospitalized nursing facility residents. Am J Geriatr Psychiatry 2001;9(1):72–7.
28. Marcantonio E, Ta T, Duthie E, et al. Delirium severity and psychomotor types: their relationship with outcomes after hip fracture repair. J Am Geriatr Soc 2002;50(5):850–7.

29. Pandharipande P, Cotton BA, Shintani A, et al. Motoric subtypes of delirium in mechanically ventilated surgical and trauma intensive care unit patients. Intensive Care Med 2007;33(10):1726–31.

30. Ross CA. CNS arousal systems: possible role in delirium. Int Psychogeriatr 1991;3(2):353–71.

31. Ross CA, Peyser CE, Shapiro I, et al. Delirium: phenomenologic and etiologic subtypes. Int Psychogeriatr 1991;3(2):135–47.

32. O'Keeffe ST, Lavan JN. Clinical significance of delirium subtypes in older people. Age Ageing 1999;28(2):115–9.

33. Kiely DK, Jones RN, Bergmann MA, et al. Association between psychomotor activity delirium subtypes and mortality among newly admitted post-acute facility patients. J Gerontol A Biol Sci Med Sci 2007;62(2):174–9.

34. Boller F, Verny M, Hugonot-Diener L, et al. Clinical features and assessment of severe dementia. A review. Eur J Neurol 2002;9(2):125–36.

35. Marcantonio ER, Simon SE, Bergmann MA, et al. Delirium symptoms in post-acute care: prevalent, persistent, and associated with poor functional recovery. J Am Geriatr Soc 2003;51(1):4–9.

36. Levkoff SE, Evans DA, Liptzin B, et al. Delirium. The occurrence and persistence of symptoms among elderly hospitalized patients. Arch Intern Med 1992;152(2): 334–40.

37. McKeith IG, Galasko D, Kosaka K, et al. Consensus guidelines for the clinical and pathologic diagnosis of dementia with Lewy bodies (DLB): report of the consortium on DLB international workshop. Neurology 1996;47(5):1113–24.

38. Smith E, Delargy M. Locked-in syndrome. BMJ 2005;330(7488):406–9.

39. Wijdicks EF, Nichols DA, Thielen KR, et al. Intra-arterial thrombolysis in acute basilar artery thromboembolism: the initial Mayo Clinic experience. Mayo Clin Proc 1997;72(11):1005–13.

40. Zehtabchi S, Abdel Baki SG, Malhotra S, et al. Nonconvulsive seizures in patients presenting with altered mental status: an evidence-based review. Epilepsy Behav 2011;22(2):139–43.

41. Inouye SK, Viscoli CM, Horwitz RI, et al. A predictive model for delirium in hospitalized elderly medical patients based on admission characteristics. Ann Intern Med 1993;119(6):474–81.

42. Inouye SK, Charpentier PA. Precipitating factors for delirium in hospitalized elderly persons. Predictive model and interrelationship with baseline vulnerability. JAMA 1996;275(11):852–7.

43. Inouye SK. Predisposing and precipitating factors for delirium in hospitalized older patients. Dement Geriatr Cogn Disord 1999;10(5):393–400.

44. Han JH, Morandi A, Ely W, et al. Delirium in the nursing home patients seen in the emergency department. J Am Geriatr Soc 2009;57(5):889–94.

45. Elie M, Cole MG, Primeau FJ, et al. Delirium risk factors in elderly hospitalized patients. J Gen Intern Med 1998;13(3):204–12.

46. Pun BT, Ely EW. The importance of diagnosing and managing ICU delirium. Chest 2007;132(2):624–36.

47. Practice guideline for the treatment of patients with delirium. American Psychiatric Association. Am J Psychiatry 1999;156(Suppl 5):1–20.

48. Fearing MA, Inouye SK. Delirium. In: Blazer DG, Steffens DC, editors. The American psychiatric publishing textbook of geriatric psychiatry. 4th edition. Washington, DC: American Psychiatric Publishing; 2009. p. 229–42.

49. Schor JD, Levkoff SE, Lipsitz LA, et al. Risk factors for delirium in hospitalized elderly. JAMA 1992;267(6):827–31.

50. Marcantonio ER, Goldman L, Mangione CM, et al. A clinical prediction rule for delirium after elective noncardiac surgery. JAMA 1994;271(2):134–9.

51. Gustafson Y, Berggren D, Brannstrom B, et al. Acute confusional states in elderly patients treated for femoral neck fracture. J Am Geriatr Soc 1988; 36(6):525–30.

52. Jitapunkul S, Pillay I, Ebrahim S. Delirium in newly admitted elderly patients: a prospective study. Q J Med 1992;83(300):307–14.

53. Kolbeinsson H, Jonsson A. Delirium and dementia in acute medical admissions of elderly patients in Iceland. Acta Psychiatr Scand 1993;87(2):123–7.

54. Rockwood K. Acute confusion in elderly medical patients. J Am Geriatr Soc 1989;37(2):150–4.

55. Pompei P, Foreman M, Rudberg MA, et al. Delirium in hospitalized older persons: outcomes and predictors. J Am Geriatr Soc 1994;42(8):809–15.

56. Voyer P, Cole MG, McCusker J, et al. Prevalence and symptoms of delirium superimposed on dementia. Clin Nurs Res 2006;15(1):46–66.

57. Jones RN, Yang FM, Zhang Y, et al. Does educational attainment contribute to risk for delirium? A potential role for cognitive reserve. J Gerontol A Biol Sci Med Sci 2006;61(12):1307–11.

58. Francis J, Martin D, Kapoor WN. A prospective study of delirium in hospitalized elderly. JAMA 1990;263(8):1097–101.

59. Kennedy M, Enander RA, Wolfe RE, et al. Identification of delirium in elderly emergency department patients. Acad Emerg Med 2012;19(Suppl 1):S147.

60. Rahkonen T, Makela H, Paanila S, et al. Delirium in elderly people without severe predisposing disorders: etiology and 1-year prognosis after discharge. Int Psychogeriatr 2000;12(4):473–81.

61. George J, Bleasdale S, Singleton SJ. Causes and prognosis of delirium in elderly patients admitted to a district general hospital. Age Ageing 1997; 26(6):423–7.

62. Wahlund L, Bjorlin GA. Delirium in clinical practice: experiences from a specialized delirium ward. Dement Geriatr Cogn Disord 1999;10(5):389–92.

63. Koponen H, Stenback U, Mattila E, et al. Delirium among elderly persons admitted to a psychiatric hospital: clinical course during the acute stage and one-year follow-up. Acta Psychiatr Scand 1989;79(6):579–85.

64. Foreman MD. Confusion in the hospitalized elderly: incidence, onset, and associated factors. Res Nurs Health 1989;12(1):21–9.

65. El-Kaissi S, Kotowicz MA, Berk M, et al. Acute delirium in the setting of primary hypothyroidism: the role of thyroid hormone replacement therapy. Thyroid 2005; 15(9):1099–101.

66. Isbell H, Fraser HF, Wikler A, et al. An experimental study of the etiology of rum fits and delirium tremens. Q J Stud Alcohol 1955;16(1):1–33.

67. Fleischhacker WW, Barnas C, Hackenberg B. Epidemiology of benzodiazepine dependence. Acta Psychiatr Scand 1986;74(1):80–3.

68. Fruensgaard K. Withdrawal psychosis: a study of 30 consecutive cases. Acta Psychiatr Scand 1976;53(2):105–18.

69. Bayer AJ, Chadha JS, Farag RR, et al. Changing presentation of myocardial infarction with increasing old age. J Am Geriatr Soc 1986;34(4):263–6.

70. Lynch EP, Lazor MA, Gellis JE, et al. The impact of postoperative pain on the development of postoperative delirium. Anesth Analg 1998;86(4):781–5.

71. Vaurio LE, Sands LP, Wang Y, et al. Postoperative delirium: the importance of pain and pain management. Anesth Analg 2006;102(4):1267–73.

72. Morrison RS, Magaziner J, Gilbert M, et al. Relationship between pain and opioid analgesics on the development of delirium following hip fracture. J Gerontol A Biol Sci Med Sci 2003;58(1):M76–81.
73. Caplan GA, Cassem NH, Murray GB. Delirium. In: Stern TA, editor. Massachusetts general hospital comprehensive clinical psychiatry. 1st edition. Philadelphia: Mosby/Elsevier; 2008. p. xvii, p. 1273.
74. Clegg A, Young JB. Which medications to avoid in people at risk of delirium: a systematic review. Age Ageing 2011;40(1):23–9.
75. Marcantonio ER, Juarez G, Goldman L, et al. The relationship of postoperative delirium with psychoactive medications. JAMA 1994;272(19):1518–22.
76. Adunsky A, Levy R, Heim M, et al. Meperidine analgesia and delirium in aged hip fracture patients. Arch Gerontol Geriatr 2002;35(3):253–9.
77. Pandharipande P, Shintani A, Peterson J, et al. Lorazepam is an independent risk factor for transitioning to delirium in intensive care unit patients. Anesthesiology 2006;104(1):21–6.
78. Dubois MJ, Bergeron N, Dumont M, et al. Delirium in an intensive care unit: a study of risk factors. Intensive Care Med 2001;27(8):1297–304.
79. Tune LE. Anticholinergic effects of medication in elderly patients. J Clin Psychiatry 2001;62(Suppl 21):11–4.
80. Caeiro L, Ferro JM, Claro MI, et al. Delirium in acute stroke: a preliminary study of the role of anticholinergic medications. Eur J Neurol 2004;11(10): 699–704.
81. Han L, McCusker J, Cole M, et al. Use of medications with anticholinergic effect predicts clinical severity of delirium symptoms in older medical inpatients. Arch Intern Med 2001;161(8):1099–105.
82. Agostini JV, Leo-Summers LS, Inouye SK. Cognitive and other adverse effects of diphenhydramine use in hospitalized older patients. Arch Intern Med 2001; 161(17):2091–7.
83. Luukkanen MJ, Uusvaara J, Laurila JV, et al. Anticholinergic drugs and their effects on delirium and mortality in the elderly. Dement Geriatr Cogn Dis Extra 2011;1(1):43–50.
84. Campbell N, Perkins A, Hui S, et al. Association between prescribing of anticholinergic medications and incident delirium: a cohort study. J Am Geriatr Soc 2011;59(Suppl 2):S277–81.
85. American Geriatrics Society 2012 Beers Criteria Update Expert Panel. American Geriatrics Society updated Beers Criteria for potentially inappropriate medication use in older adults. J Am Geriatr Soc 2012;60(4):616–31.
86. Alagiakrishnan K, Wiens CA. An approach to drug induced delirium in the elderly. Postgrad Med J 2004;80(945):388–93.
87. Teres D, Brown RB, Lemeshow S. Predicting mortality of intensive care unit patients. The importance of coma. Crit Care Med 1982;10(2):86–95.
88. Jennett B, Bond M. Assessment of outcome after severe brain damage. Lancet 1975;1(7905):480–4.
89. Levy DE, Caronna JJ, Singer BH, et al. Predicting outcome from hypoxic-ischemic coma. JAMA 1985;253(10):1420–6.
90. Tuhrim S, Dambrosia JM, Price TR, et al. Prediction of intracerebral hemorrhage survival. Ann Neurol 1988;24(2):258–63.
91. Booth CM, Boone RH, Tomlinson G, et al. Is this patient dead, vegetative, or severely neurologically impaired? Assessing outcome for comatose survivors of cardiac arrest. JAMA 2004;291(7):870–9.

92. Witlox J, Eurelings LS, de Jonghe JF, et al. Delirium in elderly patients and the risk of postdischarge mortality, institutionalization, and dementia: a meta-analysis. JAMA 2010;304(4):443–51.

93. Fong TG, Jones RN, Shi P, et al. Delirium accelerates cognitive decline in Alzheimer disease. Neurology 2009;72(18):1570–5.

94. Gross AL, Jones RN, Habtemariam DA, et al. Delirium and long-term cognitive trajectory among persons with dementia. Arch Intern Med 2012;172:1–8.

95. Inouye SK, Rushing JT, Foreman MD, et al. Does delirium contribute to poor hospital outcomes? A three-site epidemiologic study. J Gen Intern Med 1998; 13(4):234–42.

96. Leslie DL, Marcantonio ER, Zhang Y, et al. One-year health care costs associated with delirium in the elderly population. Arch Intern Med 2008; 168(1):27–32.

97. Gonzalez M, Martinez G, Calderon J, et al. Impact of delirium on short-term mortality in elderly inpatients: a prospective cohort study. Psychosomatics 2009;50(3):234–8.

98. Grover S, Shah R. Distress due to delirium experience. Gen Hosp Psychiatry 2011;33(6):637–9.

99. Bruera E, Bush SH, Willey J, et al. Impact of delirium and recall on the level of distress in patients with advanced cancer and their family caregivers. Cancer 2009;115(9):2004–12.

100. Han JH, Eden S, Shintani A, et al. Delirium in older emergency department patients is an independent predictor of hospital length of stay. Acad Emerg Med 2011;18(5):451–7.

101. O'Keeffe S, Lavan J. The prognostic significance of delirium in older hospital patients. J Am Geriatr Soc 1997;45(2):174–8.

102. McCusker J, Cole M, Abrahamowicz M, et al. Delirium predicts 12-month mortality. Arch Intern Med 2002;162(4):457–63.

103. Manos PJ, Wu R. The duration of delirium in medical and postoperative patients referred for psychiatric consultation. Ann Clin Psychiatry 1997;9(4):219–26.

104. Sirois F. Delirium: 100 cases. Can J Psychiatry 1988;33(5):375–8.

105. McCusker J, Cole M, Dendukuri N, et al. The course of delirium in older medical inpatients: a prospective study. J Gen Intern Med 2003;18(9):696–704.

106. Han JH, Shintani A, Eden S, et al. Delirium in the emergency department: an independent predictor of death within 6 months. Ann Emerg Med 2010;56(3): 244–52.

107. Vida S, Galbaud du Fort G, Kakuma R, et al. An 18-month prospective cohort study of functional outcome of delirium in elderly patients: activities of daily living. Int Psychogeriatr 2006;18(4):681–700.

108. Sanders AB. Missed delirium in older emergency department patients: a quality-of-care problem. Ann Emerg Med 2002;39(3):338–41.

109. Han JH, Bryce SN, Ely EW, et al. The effect of cognitive impairment on the accuracy of the presenting complaint and discharge instruction comprehension in older emergency department patients. Ann Emerg Med 2011;57(6): 662–71. e662.

110. Reeves RR, Parker JD, Burke RS, et al. Inappropriate psychiatric admission of elderly patients with unrecognized delirium. South Med J 2010;103(2):111–5.

111. Clarke C, Friedman SM, Shi K, et al. Emergency department discharge instructions comprehension and compliance study. CJEM 2005;7(1):5–11.

112. Teasdale G, Jennett B. Assessment of coma and impaired consciousness. A practical scale. Lancet 1974;2(7872):81–4.

113. Sacco RL, VanGool R, Mohr JP, et al. Nontraumatic coma. Glasgow Coma Score and coma etiology as predictors of 2-week outcome. Arch Neurol 1990;47(11): 1181–4.

114. Bastos PG, Sun X, Wagner DP, et al. Glasgow Coma Scale score in the evaluation of outcome in the intensive care unit: findings from the acute physiology and chronic health evaluation III study. Crit Care Med 1993;21(10):1459–65.

115. Gill MR, Reiley DG, Green SM. Interrater reliability of Glasgow Coma Scale scores in the emergency department. Ann Emerg Med 2004;43(2):215–23.

116. Wijdicks EF, Bamlet WR, Maramattom BV, et al. Validation of a new coma scale: the FOUR score. Ann Neurol 2005;58(4):585–93.

117. McNarry AF, Goldhill DR. Simple bedside assessment of level of consciousness: comparison of two simple assessment scales with the Glasgow Coma Scale. Anaesthesia 2004;59(1):34–7.

118. Terrell KM, Hustey FM, Hwang U, et al. Quality indicators for geriatric emergency care. Acad Emerg Med 2009;16(5):441–9.

119. Hogan TM, Losman ED, Carpenter CR, et al. Development of geriatric competencies for emergency medicine residents using an expert consensus process. Acad Emerg Med 2010;17(3):316–24.

120. Inouye SK, van Dyck CH, Alessi CA, et al. Clarifying confusion: the confusion assessment method. A new method for detection of delirium. Ann Intern Med 1990;113(12):941–8.

121. Wong CL, Holroyd-Leduc J, Simel DL, et al. Does this patient have delirium?: value of bedside instruments. JAMA 2010;304(7):779–86.

122. Carpenter CR, DesPain B, Keeling TN, et al. The Six-Item Screener and AD8 for the detection of cognitive impairment in geriatric emergency department patients. Ann Emerg Med 2011;57(6):653–61.

123. Blazer DG, van Nieuwenhuizen AO. Evidence for the diagnostic criteria of delirium: an update. Curr Opin Psychiatry 2012;25(3):239–43.

124. Inouye SK. Delirium in hospitalized older patients. Clin Geriatr Med 1998;14(4): 745–64.

125. Fabbri RM, Moreira MA, Garrido R, et al. Validity and reliability of the Portuguese version of the confusion assessment method (CAM) for the detection of delirium in the elderly. Arq Neuropsiquiatr 2001;59(2-A):175–9.

126. Inouye SK. The Confusion Assessment Method (CAM): training manual and coding guide. New Haven, CT: Yale University School of Medicine; 2009.

127. Young RS, Arseven A. Diagnosing delirium. JAMA 2010;304(19):2125–6 [author reply: 2126–7].

128. Wei LA, Fearing MA, Sternberg EJ, et al. The confusion assessment method: a systematic review of current usage. J Am Geriatr Soc 2008;56(5):823–30.

129. Lemiengre J, Nelis T, Joosten E, et al. Detection of delirium by bedside nurses using the confusion assessment method. J Am Geriatr Soc 2006;54(4):685–9.

130. Ely EW, Inouye SK, Bernard GR, et al. Delirium in mechanically ventilated patients: validity and reliability of the confusion assessment method for the intensive care unit (CAM-ICU). JAMA 2001;286(21):2703–10.

131. Neufeld KJ, Hayat MJ, Coughlin JM, et al. Evaluation of two intensive care delirium screening tools for non-critically ill hospitalized patients. Psychosomatics 2011;52(2):133–40.

132. Mitasova A, Kostalova M, Bednarik J, et al. Poststroke delirium incidence and outcomes: validation of the Confusion Assessment Method for the Intensive Care Unit (CAM-ICU). Crit Care Med 2012;40(2):484–90.

133. Kean J, Trzepacz PT, Murray LL, et al. Initial validation of a brief provisional diagnostic scale for delirium. Brain Inj 2010;24(10):1222–30.

134. Chester JG, Beth Harrington M, Rudolph JL. Serial administration of a modified Richmond Agitation and Sedation Scale for delirium screening. J Hosp Med 2011;7(5):450–3.

135. Zimitat C, Nixon PF. Glucose loading precipitates acute encephalopathy in thiamin-deficient rats. Metab Brain Dis 1999;14(1):1–20.

136. Mazer M, Deroos F, Hollander JE, et al. Medication history taking in emergency department triage is inaccurate and incomplete. Acad Emerg Med 2011;18(1):102–4.

137. Staroselsky M, Volk LA, Tsurikova R, et al. An effort to improve electronic health record medication list accuracy between visits: patients' and physicians' response. Int J Med Inf 2008;77(3):153–60.

138. Finlayson RE, Davis LJ Jr. Prescription drug dependence in the elderly population: demographic and clinical features of 100 inpatients. Mayo Clin Proc 1994;69(12):1137–45.

139. Blazer DG, Wu LT. The epidemiology of substance use and disorders among middle aged and elderly community adults: national survey on drug use and health. Am J Geriatr Psychiatry 2009;17(3):237–45.

140. Uguz F, Kayrak M, Cicek E, et al. Delirium following acute myocardial infarction: incidence, clinical profiles, and predictors. Perspect Psychiatr Care 2010;46(2):135–42.

141. Warshaw G, Tanzer F. The effectiveness of lumbar puncture in the evaluation of delirium and fever in the hospitalized elderly. Arch Fam Med 1993;2(3):293–7.

142. Metersky ML, Williams A, Rafanan AL. Retrospective analysis: are fever and altered mental status indications for lumbar puncture in a hospitalized patient who has not undergone neurosurgery? Clin Infect Dis 1997;25(2):285–8.

143. Moeller KE, Lee KC, Kissack JC. Urine drug screening: practical guide for clinicians. Mayo Clin Proc 2008;83(1):66–76.

144. Hardy JE, Brennan N. Computerized tomography of the brain for elderly patients presenting to the emergency department with acute confusion. Emerg Med Australas 2008;20(5):420–4.

145. Mesulam MM, Waxman SG, Geschwind N, et al. Acute confusional states with right middle cerebral artery infarctions. J Neurol Neurosurg Psychiatry 1976;39(1):84–9.

146. Ziai WC, Schlattman D, Llinas R, et al. Emergent EEG in the emergency department in patients with altered mental states. Clin Neurophysiol 2012;123(5):910–7.

147. Agarwal N, Naganananda MS, Rahman SM, et al. Portable cost-effective EEG data acquisition system. J Med Eng Technol 2011;35(3–4):185–90.

148. Inouye SK, Bogardus ST Jr, Charpentier PA, et al. A multicomponent intervention to prevent delirium in hospitalized older patients. N Engl J Med 1999;340(9):669–76.

149. Flaherty JH, Little MO. Matching the environment to patients with delirium: lessons learned from the delirium room, a restraint-free environment for older hospitalized adults with delirium. J Am Geriatr Soc 2011;59(Suppl 2):S295–300.

150. Holroyd-Leduc JM, Sen S, Bertenthal D, et al. The relationship of indwelling urinary catheters to death, length of hospital stay, functional decline, and nursing home admission in hospitalized older medical patients. J Am Geriatr Soc 2007;55(2):227–33.

151. National Institute of Heath and Clinical Excellence. Delirium: diagnosis, prevention, and management. (Clinical guideline 103). 2010. Available at: http://publications.nice.org.uk/delirium-cg103. Accessed June 21, 2012.

152. Breitbart W, Marotta R, Platt MM, et al. A double-blind trial of haloperidol, chlorpromazine, and lorazepam in the treatment of delirium in hospitalized AIDS patients. Am J Psychiatry 1996;153(2):231–7.
153. Flaherty JH, Gonzales JP, Dong B. Antipsychotics in the treatment of delirium in older hospitalized adults: a systematic review. J Am Geriatr Soc 2011;59: S269–76.
154. Lonergan E, Britton AM, Luxenberg J, et al. Antipsychotics for delirium. Cochrane Database Syst Rev 2007;(2):CD005594.
155. Hu H, Deng W, Yang H. A prospective random control study comparison of olanzapine and haloperidol in senile delirium. Chongqing Medical Journal 2004;8:1234–7.
156. Hassaballa HA, Balk RA. Torsade de pointes associated with the administration of intravenous haloperidol: a review of the literature and practical guidelines for use. Expert Opin Drug Saf 2003;2(6):543–7.
157. Ozbolt LB, Paniagua MA, Kaiser RM. Atypical antipsychotics for the treatment of delirious elders. J Am Med Dir Assoc 2008;9(1):18–28.
158. Breitbart W, Tremblay A, Gibson C. An open trial of olanzapine for the treatment of delirium in hospitalized cancer patients. Psychosomatics 2002;43(3):175–82.
159. Tahir TA, Eeles E, Karapareddy V, et al. A randomized controlled trial of quetiapine versus placebo in the treatment of delirium. J Psychosom Res 2010;69(5): 485–90.
160. Ballard C, Kahn Z, Corbett A. Treatment of dementia with Lewy bodies and Parkinson's disease dementia. Drugs Aging 2011;28(10):769–77.
161. Komossa K, Rummel-Kluge C, Schmid F, et al. Quetiapine versus other atypical antipsychotics for schizophrenia. Cochrane Database Syst Rev 2010;(1): CD006625.
162. Mayo-Smith MF, Beecher LH, Fischer TL, et al. Management of alcohol withdrawal delirium. An evidence-based practice guideline. Arch Intern Med 2004;164(13):1405–12.
163. Tollefson GD, Montague-Clouse J, Lancaster SP. The relationship of serum anticholinergic activity to mental status performance in an elderly nursing home population. J Neuropsychiatry Clin Neurosci 1991;3(3):314–9.
164. Catalano G, Catalano MC, Alberts VA. Famotidine-associated delirium. A series of six cases. Psychosomatics 1996;37(4):349–55.
165. Naughton BJ, Saltzman S, Ramadan F, et al. A multifactorial intervention to reduce prevalence of delirium and shorten hospital length of stay. J Am Geriatr Soc 2005;53(1):18–23.
166. Flaherty JH, Steele DK, Chibnall JT, et al. An ACE unit with a delirium room may improve function and equalize length of stay among older delirious medical inpatients. J Gerontol A Biol Sci Med Sci 2010;65(12):1387–92.
167. Lundstrom M, Edlund A, Karlsson S, et al. A multifactorial intervention program reduces the duration of delirium, length of hospitalization, and mortality in delirious patients. J Am Geriatr Soc 2005;53(4):622–8.
168. Milisen K, Lemiengre J, Braes T, et al. Multicomponent intervention strategies for managing delirium in hospitalized older people: systematic review. J Adv Nurs 2005;52(1):79–90.
169. Pitkala KH, Laurila JV, Strandberg TE, et al. Multicomponent geriatric intervention for elderly inpatients with delirium: effects on costs and health-related quality of life. J Gerontol A Biol Sci Med Sci 2008;63(1):56–61.
170. Pitkala KH, Laurila JV, Strandberg TE, et al. Multicomponent geriatric intervention for elderly inpatients with delirium: a randomized, controlled trial. J Gerontol A Biol Sci Med Sci 2006;61(2):176–81.

171. Vasilevskis EE, Morandi A, Boehm L, et al. Delirium and sedation recognition using validated instruments: reliability of bedside intensive care unit nursing assessments from 2007 to 2010. J Am Geriatr Soc 2011;59(Suppl 2):S249–55.
172. O'Keeffe ST, Mulkerrin EC, Nayeem K, et al. Use of serial mini-mental state examinations to diagnose and monitor delirium in elderly hospital patients. J Am Geriatr Soc 2005;53(5):867–70.
173. Wilber ST, Carpenter CR, Hustey FM. The six-item screener to detect cognitive impairment in older emergency department patients. Acad Emerg Med 2008; 15(7):613–6.
174. Wilber ST, Lofgren SD, Mager TG, et al. An evaluation of two screening tools for cognitive impairment in older emergency department patients. Acad Emerg Med 2005;12(7):612–6.
175. Carpenter CR, Bassett ER, Fischer GM, et al. Four sensitive screening tools to detect cognitive dysfunction in geriatric emergency department patients: brief Alzheimer's screen, short Blessed test, Ottawa 3DY, and the caregiver-completed AD8. Acad Emerg Med 2011;18(4):374–84.
176. Available at: http://www.americandeliriumsociety.org/About_ADS.html. Accessed September 10, 2012.

Trauma in the Older Adult
Epidemiology and Evolving Geriatric Trauma Principles

Stephanie Bonne, MD, Douglas J.E. Schuerer, MD*

KEYWORDS

- Geriatric • Trauma • Fractures • Falls

KEY POINTS

- From the initial time of injury, the overall experience of an elderly person who sustains a traumatic injury can be very different from that of a younger patient with trauma, and special consideration should be made to properly triage and treat the geriatric patient with trauma.
- Once a traumatic event occurs, there are several comorbidities that complicate recovery from the trauma. Greater than 50% of the geriatric trauma population has underlying hypertension, and greater than 30% have heart disease.
- The widespread use of medications and polypharmacy adds to the challenge of evaluating and treating the elderly patient with trauma. Older patients may be using medications, such as β-blockers, that will mask abnormal vital signs, or may have pacemakers in place, which can further confound the primary survey.

There is little debate that the world's population continues to age,[1,2] and as such there are increasing numbers of older patients presenting with traumatic injuries than in the past. The current population of both the United States and the developed world is aging, creating a new subset of patients with trauma, the geriatric patient with trauma. If we are to study this population, we must quantitatively define it. In the case of trauma, recent data suggest that mortality as adjusted for injury severity scale (ISS) increases at the age of 70 years, defining the population older than 70 as distinct from those younger than 70 years, and making the age of 70 the cutoff at which to consider a patient with trauma elderly or geriatric.[3] This notion is distinct from Advanced Trauma Life Support (ATLS) teaching, which recommends transport to a trauma center of any patient older than 55 years, or the Eastern Association for the Surgery of Trauma (EAST) guidelines, which recommend considering any patient

Washington University in St Louis, 660 South Euclid Avenue, Campus Box 8109, St Louis, MO 63110, USA
* Corresponding author.
E-mail address: schuererd@wudosis.wustl.edu

Clin Geriatr Med 29 (2013) 137–150
http://dx.doi.org/10.1016/j.cger.2012.10.008
0749-0690/13/$ – see front matter © 2013 Elsevier Inc. All rights reserved.
geriatric.theclinics.com

older than 65 years as elderly.[4,5] Although there is no consensus on an age cutoff for a patient with trauma to be considered elderly, the age of 65 is most often used when considering a patient "elderly" or "geriatric" in the trauma literature. It is well recognized that the geriatric trauma population requires special consideration with regard to diagnosis and treatment, and it is important for the trauma clinician to be aware of the special needs of these patients.

EPIDEMIOLOGY

By 2050, it is expected that there will be nearly 90 million adults older than 65 years living in the United States, representing more than one-fifth of the population.[6] In addition to the increase in the volume of the geriatric population, one can expect more injuries to occur in this population as they continue to live more independent and active lifestyles. At present, patients older than 65 years account for 23% of all trauma admissions, and trauma represents the fifth leading cause of death in this population.[7,8] Because of the high prevalence of multiple comorbidities in the elderly, there is an increased likelihood of death or severe disability following trauma.[8] Up to one-third of all patients presenting with an ISS greater than 15 can be expected to die before leaving the hospital.[9] In addition, the economic costs, as well as the societal cost and loss of life, are higher following trauma to an elderly patient. Falls are the leading cause of trauma in the elderly. There is approximately a one-third risk of fall for geriatric adults each year.[10] With an average hospital cost of $18,000 (United States, 2012) per fall, and further costs associated with long-term nursing care following trauma, the economic implication of all trauma, but specifically of standing level falls, to the elderly is astonishing.[11,12] Looking forward, the social and economic implications of the expected increase in geriatric trauma cannot be overlooked, and clinicians must continue to strive toward a more standardized and evidence-based approach to the diagnosis and treatment of these patients.

MECHANISMS OF GERIATRIC TRAUMA

Several factors place the geriatric population at particular risk for traumatic events, and for subsequent delayed recovery from trauma. Conditions that predispose patients to incurring trauma are seen in higher prevalence in the older population. Weakness or generalized deconditioning resulting from chronic illnesses can lead to an increased rate of falls or other accidents in these patients. Loss of visual acuity, balance and gait instability, slowed reaction times, and cognitive impairments are also important disabilities that may lead to an increased incidence of traumatic events in the elderly. Often these issues are not recognized before trauma, and cognitive dysfunction can be seen up to 35% of the time in the geriatric visitor to the emergency department, but is only recognized 6% of the time.[13] Trauma itself is also an increased risk factor for future traumas, with elderly patients who have sustained trauma in the past being 3 times more likely to have a future traumatic event.[14] Because this particular constellation of problems is seen in the elderly, prevention of geriatric trauma should be addressed by all clinicians caring for a geriatric patient. Trauma prevention in patients who are at high risk because of the aforementioned disabilities should be addressed by the geriatric primary care physician (**Fig. 1**).

The mechanisms of trauma are not unique to this particular population, but because geriatric trauma presents at such a higher rate than in the younger population, they can be considered to be different mechanisms than those observed younger patients with trauma. Unlike their younger counterparts, elderly patients with trauma usually sustain blunt trauma rather than penetrating trauma. Falls

%

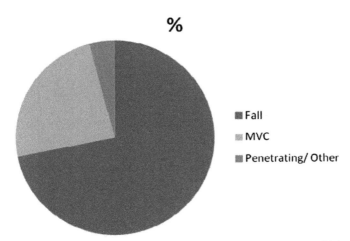

■ Fall

▒ MVC

■ Penetrating/ Other

Fig. 1. Pie chart of injury mechanism in the elderly patient. MVC, motor vehicle accident.

account for nearly three-quarters of all traumas in the geriatric population, with motor vehicle accidents accounting for nearly all of the remaining 25% of injuries. Penetrating trauma and other mechanisms make up only 4% of total trauma in the geriatric population.[9] Among the elderly patients who fall, nearly 90% experience simple falls, such as falls from standing. Despite being simple mechanisms, the multiple comorbidities in the elderly population, along with the need for rehabilitation, make falls a significant medical and economic event in the life of these patients.[15] Falls associated with blunt cerebral injury and long bone fractures lead to the greatest morbidity and mortality.[7,8] About one-quarter of all elderly victims of motor vehicle accidents sustain chest trauma, such as flail chest and rib fractures, which can complicate preexisting cardiopulmonary disease and lead to pneumonia or respiratory failure, complications which are known to have particularly high morbidity and mortality.[16] Car accidents also cause mortality at almost double the rate for the elderly as for their younger counterparts when adjusted for injury severity.[16] Finally, although penetrating trauma remains rare in the elderly population, it is associated with higher morbidity, longer stays in the intensive care unit (ICU), and longer overall hospital stays when compared with younger patients.[17] When caring for a geriatric patient with trauma after a fall or motor vehicle accident, it is important to be aware of the most likely injuries and injury patterns, reviewed herein. These injury patterns may vary from those seen to arise from the same mechanism in a younger patient, so it is important to be aware of the particular injury patterns seen in the elderly so that occult injuries are not missed.

TRIAGE AND EVALUATION OF THE GERIATRIC PATIENT WITH TRAUMA

From the initial time of injury, the overall experience of an elderly person who sustains a traumatic injury can be very different from that of a younger patient with trauma, and special consideration should be given to proper triage and treatment of the geriatric patient with trauma. Nursing homes or assisted care facilities, where elderly patients often reside, are a unique location, where health care workers are available and may attempt to treat a traumatic event on site. However, this can actually delay the trauma evaluation of a patient who might otherwise be taken to an emergency department sooner if they reside in the community. Likewise, families or other laypersons may underestimate the severity of a traumatic event to their elderly family member, because the mechanism may seem trivial or their loved one may not initially show signs and symptoms of having a major underlying injury. Once the emergency medical services (EMS) system is activated, it is critical for the emergency responder to appropriately evaluate and triage the patient. For nearly 20 years it has been recognized that elderly patients are consistently undertriaged to major trauma centers, possibly because emergency responders do not recognize potential major injuries or are not fully aware of all the potential comorbidities in the elderly patient, or because of potential age bias on the part of the responders.[18,19] Undertriage is particularly troublesome because trauma outcomes with regard to both morbidity and mortality have been shown to be improved when the geriatric patient is taken immediately to a high-level trauma center.[20] In addition to undertriage, it has been shown that geriatric patients who are transferred to a trauma center but do not meet trauma activation criteria on initial evaluation, will often have occult injuries, or their comorbid conditions will act in synergy with their traumatic event to lead to higher morbidities for that particular injury.[21,22] When adjusted for injury severity, geriatric patients have consistently higher levels of morbidity and mortality across all levels of injury.[23] This fact has led many trauma surgeons to advocate for age alone to be a criterion for activation of the trauma system and transfer to a Level 1 trauma center, although the age that should be the threshold for such activation is debated.[21,23] Level 1 trauma centers can be identified at www.traumamaps.org. Current guidelines suggest that age alone, in the absence of any diagnosable injury, is insufficient for activation of the trauma team; however, the threshold for activation should be lower in patients who show hemodynamic instability or any potentially life-threatening injuries, such as severe fractures, abdominal trauma, or chest trauma.[3] In addition to improved outcomes from immediate evaluation at a higher-level trauma center, geriatric patients may also benefit from a dedicated geriatric trauma service, which may be increasingly found at higher-level trauma centers or academic centers (**Fig. 2**).[24]

Once an elderly patient arrives at a trauma center, the staff must be careful to evaluate the geriatric patient as is appropriate for their advancing age. Vital signs and physical examination can be deceptive in these patients, who may exhibit examination characteristics very different from those of younger patients. Although the ATLS protocol should be followed for geriatric patients just as it is for younger patients, there are some differences in the normal physiology of elderly patients that will make their evaluation and treatment more challenging. Even among patients who are not taking

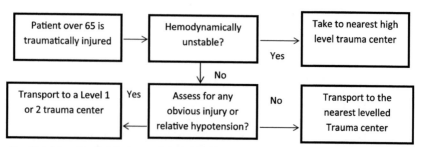

Fig. 2. Algorithm for field triage of the elderly patient with trauma. Current triage guidelines suggest transfer to a trauma center provides optimal care. Those with obvious injury or relative hypotension (low normal blood pressure but very low for patients with preexisting hypertension) should be triaged to a higher-level trauma center, depending on state regulations.

confounding medications, vital signs can be falsely reassuring. Increased mortality has been shown among elderly patients with heart rates greater than 90 beats/min and systolic blood pressure less than 110 mm Hg, whereas the same increase in mortality is not seen until 130 beats/min and 95 mm Hg in younger patients.[25] Elderly patients also subjectively report less pain for the same severity of injury than do their younger counterparts, potentially masking injuries or falsely reassuring staff that an injury is less severe than it actually is.[26] Mental status examinations and Glasgow Coma Scale (GCS) scoring can be particularly difficult in the geriatric patient, who may have preexisting cognitive deficits, hearing impairment, or other factors that can confound these examinations.[27] Clinical neurologic examination has also been shown to be unreliable in detecting significant hemorrhage in patients with minor head trauma.[28] The difficulty in using normal clinical judgment and assessment in elderly patients has led many emergency medicine and trauma surgeons to advocate for a low threshold of reliability in ancillary studies on the geriatric patient with trauma.[27]

COMORBIDITIES IN GERIATRIC TRAUMA

Once a traumatic event occurs, several comorbidities complicate recovery from the trauma. Greater than 50% of the geriatric trauma population has underlying hypertension, and greater than 30% has heart disease.[7] Other conditions that can complicate evaluation and management of the patient with trauma include diabetes, previous cerebrovascular events, chronic obstructive pulmonary disease (COPD), dementia, arrhythmias, and endocrine disorders; all of which are present in greater than 10% of the geriatric trauma population.[7] Other common diseases in the elderly, such as community-acquired infections, cancers, and chronic renal failure, also lead to increased risk of poor outcomes following trauma.[9,29] The comorbid conditions that confer the highest risk of mortality in the geriatric population are hepatic disease, renal insufficiency, and cancer.[30] The presence of congestive heart failure, particularly in patients who take β-blockers or are anticoagulated, can confer a 5- to 10-fold increased risk of death following trauma.[31] Because the geriatric population is generally less healthy at baseline, they are at increased risk of certain types of trauma and at increased risk of in-hospital complications once a trauma has occurred. Comorbid conditions, therefore, become a major factor in the evaluation and treatment of the elderly patient with trauma. Closely related to this are the medications a patient with trauma may be taking for the aforementioned comorbidities.

The widespread use of medications and polypharmacy adds to the challenge of evaluating and treating the elderly patient with trauma. Older patients may be using medications, such as β-blockers, that will mask abnormal vital signs, or may have pacemakers in place, which can further confound the primary survey. Preinjury β-blocker use does confer an increased risk of mortality, particularly when confounded with warfarin or other cardiac medications.[27] This risk may be due to under-recognition of tachycardia owing to β-blocker use, conferring a falsely reassuring clinical picture. In the secondary survey, geriatric patients may bleed more rapidly from seemingly minor wounds because of widespread use of anticoagulants and anti-platelet agents. Because falls and head trauma comprise such a large percentage of total trauma in the elderly, anticoagulation becomes a significant problem that the emergency or trauma clinician can expect to encounter often.

In addition to cardiac medications and anticoagulation, other medications can confound the treatment of trauma. Steroids, often prescribed for COPD in the elderly, can cause reduced wound healing or can lead to clinical adrenal insufficiency in the critically ill patient, and have been shown independently to lead to a 1.6- to 5-fold increased incidence of death in the geriatric trauma population.[26] Antipsychotics may render neurologic examinations unreliable, and antidopaminergic agents used for Parkinson disease may change the neurologic examination of the extremities. Eye drops or systemic medications taken for glaucoma may alter the pupillary examination, as may corneal or other eye implants. It is crucial to document the pupillary examination on arrival, and document any ophthalmologic history to avoid confusion among care providers during the patient's hospitalization. In addition to taking into account the patient's home medications when evaluating the patient, it is important to consider which home medications are necessary to continue during the stay in hospital. Patients may exhibit adverse effects to the sudden discontinuation of antidepressants, antipsychotic agents, and in particular to antidopaminergic agents. In short, the polypharmacy seen more often in the elderly must be carefully considered, from the point of initial evaluation through the entire treatment course of the geriatric patient, so as not to miss occult injuries or to cause additional clinical problems by discontinuing a chronic medication (**Table 1**).

PATTERNS OF INJURY AND SPECIFIC INJURIES

In addition to global considerations of geriatric patients, there are special considerations for each injury. In the case of head-injured patients, there is a linear relationship

Table 1
Physiologic and functional preexisting differences in the older adult

Organ System	Normal	Potential Differences in the Older Patient
Vital signs	Increased mortality if HR >130 beats/min or SBP <95 mm Hg	Increased mortality if HR >90 beats/min or SBP <110 mm Hg
Neurologic	No baseline deficits	Baseline deficits (dementia, stroke, hearing loss) Report less pain for equivalent injuries, potentially limiting injury discovery
Cardiovascular	No baseline deficits, no hypertension No cardiac medications	Baseline hypertension Medications that affect blood pressure and heart rate (β-blocker, calcium-channel blocker, amiodarone) History of heart failure
Pulmonary	Normal functional residual capacity Potential smoker	Decreased functional residual capacity Chronic obstructive pulmonary disease
Renal	Normal renal function	Decreased glomerular filtration rate
Coagulation	Normal coagulation status	On blood-thinning medications including ASA, warfarin, and platelet inhibitors
Skeletal	Normal bone density	Osteoporosis, leading to easier fracture rate
Medications	Minimal medications	Polypharmacy that can change mental, hemodynamic, renal, and coagulation status

Abbreviations: ASA, acetylsalicylic acid; HR, heart rate; SBP, systolic blood pressure.

between age and mortality following head injury, such that even within the population older than 65 there is increased risk of death with increasing age.[32] Among those patients who do not die from their head trauma, poor outcomes are common and also increase with increasing age.[33] These patients may present with a very mild mechanism for head injury or may have few hard neurologic signs, such as neurologic deficits, weakness, or altered mental status, on initial evaluation, but may still have very significant underlying subdural or epidural hematomas.[34] The widespread use of anticoagulation in the elderly population has led to a large body of literature evaluating the effects of anticoagulation on the patient with trauma. Some studies have shown an increased risk of mortality with warfarin use in all patients with trauma, whereas other students show that in the absence of head trauma, warfarin use does not lead to increased mortality in the patient with trauma.[31,35] However, if the elderly patient with head trauma is taking warfarin, there is a significantly increased risk of fatal intracranial hemorrhage.[31] Patients who are anticoagulated on arrival, particularly those with head trauma, should be rapidly corrected, and there should be a low threshold to repeat brain imaging with any clinical neurologic change.[36] The GCS is an unreliable clinical tool in this scenario, and rapid and repeated use of computed tomography (CT) of the head becomes the essential means of identifying increased intracranial pressure in this scenario.[37] In the case where medical history is unavailable or unreliable, there should be a low threshold for the use of head CT in the elderly population, because of both the high prevalence of occult injuries and the rising prevalence of anticoagulant use.[34] Common rules such as the NEXUS-II specifically rule out patients older than 65 when determining who does not need a CT.[38] Even with use of intracranial pressure (ICP) monitoring and careful pharmacologic management of ICP, elderly patients have poorer autoregulatory mechanisms, which subsequently lead to a 30% decrease in the Glasgow Outcome Score after head injury in comparison with their younger counterparts.[39]

In the case of cervical spine injuries, elderly patients have mechanisms and risks for spine injury similar to those of their younger counterparts; however, the prevalence of cervical stenosis or degenerative spine disease is more common in this population. Also, there is little need to consider future cancer risk from radiation in the elderly patient. Common predictors of cervical spine injury include focal neurologic deficits, concomitant head injury, and high energy mechanism. Although similar predictors are seen in the younger population, the older population requires its own risk stratification to guide clinicians to suspect cervical spine fractures, because an apparently lesser injury can be so much more devastating in the older population.[40] One can expect a lower energy mechanism, such as a fall from standing, to cause greater injury to an elderly patient, because of the higher likelihood that the patient has preexisting degenerative spine disease or cervical stenosis. Also, because the elderly patient is most likely a victim of blunt trauma, most will require cervical spine evaluation. Early spine evaluation, a low threshold for involvement of a spine service, and the careful use of cervical spine immobilization are all essential in ensuring that a low energy mechanism does not become a devastating neurologic injury.

Thoracic trauma in the elderly is most likely to be blunt, and most likely to be from a motor vehicle accident. Fractures that might seem clinically insignificant in a younger patient, such as isolated rib fractures or clavicle fractures, may represent significant force and be associated with significantly higher morbidity in elderly patients.[8] Rib fractures in the elderly can be particularly worrisome, because of the increased morbidity and mortality associated with as few as 3 or fewer nondisplaced rib fractures. In addition, the increase in number of rib fractures increases the rate of complications.[41] Elderly patients are likely to develop pulmonary contusions or pneumonia from rib fractures, even isolated rib fractures.[42] Pneumonia following a rib fracture can be a devastating complication for an elderly patient who, at baseline, does not have the pulmonary reserve and ability to generate a forceful cough that a younger patient may have. It is essential to aggressively manage rib fractures in elderly patients, including, when indicated, epidural anesthesia and rib fixation. Pain control will help with pulmonary toilet and use of incentive spirometry (IS). Admission should be strongly considered if more than 2 rib fractures and/or IS use is found to be poor despite analgesia.

Abdominal trauma in the geriatric patient does not differ significantly from abdominal trauma in the younger patient. The same mechanisms and grades of solid organ injury apply to the older adult. Early experience with operative management for blunt abdominal trauma in the geriatric population showed poor outcomes; however, more recent studies have shown that operative management is possible and, in fact, preferable to nonoperative management based on age criteria alone, likely attributable in part to improved perioperative care and improved surgical optimization.[43,44] In fact, a patient older than 55 years will be more likely than their younger counterparts to fail nonoperative management of blunt splenic trauma.[45] Of course, in cases of penetrating abdominal trauma or bowel injury, operative exploration must be performed regardless of age criteria.

Much like the other injuries discussed, pelvic fractures in the elderly have a higher incidence of complications and mortality than in the younger population. The injury pattern of pelvic fractures in the geriatric population tends to be different to that in the younger population, specifically with a higher incidence of lateral compression fractures.[46] These fractures are more likely to cause hemorrhage that requires intervention, such as angiography.[47] The trauma surgeon should be aware that the elderly patient with a pelvic fracture may have pelvic bleeding that often otherwise goes unrecognized both clinically and radiographically on simple radiographic or CT examinations.[48] In addition, older age and concomitant long bone fracture, often seen in the elderly, impart a higher likelihood of finding occult bleeding with angiography.[49] Some investigators therefore advocate the liberal use of angiography in the geriatric population, regardless of hemodynamic stability, because of the very high incidence of occult bleeding.

The treatment of extremity orthopedic injuries among the elderly does not vary significantly from treatment of the younger population. The evaluation of concomitant neurovascular injury and the treatments of surgery, splinting, and reduction are largely the same as for the younger population. The exception is the long bone femur fracture, or hip fracture. This fracture was formerly considered a fatal event for the elderly osteoporotic patient, but with advances in pinning and plating, this is no longer true. The incidence of this injury remains high, however, as more women live well past menopause and experience osteoporosis, among other risk factors.[50] Low bone density imparts an increased risk for all types of long bone fractures, but particularly for hip fractures. It is also important to consider the surgical risk of a patient in whom operative fixation may be indicated. Should the elderly patient have multiple surgical risk factors, it may be more prudent for the orthopedic surgeon to simply splint or cast a fracture rather than expose the patient to the risk of anesthesia. This approach needs to be carefully considered in juxtaposition to the patient's functional goals and outcomes, and the potential risks of deep vein thrombosis or occupational deconditioning if the patient is unable to use the extremity for a period of time. Although orthopedic management may not be drastically different for the elderly patient with trauma, careful medical management must be considered for the geriatric patient (**Fig. 3**).

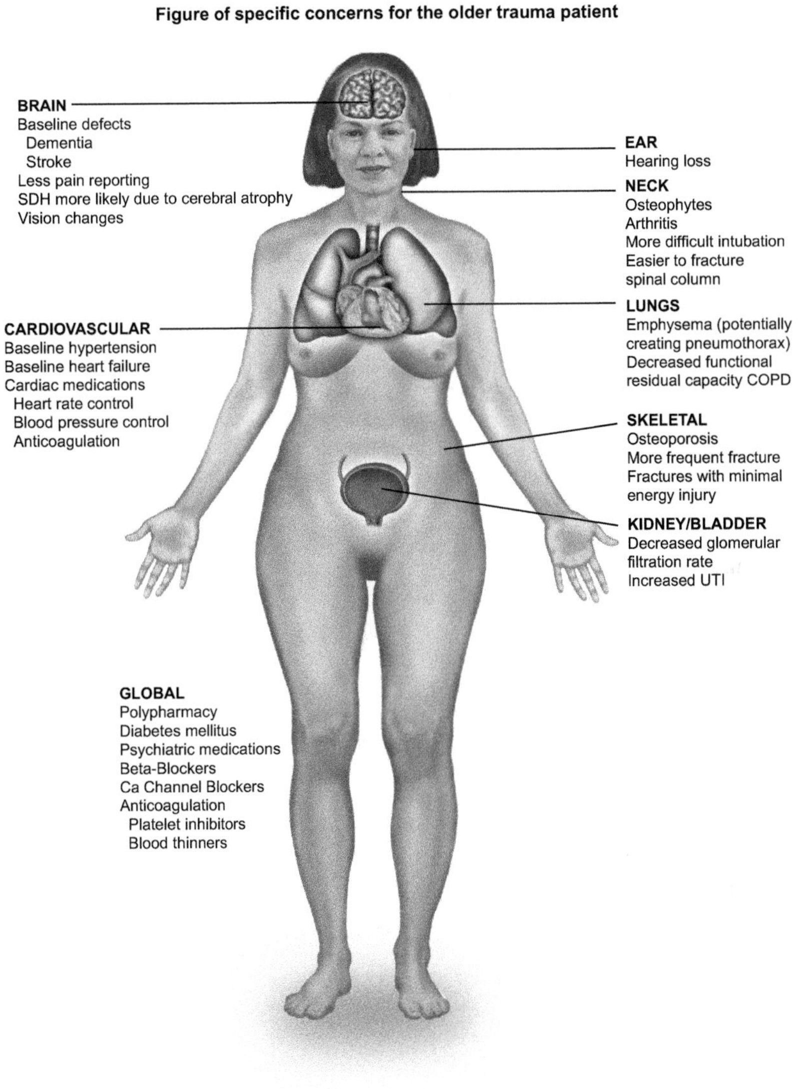

Figure of specific concerns for the older trauma patient

BRAIN
Baseline defects
  Dementia
  Stroke
Less pain reporting
SDH more likely due to cerebral atrophy
Vision changes

EAR
Hearing loss

NECK
Osteophytes
Arthritis
More difficult intubation
Easier to fracture
spinal column

LUNGS
Emphysema (potentially
creating pneumothorax)
Decreased functional
residual capacity COPD

CARDIOVASCULAR
Baseline hypertension
Baseline heart failure
Cardiac medications
  Heart rate control
  Blood pressure control
  Anticoagulation

SKELETAL
Osteoporosis
More frequent fracture
Fractures with minimal
energy injury

KIDNEY/BLADDER
Decreased glomerular
filtration rate
Increased UTI

GLOBAL
Polypharmacy
Diabetes mellitus
Psychiatric medications
Beta-Blockers
Ca Channel Blockers
Anticoagulation
  Platelet inhibitors
  Blood thinners

Fig. 3. Specific concerns for the older trauma patient.

INTENSIVE CARE MANAGEMENT OF GERIATRIC PATIENTS WITH TRAUMA

Once a patient's management course has been set, or their injuries have been definitively managed, the patient may require a course of treatment in the ICU. Intensive care medicine for the elderly patient, and specifically the elderly patient with trauma, differs from that for younger patients. Patients older than 65 years have a significantly greater mortality rate when matched for injury severity and comorbidities. This situation actually leads to decreased use of ICU resources, as many elderly patients will die before reaching the ICU and thus use little or no ICU resources.[51] Once resuscitation has begun, it is clear that the geriatric population has less physiologic reserve and therefore requires more rapid, yet judicious, treatment.[52] In addition, patients who are stable on initial evaluation will often have measureable hemodynamic compromise when invasive monitoring has been performed.[53] This occult hemodynamic compromise can present a unique challenge to the clinician who does not retain a high index of suspicion. Renal function in the elderly patient will differ from that in the younger patient owing to decreased renal blood flow and declining renal mass, therefore urine output alone is a poor clinical indicator of resuscitation. Creatinine clearance also becomes a much more important marker of renal function because creatinine alone can be deceptive in the elderly patient with lower muscle mass.[54] Although there has been insufficient evidence to suggest the routine use of pulmonary artery catheters in this population, the judicious use of invasive monitoring is warranted in the patient with an unclear clinical picture. Newer studies have shown a benefit to elderly patients who receive pulmonary artery catheter monitoring, and this monitoring has been shown to be low risk.[55,56] Even though there are no specific end points for resuscitation in these patients, the optimization of cardiac index and the use of base deficit as a measure of the status of resuscitation may be useful to the clinician.[57] It remains the clinician's choice to place an invasive line in a patient who is thought to warrant one; however, it can be beneficial in guiding the resuscitation of the older patient with trauma.

In addition to the hemodynamic changes seen in the elderly, the pulmonary mechanics of the elderly individual vary significantly from those of younger patients, leading to challenges in ventilator management in the older population. Elderly patients with trauma have a distinct increase in the vulnerability to pulmonary complications after trauma, owing to the decrease in their pulmonary reserve.[58] The ability of a nonventilated older patient to compensate for metabolic disturbances is decreased, which may cloud the clinical picture for the clinician because the patient may have a normal respiratory rate while becoming progressively hypoxic and hypercarbic.[59] In addition, when matched for injury severity, elderly patients are more likely to develop nosocomial infections, such as pneumonia, which in turn lead to longer length of stay in the ICU and hospital, and a higher mortality.[60] To reduce these complications, early and aggressive treatment of injuries, pulmonary toilet, pain control, and early mobilization must be implemented to give such fragile patients the best opportunity for a good outcome.

It is known that elderly patients have a higher morbidity and mortality following trauma than younger patients, which may lead to different recommendations regarding continuing care and withdrawal of care by clinicians. Elderly patients may not have the reserve to survive a long hospitalization following trauma, nor may they be able to participate in intensive rehabilitation following neurologic or orthopedic injuries. These patients may be intubated, sedated, confused, or delirious following their injuries, and therefore may be unable to participate in conversations regarding their goals of care. The discussion a clinician has with the patient's family must therefore take into consideration the increased length of stay, increased complications, and long recovery time associated with an elderly patient following trauma.[61] Because the majority of these patients will survive their injuries, a frank discussion of rehabilitation expectations, disposition, and other outcomes besides mortality is key to patient and family understanding of the severity of injury.[62]

THE TRAUMA TEAM FOR GERIATRIC PATIENTS

The unique difficulties of caring for the patient with trauma have led to the development of trauma teams for geriatric patients at many institutions. While still awaiting good data, the concept is to treat this population as a distinct specialty. In the past such patients may have end up with the orthopedic, medicine, or trauma service.

Although each specialty does its part well, often it may not as accurately address the other medical issues. For instance, the medical practitioner will likely address the cardiac problems, but may not as aggressively treat a few rib fractures. In such a situation the patient would benefit from a traumatologist as well.

To improve on the old system, a trauma team for geriatric patients should be staffed with interested individuals from each of the disciplines, along with mid-level providers to bring the consistency needed in treating these individuals. Protocols to address well-proven strategies should be written, created, and followed. Early involvement with anesthesia and prevetted anesthesia workups should take place, limiting delays to the operating room for unnecessarily thorough medical clearance. These teams should be led by geriatric traumatologists, who have experience in leading a multidisciplinary team, and should include orthopedic surgeons and neurosurgeons, geriatricians, dedicated therapists, social workers, dieticians, and others, all experienced in treating and appropriately dispositioning such patients. While an inpatient, home health could also perform evaluation of fall hazards to help prevent future injuries. In short, the team approach used in the ICU should be used to improve patient outcomes.

OUTCOMES IN GERIATRIC TRAUMA

As geriatric patients are studied, improvement in care of their trauma can be expected. Although geriatric patients have a higher mortality owing to multiple factors already discussed, the patients who do survive will eventually achieve some level of functional outcome following trauma. Their comorbidities, while playing a role in their survival and recovery, do not appear to affect their overall outcome.[63] For example, although geriatric brain-injured patients have a longer recovery time and require more inpatient care, they will generally improve in functional status and eventually reach the same rehabilitation goals as their younger counterparts.[64] These results, however, are age dependent, with geriatric patients older than 80 years having poorer functional outcomes than those aged 65 to 80.[65] There are also promising results regarding long-term survival following trauma, with long-term survival of several years after trauma for geriatric patients who are discharged from hospital.[66] Such lead data should inspire optimism in the clinician caring for the geriatric patient with trauma, who can be confident that in most patients, survival and functional outcomes will be good should the patient survive hospitalization. The effort spent, therefore, in caring for and rehabilitating the older patient with trauma is not in vain, and provides good quality of life and longer quality time for these patients.

Future research that will likely yield improvement for the elderly patient must focus on early recognition of instability and on falls, which make up approximately 75% of trauma in elderly patients. Efforts in early recognition have included triaging the elderly to trauma centers, but proof that this prospectively improves survival is not yet available. Also, research that helps EMS recognition of relative hypotension, and thus triages the patient appropriately, may improve survival. However, research that works toward reducing the incidence of falls, especially recurrent falls, and determining risk of falls of this population, will begin to address the single largest reason for injury in this population.

In conclusion, elderly patients with trauma must be triaged, evaluated, and treated differently to their younger counterparts. We must learn, as we did with children, that older adults have unique physiologic and structural differences that leave them at an increased risk of mortality from even minor trauma. Early recognition of these differences can lead to a better mortality rate and a more productive recovery after trauma.

REFERENCES

1. O'Neill S, Brady RR, Kerssens JJ, et al. Mortality associated with traumatic injuries in the elderly: a population based study. Arch Gerontol Geriatr 2012;54(3):e426–30.
2. Lustenberger T, Talving P, Schnüriger B, et al. Impact of advanced age on outcomes following damage control interventions for trauma. World J Surg 2012; 36(1):208–15.
3. Caterino JM, Valasek T, Werman HA. Identification of an age cutoff for increased mortality in patients with elderly trauma. Am J Emerg Med 2010;28:151–8.
4. American College of Surgeons Committee on Trauma. Geriatric trauma. In: ATLS: student course manual. 8th edition. Chicago: ACLS; 2008. p. 247–57.
5. The Eastern Association for the Surgery of Trauma. Geriatric trauma (update). Available at: http://www.east.org/resources/treatment-guidelines/geriatric-trauma-(update). Accessed July 20, 2012.
6. The Department of Health and Human Services, Administration on Ageing. Projected future growth of the older population. Available at: http://www.aoa.gov/aoaroot/aging_statistics/future_growth/future_growth.aspx#age. Accessed July 20, 2012.
7. Thompson HJ, McCormick WC, Kagan SH. Traumatic brain injury in older adults: epidemiology, outcomes, and future implications. J Am Geriatr Soc 2006;54:1590–5.
8. Keller JM, Sciadini MF, Sincalir E, et al. Geriatric trauma: demographics, injuries and mortality. J Orthop Trauma 2012;26(9):e161–5.
9. Labib N, Nouh T, Winocour S, et al. Severely injured geriatric population: morbidity, mortality and risk factors. J Trauma 2011;71:1908–14.
10. Ganz DA, Bao Y, Shekelle PE, et al. Will my patient fall? JAMA 2007;297:77–86.
11. Roudsari BS, Ebel BE, Corso PS, et al. The acute medical care costs of fall-related injuries among the US older adults. Injury 2005;36:1316–22.
12. Hartholt KA, Polinder S, Van der Cammen TJ, et al. Costs of falls in an ageing population: a nationwide study from the Netherlands (2007-2009). Injury 2012; 43:1199–203.
13. Carpenter CR, DesPain B, Keeling TN, et al. The Six-Item Screener and AD8 for the detection of cognitive impairment in geriatric emergency department patients. Ann Emerg Med 2011;57(6):653–61.
14. McGwin G, May AK, Melton SM, et al. Recurrent trauma in elderly patients. Arch Surg 2001;136:197–203.
15. Siracuse JJ, Odell DD, Gondek SP, et al. Health care and socioeconomic impact of falls in the elderly. Am J Surg 2012;203:335–8.
16. Lee WY, Cameron PA, Bailey MJ. Road traffic injuries in the elderly. Emerg Med J 2005;23:42–6.
17. Nagy KK, Smith RF, Roberts RR, et al. Prognosis of penetrating trauma in elderly patients: a comparison with younger patients. J Trauma 2000;49:190–3.
18. Phillips S, Rond PC 3rd, Kelly SM, et al. The failure of triage criteria to identify geriatric patients with trauma: results from the Florida trauma triage study. J Trauma 1996;40:278–83.
19. Chang DC, Bass RR, Cornwell EE, et al. Undertriage of elderly trauma patients to state-designated trauma centers. Arch Surg 2008;8:776–81.
20. Meldon SW, Reilly M, Drew BL, et al. Trauma in the very elderly: a community-based study of outcomes at trauma and nontrauma centers. J Trauma 2002;52: 79–84.
21. Demetriades D, Sava J, Alo K, et al. Old age as a criterion for trauma team activation. J Trauma 2001;51:754–7.

22. Lehmann R, Beekley A, Casey L, et al. The impact of advanced age on trauma triage decisions and outcomes: a statewide analysis. Am J Surg 2009;197:571–4.
23. Shifflette VK, Lorenzo M, Mangram AJ, et al. Should age be a factor to change from a Level II to a Level I trauma activation? J Trauma 2010;69:88–92.
24. Mangram AJ, Mitchell CD, Shifflette VK, et al. Geriatric trauma service: a one-year experience. J Trauma Acute Care Surg 2012;72(1):119–22.
25. Hefferman DS, Thakkar RK, Monahan SF, et al. Normal presenting vital signs are unreliable in geriatric blunt trauma victims. J Trauma 2010;69:813–20.
26. Gibson SJ, Helme RD. Age-related differences in pain perception and report. Clin Geriatr Med 2001;17:433–56.
27. Zuercher M, Ummenhofer W, Baltussen A, et al. The use of Glasgow Coma Scale in injury assessment: a critical review. Brain Inj 2009;23(5):371–84.
28. Mack LR, Chan SB, Silva JC, et al. The use of head computed tomography in elderly patients sustaining minor head trauma. J Emerg Med 2003;24:157–62.
29. Bochicchio GV, Joshi M, Scalea T. Community-acquired infections in the geriatric trauma population. Shock 2000;14:338–42.
30. Grossman MD, Miller D, Scaff DW, et al. When is an elder old? Effect of preexisting conditions on mortality in geriatric trauma. J Trauma 2002;52:242–6.
31. Ferraris VA, Ferraris SP, Saha SP. The relationship between mortality and preexisting cardiac disease in 5,971 trauma patients. J Trauma 2010;69(3):645–52.
32. Hukkelhoven CW, Steyerberg EW, Rampen AJ, et al. Patient age and outcome following severe traumatic brain injury: an analysis of 5600 patients. J Neurosurg 2003;99:666–73.
33. Mosenthal AC, Lavery RF, Addis M, et al. Isolated traumatic brain injury: age is an independent predictor of mortality and early outcome. J Trauma 2002;52:907–11.
34. Rathlev N, Medzon R, Lowery D, et al. Intracranial pathology in the elderly with mild head injury. Acad Emerg Med 2006;13:302–7.
35. Mina AA, Knipfer JF, Park DY, et al. Intracranial complications of preinjury anticoagulation in trauma patients with head injury. J Trauma 2002;53:668–72.
36. Cohen DB, Rinker C, Wilberger JE. Traumatic brain injury in anticoagulated patients. J Trauma 2006;60:553–7.
37. Ivascu FA, Howells FA, Junn FS, et al. Rapid warfarin reversal in anticoagulated patients with traumatic intracranial hemorrhage reduces hemorrhage progression and mortality. J Trauma 2005;59:1131–7.
38. Mower WR, Hoffman JR, Herbert M, et al. NEXUS II Investigators. Developing a decision instrument to guide computed tomographic imaging of blunt head injury patients. J Trauma 2005;59(4):954–9.
39. Czosnyka M, Balestreri M, Steiner L, et al. Age, intracranial pressure, autoregulation, and outcome after brain trauma. J Neurosurg 2005;102:450–4.
40. Bub LD, Blackmore CC, Mann FA, et al. Cervical spine fractures in patients 65 years and older: a clinical prediction rule for blunt trauma. Radiology 2005;234(1):143–9.
41. Battle CE, Hutchings H, Evans PA. Risk factors that predict mortality in patients with blunt chest wall trauma: a systematic review and meta-analysis. Injury 2012;43(1):8–17.
42. Elmistekawy EM, Hammad AA. Isolated rib fractures in geriatric patients. Ann Thorac Med 2007;2(4):166–8.
43. Falimirski ME, Provost D. Nonsurgical management of solid abdominal organ injury in patients over 55 years of age. Am Surg 2000;66:631–5.
44. Myers JG, Dent DL, Stewart RM, et al. Blunt splenic injuries: dedicated trauma surgeons can achieve a high rate of nonoperative success in patients of all ages. J Trauma 2000;48:801–5.

45. Harbrecht BG, Peitzman AB, Rivera L, et al. Contribution of age and gender to outcome of blunt splenic injury in adults: multicenter study of the eastern association for the surgery of trauma. J Trauma 2001;51:887–95.
46. O'Brien DP, Luchette FA, Pereira SJ, et al. Pelvic fracture in the elderly is associated with increased mortality. Surgery 2002;132:710–4.
47. Henry SM, Pollack AN, Jones AL, et al. Pelvic fracture in geriatric patients: a distinct clinical entity. J Trauma 2002;53:15–20.
48. Kimbrell BJ, Velmahos GC, Chan LS, et al. Angiographic embolization for pelvic fractures in older patients. Arch Surg 2004;139:728–32.
49. Velmahos GC, Toutouzas KG, Vassiliu P, et al. A prospective study on the safety and efficacy of angiographic embolization for pelvic and visceral injuries. J Trauma 2002;53:303–8.
50. Cummings SR, Melton LJ. Epidemiology and outcomes of osteoporotic fractures. Lancet 2002;359:1761–7.
51. Taylor MD, Tracy JK, Meyer W, et al. Trauma in the elderly: intensive care unit resource use and outcome. J Trauma 2002;53:407–14.
52. Schulman AM, Claridge JA, Young JS. Young vs old: factors affecting mortality after blunt traumatic injury. Am Surg 2002;68:942–7.
53. Scalea TM, Simon HM, Duncan AO, et al. Geriatric blunt multiple trauma: improved survival with invasive monitoring. J Trauma 1990;30:129–36.
54. Fairman R, Rombeau JL. Physiologic problems in the elderly surgical patient. In: Miller TA, Rowlands BJ, editors. Physiologic basis of modern surgical care. St Louis (MO): CV Mosby; 1988. p. 1108–17.
55. Friese RS, Shafi S, Gentilello LM. Pulmonary artery catheter use is associated with reduced mortality in severely injured patients: a national trauma data bank analysis of 53,312 patients. Crit Care Med 2006;34(6):1597–601.
56. Brown CV, Shoemaker WC, Wo CC, et al. Is noninvasive hemodynamic monitoring appropriate for the elderly critically injured patient? J Trauma 2005;58:102–7.
57. Jacons DG, Plaisier BR, Barie PS, et al. Practice management guidelines for geriatric trauma: the EAST practice management guidelines work group. J Trauma 2003;54:391–416.
58. Epstein CD, Peerless J, Martin J, et al. Oxygen transport and organ dysfunction in the older trauma patient. Heart Lung 2002;31:315–26.
59. Sharma G, Goodwin J. Effect of aging on respiratory system physiology and immunology. Clin Interv Aging 2006;1:253–60.
60. Bochicchio GV, Joshi M, Knorr KM, et al. Impact of nosocomial infection in trauma: does age make a difference? J Trauma 2001;50:612–7.
61. Schecter WP. Withdrawing and withholding life support in geriatric surgical patients. Ethical considerations. Surg Clin North Am 1994;74:245–59.
62. Richmond TS, Kauder D, Strumpf N, et al. Characteristics and outcomes of serious traumatic injury in older adults. J Am Geriatr Soc 2002;50:215–22.
63. Ferrera PC, Bartfield JM, D'Andrea CC. Outcomes of admitted geriatric trauma victims. Am J Emerg Med 2000;18:575–80.
64. Mosenthal AC, Livingston DH, Lavery RF, et al. The effect of age on functional outcome in mild traumatic brain injury: 6-month report of a prospective multicenter trial. J Trauma 2004;56:1042–8.
65. Grossman M, Scaff DW, Miller D, et al. Functional outcomes in octogenarian trauma. J Trauma 2003;55:26–32.
66. Grossman MD, Ofurum U, Stehly CD, et al. Long-term survival after major trauma in geriatric patients: the glass is half-full. J Trauma Acute Care Surg 2012;72:1181–5.

Acute Pain Management in Older Adults in the Emergency Department

Ula Hwang, MD, MPH[a,b,c,*], Timothy F. Platts-Mills, MD[d,e]

KEYWORDS

- Pain • Geriatrics • Emergency medicine • Pain assessment • Analgesics

KEY POINTS

- Effective treatment of acute pain in older patients is a common challenge faced by emergency providers.
- Because older adults are at increased risk for adverse events associated with systemic analgesics, pain treatment must proceed cautiously.
- Essential elements to quality acute pain care include an early initial assessment for the presence of pain, selection of an analgesic based on patient-specific risks and preferences, and frequent reassessments and retreatments as needed.

INTRODUCTION

Acute pain is a common reason for emergency department (ED) visits among older adults.[1] Effective treatment of acute pain is important for the relief of suffering and because unrelieved acute pain is associated with poorer outcomes during hospitalization, including persistent pain, longer hospital lengths of stay, missed or shortened physical therapy sessions, delays to ambulation, and delirium.[2–7] Despite the frequency with which this problem is encountered and the importance of effective pain treatment, disparities in pain care continue to exist for older adults when compared with younger adults as evidenced by high rates of pain at the end of the ED visit and lower rates of

Disclosure: See last page of article.
a Department of Emergency Medicine, Mount Sinai School of Medicine, New York, NY, USA;
b Brookdale Department of Geriatrics and Palliative Medicine, Mount Sinai School of Medicine, New York, NY, USA; c Geriatric Research, Education and Clinical Center, James J. Peters Veterans Affairs Medical Center, Bronx, NY, USA; d Department of Emergency Medicine, University of North Carolina Chapel Hill, Chapel Hill, NC, USA; e Department of Anesthesiology, University of North Carolina Chapel Hill, Chapel Hill, NC, USA
* Corresponding author. Department of Emergency Medicine, One Gustave L. Levy Place, Box 1620, New York, NY 10029.
E-mail address: ula.hwang@mountsinai.org

Clin Geriatr Med 29 (2013) 151–164
http://dx.doi.org/10.1016/j.cger.2012.10.006
0749-0690/13/$ – see front matter Published by Elsevier Inc.
geriatric.theclinics.com

treatment for older versus younger adults.[1,8–16] Although increased attention to this issue has resulted in some improvement in pain care documentation and use of analgesic in older adults,[17,18] older adults with acute pain are up to 20% less likely to receive treatment[1] than younger patients and still often leave the ED with pain.

The optimal management of acute pain in older adults requires an iterative process of treatment and assessment. This is true for all individuals with acute pain, but particularly so for older adults because of the increased risk of adverse events. Thus, reassessment of pain is as important as providing initial treatment, and failure to reassess pain is a common cause of under-treatment of pain in older adults.[19] Adverse events associated with analgesic treatment in older adults include over-sedation, respiratory depression, acute kidney injury, and gastrointestinal bleeding. Older adults are at increased risk for these events for several reasons: Polypharmacy increases risk for drug–drug interactions; physiologic changes and higher rates of chronic medical problems decrease drug metabolism and clearance; and higher rates of pretreatment functional impairments (physical and cognitive) lower the threshold at which patients may experience symptoms such as loss of balance. Thus, systemic analgesics must be used with caution in older adults.

Goals of Acute Pain Care Management

Goals of care should include early initial assessment of pain, selection of an analgesic based on patient-specific risks and preferences, and effective reduction in pain. Because of the increased risk of adverse drug events, the maxim "start low and go slow" is recommended when dosing analgesics for older adults. Careful titration with frequent reassessment allows for optimal and safe acute pain care in older adults.[20]

Pain Assessment

Older adults are less likely to have documented pain assessments in the ED,[13] despite studies that demonstrate that documentation of pain scores improves analgesic administration patterns in the ED.[21] Potential barriers to assessing and treating pain include patient limitations in the ability to report pain symptoms owing to cognitive and functional impairments and provider limitations in knowledge as well as misconceptions about the value of treating pain in older patients.[22,23] The need for titration of analgesic dosing requires frequent assessment and reassessment of pain in older adults. Thus, the assessment of pain is critical for the safe and effective treatment of acute pain.

Pain scores

Numerous pain assessment methods have been described and studied in older adults.[24] For patients who are cognitively intact, the verbal Numeric Rating Scale is the easiest, most commonly administered method of assessing pain, and preferred by patients.[25,26] The Verbal Descriptor Scale may serve as a more sensitive and reliable instrument for measuring pain in older adults than the Numeric Rating Scale,[26] but the marginal benefit of using a descriptor scale rather than a Numeric Rating Scale in cognitively intact older adults is unclear. For the Numeric Rating Scale and Verbal Descriptor Scale, see **Fig. 1**.

The assessment of pain in older adults with cognitive impairment generally combines information from multiple sources: Patient self-report, searches for potential

NRS: 0 1 2 3 4 5 6 7 8 9 10 [0, no pain; 10, worst pain ever experienced]

VDS[29]: no pain, mild pain, moderate pain, severe pain, extreme pain, most intense pain imaginable

Fig. 1. Numerical rating and verbal descriptor scales for pain.

causes of pain, observations of the patient's facial expressions and behaviors, surrogate reports, and a trial of analgesic therapy.[27,28] These tools include the Abbey Pain Scale (Abbey),[29] Assessment of Discomfort in Dementia protocol,[30] Checklist of Nonverbal Pain Indicators,[31] Noncommunicative Patient's Pain Assessment Instrument,[32] Pain Assessment Checklist for Seniors with Limited Ability to Communicate (PACSLAC[33] and PACSLAC-D-Revised[34]), Pain Assessment in Advanced Dementia,[35] the Critical Care Pain Observation Tool (CPOT),[36] and the Algoplus (**Fig. 2**).[37] Advantages and disadvantages of each of these are provided in **Table 1** based on a modified summary by Bjoro and colleagues.[38] Unfortunately, no single pain scale has been identified to be superior for assessing pain in older adults with limited communication ability, nor have any been developed or validated specifically for the ED setting. Choice of preferred pain assessment may ultimately be determined by feasibility and ease of quickly administering and assessing pain levels in the busy ED environment. More important than which scale is used is that an effort should be made to assess pain in all cognitively impaired patients and treat it when present.

Treatment

Patient goals of pain care

Incorporating patient preferences and goals of care for treatment and pain relief are also priorities of quality geriatric patient care.[39,40] Pain control in older adults almost always involves a balance between pain relief and the risk of unwanted side effects. An open discussion with the patient about their goals and expectations for pain relief can help the provider to understand the manner and degree to which the pain causes problems for the patient and what they perceive to be their risks of various side effects. A shared decision-making effort may result in greater satisfaction with the analgesic choice and improved pain reduction.[41] Among patients with acute severe pain, most patients desire that pain be treated in the ED, would like to be treated early on, and are agreeable to having a nurse administering medication before physician evaluation, but prefer pain control without sedation.[42] Because physician prescribed treatment of pain in the ED is often slow and worsened by ED crowding,[43,44] these preferences support the use of protocols for nurse-administered analgesia. However, nurse-administered analgesia in older adults should initiate treatment with a lower starting dose than for younger patients. A titrated approach will aid providers and patients in finding an appropriate balance between pain control and risk of side effects such as sedation.

Analgesic Options

No guidelines currently exist regarding acute analgesic treatment and dosing for older adults. Evidence-based guidelines in pain treatment for older adults have primarily

Score each grouped item YES / NO for *presence* or *absence*   *YES / NO*

1. Facial expressions: frowning, grimacing, wincing, clenching teeth, unexpressive
2. Look: inattentive, blank stare, distant or imploring, teary-eyed, closed eyes
3. Complaints: "ow-ouch", "that hurts", groaning, screaming
4. Body position: Withdrawn, guarded, refuses to move, frozen posture
5. Atypical behaviors: agitations, aggressivity, grabbing onto something or someone

TOTAL YES   /5

Fig. 2. Algoplus pain scale: Acute pain behavior scale for older persons with inability to communicate verbally. (*Adapted from* Rat P, Jouve E, Pickering G, et al. Validation of an acute pain-behavior scale for older persons with inability to communicate verbally: algoplus. Eur J Pain 2011;15(2):198.e191–10; with permission.)

Table 1
Comparison of pain scales for patients with cognitive impairment or limited ability to communicate

Pain Scale	Objectives/Metrics of Scale	Validation Sample	Advantages (in the ED)	Disadvantages
Abbey Pain Scale[29]	Six questions based on observation of vocalization, facial expression, body language, behavioral, and physiologic and physical changes.	Nursing home resident with end- or late-stage dementia	<1 minute to complete	—
Assessment of Discomfort in Dementia Protocol[30]	Multiple checklist observations (physical symptoms, behavioral changes, sleep changes), use of nonpharmacologic comfort measures, appropriate use of pharmacologic interventions, coordination with physicians, and documentation of care protocols.	Long-term care patients	—	Pain care protocol that focuses on both assessment of discomfort, treatment of this, and use of psychotropic medication; not ED based.
Checklist of nonverbal pain indicators[31]	Summed score of 6 nonverbal indicators (vocalizations, grimaces, bracing, rubbing, restlessness, verbal complaint) observed at rest and with movement.	Cognitively impaired and intact patients with hip fracture during transfer from bed to chair	More appropriate for pain assessment in acute care and procedural pain situations[38]	—
Noncommunicative Patient's Pain Assessment Instrument (NOPPAIN): Nursing Assistant-Administered Pain Assessment Instrument for Use in Dementia[32]	During the performance of daily care activities (laying, turning, transferring from bed; sitting, dressing, feeding, talking, bathing) scaled intensity observations of pain responses with verbal and visualized cues.	Nursing home residents	—	Less than 5 minutes to complete, observation of tasks generally not completed in the ED (bathing, dressing, etc.)

Tool	Description	Population/Setting	Advantage	Limitation
PACSLAC: Pain Assessment Checklist for Seniors with Limited Ability to Communicate[33] PACSLAC-D-Revised[34]	Observation checklist of 60 facial expressions, activity/body movement, social/personality/mood indicators, and physiologic/eating/sleeping/vocal behaviors; Abbreviated version of PACSLAC scale reduced to 24 observed items.	Patients/nursing home resident with dementia and limited ability to communicate	Seems easy to use and preferred by nurses[38]	—
PAINAD: Pain Assessment In Advanced Dementia Scale[35]	Observation of 5 items (and scaled ratings) of breathing, negative vocalizations, facial expression, body language, consolability.	Dementia special care unit	—	Requires >5 minutes observation period
CPOT: Critical-care pain observation tool[36]	Observation of 4 items (facial expression, body movements, muscle tension and compliance with ventilator or vocalization).	Adult cardiac surgical patients in the intensive care unit	<1 minute observation period	—
Algoplus[37]	Observation for presence (yes/no) of 5 items (facial expressions, look, complaints, body position, atypical behaviors).	Cross section of patients ≥65 years in EDs, acute settings, rehabilitation units, long-term care facilities	Less than 1 minute observation period, specifically designed to assess acute pain in elders with inability to communicate verbally (ICV)	—

focused on treatment of chronic or persistent pain with medication recommendations divided into short- (<6 weeks) and long-term (>6 weeks) periods.[45] For older adults with acute moderate to severe pain (pain ≥4–10 on a 0–10 scale), opioids remain the standard of care. There is insufficient evidence at present to support guidelines further characterizing which patients with acute pain are most likely to benefit from opioids versus alternative therapies including nonsteroidal anti-inflammatory drugs (NSAIDs), acetaminophen, or regional anesthesia. For a summary of analgesic options for use in the ED setting, please see **Table 2**.

Non-opioids

Acetaminophen Acetaminophen is perhaps the safest analgesic in older ED patients because of the absence of gastrointestinal, renal, and cardiovascular risks with appropriate dosing.[45] Effective for musculoskeletal pain, acetaminophen is recommend by the American Geriatric Society as a first-line agent for mild ongoing and persistent pain, with increased dosing if pain relief is not satisfactory (up to 4 mg/24 hours) before moving onto a stronger alternative.[45] Risks of hepatic toxicity with acetaminophen are minimal and have primarily been observed with long-term use.[46] Unfortunately, acetaminophen may not be as effective as NSAIDs for pain secondary to inflammatory

Table 2
Common analgesic options for use in older adults: dosing, and considerations

Analgesic	Recommended Starting Dose	Considerations
Acetaminophen (Tylenol)	325–500 mg every 4 h or 500–1,000 mg every 6 h	Recommended as first-line pharmacotherapy for pain. One of the safest analgesic profiles. Use limited by maximal daily dose of 4 g.
Ibuprofen	200 mg 3 times a day	If prescribing for prolonged periods, consider adding proton pump inhibitor to reduce gastric side effects.
Naproxen sodium	220 mg twice a day	If prescribing for prolonged periods, consider adding proton pump inhibitor to reduce gastric side effects.
Hydrocodone	2.5–5 mg every 4–6 h	Usually prescribed as a combination drug (with acetaminophen or ibuprofen) which will limit its maximal dosing.
Oxycodone	2.5–5 mg every 4–6 h	Usually prescribed as a combination drug (with acetaminophen or ibuprofen), which will limit its maximal dosing.
Morphine	Immediate release: 2.5–10 mg every 4 h Sustained release: 15 mg every 8–24 h	No maximal ceiling dose.
Hydromorphone (Dilaudid)	1–2 mg every 3–4 h	Effective for breakthrough pain (acute on chronic pain).
Tramadol (Ultram)	12.5–2.5 mg every 4–6 h	Drowsiness, constipation are still common side effects (though not as extreme as with other opioids), lowers seizure threshold.

Data from American Geriatrics Society Panel on the Pharmacologic Management of Persistent Pain in Older Persons. Pharmacologic management of persistent pain in older persons. J Am Geriatr Soc 2009;57:1331–46.

conditions,[47] and the analgesic benefit of acetaminophen is its ceiling dose that limits its effectiveness in treating severe pain.

NSAIDs All commonly used NSAIDs are on Beers list of inappropriate medications for older adults. Beers criteria[48] are a list of medications considered inappropriate for use in older adults in the nursing home, community, outpatient, and acute care settings. Initially developed in the early 1990s to assist in geriatric medication prescribing, the most recent update of Beers criteria have been compiled and reviewed by an interdisciplinary panel of experts in geriatric care, clinical pharmacology, and psychopharmacology has developed guidelines and criteria for appropriate medication use in older adults. Even short-term use of NSAIDS has been considered unacceptable in older adults with diabetes, impaired kidney function, or taking medications that may impair kidney function (diuretics, angiotensin-converting enzyme inhibitors) or metformin.[49] Both renal and gastrointestinal toxicity from NSAIDs are dose and time dependent.[50,51] The patient's risk factors for toxicities and adverse drug reactions (including renal insufficiency, congestive heart failure, hypertension, or concomitant medications such as warfarin use) and recent history of NSAID exposure should be reviewed before administering or prescribing NSAIDs.

Despite these concerns, ibuprofen and ketorolac are commonly used in the treatment of acute pain in older ED patients. Ketorolac (including its parenteral form) should not be used to treat pain secondary to its high potential for adverse gastrointestinal and renal toxicity. "Key issues in the selection of NSAID therapy are pain amelioration, cardiovascular risk, nephrotoxicity, drug interactions, and gastrointestinal toxicity."[45] Other NSAIDs, however, that may be considered for use are ibuprofen and naproxen sodium, and may be used judiciously in the acute setting for older patients who do not have contraindications to their use (decreased renal function, gastropathy, cardiovascular disease, congestive heart failure). When NSAIDs are administered, patients should be informed of the risks and warning signs of adverse effects (eg, decreased urine output, abdominal pain, nausea)[40] and initially started on lowest doses available. Gastric acid suppression with a proton pump inhibitor may also be considered if NSAIDs will be prescribed for prolonged periods (≥4 weeks) at discharge.[52]

Opioids Opioids are recommended for the treatment of moderate to severe persistent pain in older adults by the American Geriatric Society.[45] Secondary to higher fat to lean body mass ratios, older adults should have starting doses 25% to 50% lower than those used in young adults.[53] Opioids commonly used in the ED include oxycodone, morphine, and hydromorphone.[54] Oxycodone is a preferred oral agent because it has a short half-life and little to no toxic metabolites. Morphine can be used with caution, with reduced dosing in patients with renal insufficiency. Tramadol (Ultram) is an atypical opioid analgesic that, although not classified as an opioid, has weak centrally acting opioid activity. For these reasons, some patients may not find it as potent as other opioids, but concurrently it has milder respiratory, abuse potential, and constipation side effects. It may be considered as another option for individuals with moderate pain who cannot tolerate NSAID side effects but are wary about taking opioids.[55] It is metabolized by the liver via the cytochrome P450 isoenzyme and then excreted by the kidney, so cautious dosing is recommended in patients with limited liver and renal function. Doses of warfarin may also need to reduced with concomitant use. Because of neurotoxic metabolites and the presence of safer alternatives,[48] meperidine is listed as inappropriate in older adults by the Beers criteria[48] and should be avoided. Codeine should be used with caution in older adults because it has been found to have greater central nervous system side effects and be associated with increased risk of falls and hip fractures.[56,57]

Common side effects of opioid therapy include nausea/vomiting, dizziness, constipation, and somnolence. Opioid use has also been associated with an increased risk for falls and fall-related injuries in older adults.[58] Thus, the post-ED visit use of opioids in older adults ought to consider the patient's risk of falls including prior history of falls, visual impairment, need for frequent toileting, or limited ability to walk or transfer.[59] A recent study in an adult veteran population found that higher doses of opioids were associated with increased risk of overdose death.[60]

Specific opioids have been associated with specific risks. Cardiovascular effects (QT prolongation and Torsades de pointes) are more commonly seen with methadone than other opioids.[61] A review of more than 5 million Medicare/Medicaid dual enrollees found that of the opioid medications, rates of injury-related ED visits were highest for patients who had recently filled prescriptions for methadone, propoxyphene, and fentanyl.[62]

When compared with hydrocodone, codeine carries an increased cardiovascular event risk after 180 days, and oxycodone and codeine had higher all-cause mortality at 30 days.[63] In another study by the same investigators, it was found that coxibs and opioids carried greater risks for cardiovascular events (when compared with NSAIDs) and opioids had increased risks for fracture, adverse events resulting in hospitalizations, and mortality.[64] Although potentially important for decisions regarding long-term pain management, these results are based on analyses of observational data and, despite appropriate methods for adjustment, may still be confounded by indication (ie, patients with a greater risk of death being more likely to receive opioids). As a result, it remains unclear how these results should inform acute pain treatment in older adults.[65]

Nonpharmacologic strategies

Regional anesthesia Femoral nerve blocks are a feasible and effective option for acute pain owing to hip fractures. Usually, this involves administration of a long-acting local anesthetic (eg, bupivacaine) under ultrasound guidance.[66] Regional anesthesia may provide excellent pain relief without exposing the patient to side effects from systemic analgesics. A combination of regional and systemic anesthesia may also be appropriate. Unfortunately, the use of regional anesthesia is limited primarily to injuries to the face, hands, and lower legs (**Fig. 3**).

Alternate non-pharmacologic therapies

The feasibility and effectiveness of using other types of non-pharmacologic therapies including complementary alternative therapies such as acupuncture, aromatherapy, biofeedback training, and physical modalities such as heat, cold, massage, positioning, and exercise have not been studied in the ED setting. These may, however, be considered by patients as self-management strategies for use once discharged from the ED. Cognitive–behavioral therapy has been demonstrated to be effective in the treatment of chronic pain in older adults.[67–70] Whether cognitive–behavioral therapy can improve outcomes for older adults with acute pain is unknown, but patients with acute severe pain at high risk for persistent pain are, in theory, likely to benefit from early exposure to coping strategies and methods of controlling negative cognitions associated with a new pain condition.

Reassessment

The complexity and risks of managing acute pain in older adults requires frequent reassessment of pain and response to analgesic treatment. Patients should be re-assessed with 15 to 20 minutes after a dose of intravenous opioids and within 20 to 30 minutes of administration of oral analgesics. Consistent with the management of

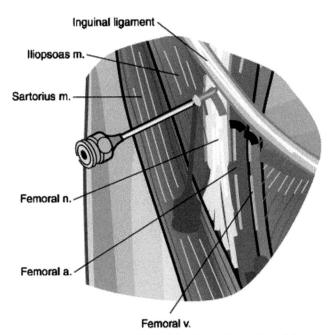

Inguinal ligament

Iliopsoas m.

Sartorius m.

Femoral n.

Femoral a.

Femoral v.

Fig. 3. Femoral nerve block. (*Adapted from* Waldman SD. Atlas of interventional pain management. 2nd edition. Philadelphia: Saunders; 2004. p. 453; with permission.)

diabetic ketoacidosis in the ED setting, where frequent measurements of patient glucose levels are necessary to appropriately manage hyperglycemia, effective management of acute pain in older adults similarly requires frequent reassessments of pain and often requires retreatment.

Geriatric ED Pain Care Quality Indicators

Quality indicators are operational metrics used to determine whether or not care is delivered well or poorly. They set a minimum standard for the care expected from clinicians. Following the Assessing Care of Vulnerable Elders quality indicator approach,[71] a task force convened by the Society for Academic Emergency Medicine and the American College of Emergency Physicians developed the following indicators to measure the quality of geriatric pain care received in the ED setting[72]:

1. Formal assessment for the presence of acute pain should be documented within 1 hour of ED arrival.
2. If a patient remains in the ED for longer than 6 hours, a second pain assessment should be documented.
3. If a patient receives pain treatment, a pain reassessment should be documented before discharge from the ED.
4. If a patient has moderate to severe pain, pain treatment should be initiated (or a reason documented why it was not initiated).
5. Meperidine (Demerol) should not be used to treat pain in older adults.
6. If a patient is prescribed opioid analgesics upon discharge from the ED, a bowel regimen should also be provided.

SUMMARY

Acute pain management in older adults is an increasingly common challenge faced by emergency clinicians. Because of the negative consequences of pain on the health and function of older adults, quality pain care is an important priority in this population. The high frequency of analgesic side effects in older adults, however, requires a cautious approach. Rigorous assessment, treatment, and reassessment of pain are the cornerstone of optimal acute pain care in older adults. Acetaminophen, NSAIDs, opioids, and non-pharmacologic options such as regional anesthesia each have a role to play in acute pain management. Understanding the limitations, contra-indications, and risks of these medications are necessary in selecting the appropriate analgesic for both ED and early outpatient treatment in older patients. Communication about risks and close outpatient follow-up with a primary physician is essential to opti-mize the safe and effective treatment of pain in older adults.

DISCLOSURE

Ula Hwang is supported by a K23 (AG031218) and R21 (AG040734) from the National Institute on Aging to study pain care for older adults in the ED setting. Dr Platts-Mills is supported by Award Number KL2 TR000084 and UL1 TR000083 from the National Center for Research Resources through the North Carolina Translational and Clinical Science Institute. The content is solely the responsibility of the authors and does not necessarily represent the official views of the National Center for Research Resources, the National Institutes of Health, or the North Carolina Translational and Clinical Science Institute.

REFERENCES

1. Platts-Mills TF, Esserman DA, Brown DL, et al. Older US emergency department patients are less likely to receive pain medication than younger patients: results from a national survey. Ann Emerg Med 2012;60(2):199–206.
2. Desbiens N, Mueller-Rizner N, Connors A, et al. Pain in the oldest-old during hospitalization and up to one year later. J Am Geriatr Soc 1997;45:1167–72.
3. Dworkin R. Which individuals with acute pain are most likely to develop a chronic pain syndrome? Pain Forum 1997;6:127–36.
4. Katz J, Jackson M, Kavanaugh B, et al. Acute pain after thoracic surgery predicts long-term post-thoracotomy pain. Clin J Pain 1996;12:50–6.
5. Morrison RS, Magaziner J, McLaughlin MA, et al. The impact of post-operative pain on outcomes following hip fracture. Pain 2003;103(3):303–11.
6. Duggleby W, Lander J. Cognitive status and postoperative pain: older adults. J Pain Symptom Manage 1994;9:19–27.
7. Lynch E, Lazor M, Gelis J, et al. The impact of postoperative pain on the devel-opment of postoperative delirium. Anesth Analg 1998;86:781–5.
8. Terrell KT, Hui SL, Castelluccio P, et al. Analgesic prescribing for patients who are discharged from an emergency department. Pain Med 2010;11:1072–7.
9. Jones J, Johnson K, McNinch M. Age as a risk factor for inadequate emergency department analgesia. Am J Emerg Med 1996;14:157–60.
10. Heins J, Heins A, Grammas M, et al. Disparities in analgesia and opioid prescribing practices for patients with musculoskeletal pain in the emergency department. J Emerg Nurs 2006;32:219–24.

11. Heins A, Grammas M, Heins JK, et al. Determinants of variation in analgesic and opioid prescribing practice in an emergency department. J Opioid Manag 2006; 2:335–40.
12. Hwang U, Richardson LD, Harris B, et al. The quality of emergency department pain care for older adult patients. J Am Geriatr Soc 2010;58:2122–8.
13. Iyer RG. Pain documentation and predictors of analgesic prescribing for elderly patients during emergency department visits. J Pain Symptom Manage 2010;41: 367–73.
14. Arendts G, Fry M. Factors associated with delay to opiate analgesia in emergency departments. J Pain 2006;7:682–6.
15. Platts-Mills TF, Esserman DA, Brown L, et al. Older US emergency department patients are less likely to receive pain medication than younger patients: results from a national survey. Ann Emerg Med 2012;60:199–206.
16. Mills AM, Edwards JM, Shofer FS, et al. Analgesia for older adults with abdominal or back pain in emergency department. West J Emerg Med 2011;12:43–50.
17. Herr K, Titler M. Acute pain assessment and pharmacological management practices for the older adult with a hip fracture: review of ED trends. J Emerg Nurs 2009;35:312–20.
18. Cinar O, Ernst R, Fosnocht D, et al. Geriatric patients may not experience increased risk of oligoanalgesia in the emergency department. Ann Emerg Med 2012;60:207–11.
19. Wells N, Pasero C, McCaffery M. Improving the quality of care through pain assessment and management. patient safety and quality: an evidence-based handbook for nurses. Rockville (MD): Agency for Healthcare Research and Quality; 2008.
20. Fine PG. Treatment guidelines for the pharmacological management of pain in older persons. Pain Med 2012;13(Suppl 2):s57–66.
21. Silka PA, Roth MM, Moreno G, et al. Pain scores improve analgesic administration patterns for trauma patients in the emergency department. Acad Emerg Med 2004;11:264–70.
22. Duignan M, Dunn V. Barriers to pain management in emergency departments. Emerg Nurse 2008;15(9):30–4.
23. Rupp T, Delaney K. Inadequate analgesia in emergency medicine. Ann Emerg Med 2004;43:494–503.
24. Hwang U, Jagoda A. Geriatric emergency analgesia. In: Thomas S, editor. Emergency department analgesia. Cambridge (UK): Cambridge University Press; 2008. p. 42–51.
25. Ware LJ, Epps CD, Herr K, et al. Evaluation of the revised faces pain scale, verbal descriptor scale, numeric rating scale, and Iowa pain thermometer in older minority adults. Pain Manag Nurs 2006;7(3):117–25.
26. Herr K, Spratt K, Mobiliy P, et al. Pain intensity assessment in older adults: use of experimental pain to compare psychometric properties and usability of selected pain scales with younger adults. Clin J Pain 2004;20:207–19.
27. Herr K, Coyne PJ, Key T, et al. Pain assessment in the nonverbal patient: position statement with clinical practice recommendations. Pain Manag Nurs 2006;7(2): 44–52.
28. Herr K, Bjoro K, Decker S. Tools for assessment of pain in nonverbal older adults with dementia: a state-of-the-science review. J Pain Symptom Manage 2006; 31(2):170–92.
29. Abbey J, Piller N, De Belllis A, et al. The Abbey pain scale: a 1-minute numerical indicator for people with end-stage dementia. Int J Palliat Nurs 2004;10(1):6–13.

30. Kovach CR, Weissman DE, Griffie J, et al. Assessment and treatment of discomfort for people with late-stage dementia. J Pain Symptom Manage 1999;18(6): 412–9.

31. Feldt KS. The Checklist of nonverbal pain indicators (CNPI). Pain Manag Nurs 2000;1:13–21.

32. Snow AL, Weber JB, O'Malley KJ, et al. NOPPAIN: a nursing assistant-administered pain assessment instrument for use in dementia. Dement Geriatr Cogn Disord 2004;17(3):240–6.

33. Fuchs-Lacelle S, Hadjistavropoulos T. Development and preliminary validation of the pain assessment checklist for seniors with limited ability to communicate (PACSLAC). Pain Manag Nurs 2004;5(1):37–49.

34. Zwakhalen SM, Hamers JP, Berger MP. Improving the clinical usefulness of a behavioural pain scale for older people with dementia. J Adv Nurs 2007;58: 493–502.

35. Warden V, Hurley AC, Volicer L. Development and psychometric evaluation of the pain assessment in advanced dementia (PAINAD) scale. J Am Med Dir Assoc 2003;4(1):9–15.

36. Gelinas C, Fillion L, Puntillo KA, et al. Validation of the critical-care pain observation tool in adult patients. Am J Crit Care 2006;15(4):420–7.

37. Rat P, Jouve E, Pickering G, et al. Validation of an acute pain-behavior scale for older persons with inability to communicate verbally: algoplus. Eur J Pain 2011; 15(2):198.e191–10.

38. Bjoro M, Herr K. Chapter 5-assessment of pain in the nonverbal and/or cognitively impaired older adults. In: Smith H, editor. Current therapy in pain. Philadelphia: Saunders Elsevier; 2009. p. 24–37.

39. Isaacs CG, Kistler C, Hunold KM, et al. Shared decision making in the selection of outpatient analgesics for older emergency department patients. Chicago: Society of Academic Emergency Medicine; 2012.

40. Bowling CB, O'Hare AM. Managing older adults with CKD: individualized versus disease-based approaches. Am J Kidney Dis 2012;59:293–302.

41. Isaacs CG, Kistler C, Hunold KM, et al. Shared decision making in the selection of outpatient analgesics for older emergency department patients. J Am Geriatr Soc, in press.

42. Beel TL, Mitchiner JC, Frederiksen SM, et al. Patient preferences regarding pain medication in the ED. Am J Emerg Med 2000;18:376–80.

43. Hwang U, Richardson LD, Sonuyi TO, et al. The effect of emergency department crowding on the management of pain in older adults with hip fracture. J Am Geriatr Soc 2006;54:270–5.

44. Pines JM, Hollander JE. Emergency department crowding is associated with poor care for patients with severe pain. Ann Emerg Med 2008;51:1–5.

45. American Geriatrics Society Panel on the Pharmacological Management of Persistent Pain in Older Persons. Pharmacological management of persistent pain in older persons. J Am Geriatr Soc 2009;57:1331–46.

46. Watkins PB, Kaplowitz N, Slattery JT, et al. Aminotransferase elevations in healthy adults receiving 4 grams of acetaminophen daily: a randomized controlled trial. JAMA 2006;296:87–93.

47. Weinecke T, Gotzsche PC. Paracetamol versus nonsteroidal anti-inflammatory drugs for rheumatoid arthritis. Cochrane Database Syst Rev 2004;(1):CD003789.

48. American Geriatrics Society 2012 Beers criteria update expert panel. American Geriatrics Society updated Beers Criteria for potentially inappropriate medication use in older adults. J Am Geriatr Soc 2012;60(4):616–31.

49. Platts-Mills TF, Richmond NL, Hunold KM, et al. Life-threatening hyperkalemia following two days of ibuprofen. Am J Emerg Med, in press.

50. Whelton A, Stout RL, Spilman PS, et al. Renal effects of ibuprofen, piroxicam, and sulindac in patients with asymptomatic renal failure. A prospective, randomized, crossover comparison. Ann Intern Med 1990;112(8):568–76.

51. Rainsford KD. Profile and mechanisms of gastrointestinal and other side effects of nonsteroidal anti-inflammatory drugs (NSAIDs). Am J Med 1999;107(6A): 27S–35S.

52. Rostom A, Dube C, Wells G, et al. Prevention of NSAID-induced gastrodudenal ulcers. Cochrane Database Syst Rev 2002;(4):CD0022960.

53. Abrahm JL. Advances in pain management for older adult patients. Clin Geriatr Med 2000;16:269–311.

54. Chang AK, Bijur PE, Baccelieri A, et al. Efficacy and safety profile of a single dose of hydromorphone compared with morphine in older adults with acute, severe pain: a prospective, randomized, double-blind clinical trial. Am J Geriatr Pharmacother 2009;7:1–10.

55. Barkin R, Barkin S, Barkin D. Perception, assessment, treatment, and management of pain in the elderly. Clin Geriatr Med 2005;21:465–90.

56. Shorr RI, Griffin MR, Daughterty JR, et al. Opioid analgesics and the risk of hip fracture in the elderly: codeine and propoxyphene. J Gerontol 1992;47: M111–5.

57. Turturro MA, Paris PM, Yealy DM, et al. Hydrocodone versus codeine in acute musculoskeletal pain. Ann Emerg Med 1991;20(10):1100–3.

58. Huang AR, Mallet L, Rochefort CM, et al. Medication-related falls in the elderly: causative factors and preventive strategies. Drugs Aging 2012;29:359–76.

59. Vassallo M, Stockdale R, Sharma JC, et al. A comparative study of the use of four fall risk assessment tools on acute medical wards. J Am Geriatr Soc 2005;53: 1034–8.

60. Bohnert AS, Valenstein M, Bair MJ, et al. Association between opioid prescribing patterns and opioid overdose-related deaths. JAMA 2011;305:1315–21.

61. Chan BK, Tam LK, Wat CY, et al. Opioids in chronic non-cancer pain. Expert Opin Pharmacother 2011;12:705–20.

62. Blackwell SA, Montgomery MA, Waldo D, et al. National study of medications associated with injury in elderly Medicare/Medicaid dual enrollees. J Am Pharm Assoc 2003;49(6):751–9.

63. Solomon DH, Rassen JA, Glynn RJ, et al. The comparative safety of opioids for nonmalignant pain in older adults. Arch Intern Med 2010;170:1979–86.

64. Solomon DH, Rassen JA, Glynn RJ, et al. The comparative safety of analgesics in older adults with arthritis. Arch Intern Med 2010;170:1968–76.

65. Hwang U, Morrison RS, Richardson LD, et al. A painful setback: misinterpretation of analgesic safety in older adults may inadvertently worsen pain care. Arch Intern Med 2011;171(12):1127.

66. Beaudoin FL, Nagdev A, Merchant RC, et al. Ultrasound-guided femoral nerve blocks in elderly patients with hip fractures. Am J Emerg Med 2010;28(1):76–81.

67. Abbasi M, Dehghani M, Keefe FJ, et al. Spouse-assisted training in pain coping skills and the outcome of multidisciplinary pain management for chronic low back pain treatment: a 1-year randomized controlled trial. Eur J Pain 2012;16(7): 1033–43.

68. Keefe FJ, Blumenthal J, Baucom D, et al. Effects of spouse-assisted coping skills training and exercise training in patients with osteoarthritic knee pain: a randomized controlled study. Pain 2004;110(3):539–49.

69. Morley S, Eccleston C, Williams A. Systematic review and meta-analysis of randomized controlled trials of cognitive behaviour therapy and behaviour therapy for chronic pain in adults, excluding headache. Pain 1999;80(1–2):1–13.

70. Waters SJ, Woodward JT, Keefe FJ. Cognitive-behavioral therapy for pain in older adults. In: Gibson SJ, Weiner DK, editors. Pain in older persons, progress in pain research and management, vol. 35. Seattle (WA): IASP Press; 2005. p. 239–61.

71. Wenger N, Shekelle P. Assessing care of vulnerable elders: ACOVE project overview. Ann Intern Med 2001;135(8 Part 2):642–6.

72. Terrell KT, Hustey FM, Hwang U, et al. Quality indicators for geriatric emergency care. Acad Emerg Med 2009;16:441–50.

Acute Visual Changes in the Elderly

Victoria M. Addis, MD[a], Heather K. DeVore, MD[b,*],
Michael E. Summerfield, MD[c]

KEYWORDS

- Vision disturbance • Vision loss • Vision change • Elderly vision

KEY POINTS

- Acute vision changes in the elderly are common and life altering.
- Chronic vision diseases may present as acute changes in vision due to a sudden awareness by patients.
- Acute vision changes can be evaluated based on unilateral versus bilateral involvement, and painful versus painless complaints.
- Changes in vision may be associated with a systemic disease process.
- High-risk ophthalmologic complaints must be recognized by the primary care provider in order to provide prompt and appropriate referral to a specialist.

INTRODUCTION

Visual changes and the loss of vision in the elderly population is a common and often life-altering condition. It is estimated that 1 in 3 elderly persons suffers from some form of loss of vision by the age of 65 years.[1] Loss of vision is often associated with a subsequent decreased ability to perform activities of daily living, a loss of independence, and an increased risk of depression.[2] In the United States, it is estimated that $8.3 billion per year is spent on medical expenses related to loss of vision and impairments in the elderly.[3] Eye-related complaints constitute 3% of visits to emergency department in the United States and 6% in the United Kingdom.[4,5] Acute loss of vision is considered a high-risk chief complaint (**Box 1**) because diagnoses are elusive, some causes have time-sensitive outcomes, and emergent evaluation by an ophthalmology specialist is required.[6]

[a] Department of Ophthalmology, MedStar Washington Hospital Center, 110 Irving Street, North West, Washington, DC 20010, USA; [b] Department of Emergency Medicine, MedStar Washington Hospital Center, Georgetown University, 110 Irving Street, North West Suite NA1177, Washington, DC 20010. USA; [c] Department of Ophthalmology, MedStar Washington Hospital Center, Georgetown University, 110 Irving Street, North West Suite 1A-1, Washington, DC 20010, USA
* Corresponding author.
E-mail address: Heather.K.DeVore@MedStar.net

Clin Geriatr Med 29 (2013) 165–180
http://dx.doi.org/10.1016/j.cger.2012.10.009
0749-0690/13/$ – see front matter © 2013 Elsevier Inc. All rights reserved.

> **Box 1**
> **High-risk ophthalmologic conditions warranting emergent consultation**
>
> - Acute loss of vision
> - Acute-angle closure glaucoma
> - Central retinal artery occlusion
> - Retinal detachment
> - Endophthalmitis
> - Optic neuritis
> - Ruptured globe
> - Lid laceration involving lid margin, nasolacrimal duct, or canaliculus
>
> *Data from* Magauran B. Conditions requiring emergency ophthalmologic consultation. In: Kahn J, Magauran B, Mattu A, editors. Ophthalmologic emergencies. Emerg Med Clin North Am 2008;(26):233–8.

Evaluation, diagnosis, and management of acute visual changes are valuable and necessary skills for the primary physician and emergency physician, given the rapidly expanding elderly population. This article reviews the evaluation of a geriatric patient presenting with vision changes, including pertinent history taking and examination specifics, recognizing time-sensitive diagnoses, classifying and managing common ophthalmic causes, and when to appropriately refer to ophthalmology or neurology. Although the main focus of this article is acute ocular disease, the differential diagnoses include chronic conditions, as occasionally patients present with an acute awareness of loss of vision only to be subsequently diagnosed with a chronic disease process (**Box 2**).

HISTORY

When an elderly patient presents complaining of visual changes, it is imperative for the physician to attempt to further qualify the symptoms. Visual perceptions may be difficult to describe for some patients, and culture and past experiences can influence a patient's perception and description of symptoms. The type of vision change is a key piece of ophthalmic history. Vision changes can represent negative or positive visual phenomena. Negative visual phenomena constitute the loss of all or part of the sensory input in one or both eyes. By contrast, positive visual phenomena are false visual images or misinterpreted sensory input. Specific descriptors might include complete loss of vision, blurry vision, flashes, floaters, distortion, double vision, or

> **Box 2**
> **Most common causes of loss of vision in the geriatric population**
>
> - Cataract
> - Age-related macular degeneration
> - Glaucoma
> - Diabetic retinopathy
>
> *Data from* Quillen DA. Common causes of vision loss in elderly patients. Am Fam Physician 1999;60(1):99–108.

dimmed vision. Monocular or binocular vision changes should be differentiated. Often a patient suffering from a loss of visual field, such as hemianopsia, may report loss of vision in one eye, whereas the condition affects part of the visual field of both eyes. Unilateral loss of vision classically represents disease anterior to the optic chiasm. Bilateral loss of vision may imply bilateral retinal or optic nerve abnormality as well as chiasmal or retrochiasmal disease.[7] The timing of vision changes can vary from transient symptoms that last fractions of a second to permanent loss. Determination of transient versus permanent symptoms is important. Vision changes can occur in isolation or in combination with other symptoms. A thorough review of systems will aid in the diagnosis. Gathering information about medical history, recent trauma, or surgery is imperative. Associated symptoms may include eye pain, headache, nausea, numbness or weakness of the face or body, changes in mental status, or hallucinations.

PHYSICAL EXAMINATION

The initial physical assessment begins with a gross inspection of the orbit, which will reveal disconjugate gaze, and obvious signs of trauma or infection. Next, the patient's best-corrected visual acuity is assessed. When possible, each eye should be tested separately at both distance and near. If the patient cannot see even the largest optotype on the vision chart (ie, the "big E"), the patient should be assessed for ability to count the examiner's fingers, see the examiner's hand movements, or perceive light. If the patient is unable to see light, the vision should be recorded as "no light perception."

Pupillary testing should be performed next. In dim light, the patient should be asked to fixate at distance. The examiner uses a bright light source to stimulate the right eye for several seconds. The amount of pupil constriction should be documented. The same test is repeated for the left eye. The examiner should then test for an afferent papillary defect by "swinging" the light between the right and left eyes several times. The light should be held to stimulate each eye for several seconds. The normal result is for the pupil to remain equally constricted as the light moves from eye to eye. If the pupil dilates slightly when the light is moved to one eye, it is not getting the same afferent input and an afferent pupillary defect should be noted. This defect is a hallmark of optic nerve conduction disease.[8]

Confrontational visual-field testing is performed separately on each eye. The examiner should sit 1 m opposite the patient, and ask the patient to cover one eye and fixate on the examiner's nose. The examiner should check each of 4 quadrants of the patient's peripheral vision by presenting 1, 2, or 5 fingers in the midpoint of each quadrant of vision. If the patient is unable to see the examiner's fingers, hand motions or light may be used for quadrant testing.

The fundus examination may be evaluated initially by using a direct ophthalmoscope, which allows the examiner to visualize the fundus and provides a magnified view of the optic nerve, macula, vessels, and retina. Elderly patients who often have cataracts and miotic pupils often require dilation for a complete fundus evaluation and diagnosis. Dilating the eye is indicated when the diagnosis is unable to be made on an undilated pupil, and is often therapeutic for many inflammatory conditions. It is imperative to document a pupil examination before dilation, as this physical sign will no longer be available afterward. Thus dilation is discouraged when following pupil status is helpful, for example, in cases of head injury and monitoring for brain herniation. A contraindication to dilation is concern for acute-angle closure glaucoma, as it will precipitously worsen this condition.[9] One drop of phenylephrine 2.5% per eye is recommended for dilation, as it is short acting and vision is not affected. If the examiner is unable to obtain an adequate view with the direct ophthalmoscope, consultation with an ophthalmologist may be necessary.

Intraocular pressure can be obtained with a tonometer where available, and should be documented. It is not routinely needed in all ophthalmic evaluations, but is important in the determination of acute-angle closure glaucoma and in obtaining a baseline pressure determination in blunt ocular injury and iritis. In cases of trauma where a ruptured globe is considered, this test should be deferred. Other contraindications include infections for which a sterile tonometer cover is unavailable, corneal defects, or patients who cannot tolerate the procedure, as movement may result in corneal injury.[10]

CLASSIFICATION AND MANAGEMENT

Vision changes may be classified based on a patient's history and presentation of symptoms. Often a patient may complain of an abrupt vision change only to discover through further evaluation that there is a chronic cause and simply an acute awareness of the change by the patient. For the purposes of this review, vision changes have been classified into unilateral versus bilateral and painful versus painless, thus allowing for quick differentiation of causes of vision changes based on presentation of symptoms. Vision changes that occur in only one eye represent abnormality anterior to the chiasm, whereas simultaneous bilateral vision changes are generally postchiasmal in origin. Pain is often a sign of inflammation and may help determine etiology (**Box 3**).

Acute Awareness of Chronic Visual Changes

Cataracts
The most common cause of lens-related loss of vision is a cataract, or lens opacity. Cataracts may be unilateral or bilateral, and are acutely recognized by the patient as decreased vision, symptoms of glare, or monocular diplopia. Symptoms usually progress over months to years, but rarely can occur more rapidly. Cataract surgery should be considered when loss of vision begins to interfere with daily activities, and referral to an ophthalmologist will help determine the timing of surgery.

Age-related macular degeneration
Age-related macular degeneration (AMD) is the most common macular disease seen in the elderly population. In the Beaver Dam Eye Study, the prevalence of macular degeneration was estimated to be 7.8%.[11] This disease is most commonly seen in

---

Box 3
Algorithm for the development of differential diagnosis of loss of vision

Unilateral		Bilateral	
Painless	Painful	Painless	Painful
Corneal Dystrophy	Corneal abrasion	Cataract	Chemical exposure
Cataract	Corneal infiltrate	Stroke	Photokeratitis
PVD	Iritis/uveitis	Vascular insufficiency	
Vitreous hemorrhage	Endophthalmitis	Mass lesion	
Macular degeneration	Angle closure glaucoma	Metabolic/toxic	
Retinal detachment	Optic neuritis		
Amaurosis fugax	Cavernous sinus thrombosis		
CRAO/CRVO			
AION/NAION			
Optic neuropathy			

Abbreviations: AION, anterior ischemic optic neuropathy; CRAO, central retinal artery occlusion; CRVO, central retinal vein occlusion; NAION, nonarteritic anterior ischemic optic neuropathy; PVD, posterior vitreous detachment.

patients older than 60 years, and risk factors include family history, Caucasian race, advanced age, hyperopia, blue eyes, systemic hypertension, and smoking. Patients may complain of blurred or distorted central vision but often will retain their peripheral vision. Other complaints include difficulty reading and driving, and needing bright light or magnifying lenses to read fine print. A screening examination of the macula may be performed in the primary care setting using an Amsler grid (**Figs. 1** and **2**), and it is suggested to have patients routinely screen their vision at home. A patient may identify a new visual-field defect or area of distortion on the grid that can be subsequently evaluated by an ophthalmologist. An APD is typically not present on pupillary examination, and a fundus examination by an ophthalmologist will determine the presence and type of AMD, either nonexudative (dry) or exudative (wet). Although only 10% of patients have the exudative form of AMD, it accounts for 80% to 90% of cases of severe loss of vision caused by AMD.[12] Nonexudate AMD treatment includes antioxidant vitamin and mineral supplementations, whereas exudative AMD is often treated with intravitreal injections. Patients with AMD tend to have minimal recovery of vision despite current therapies. Extensive research currently is being done to improve treatment options, with a focus on thermal laser photocoagulation, excision, displacement or transplantation surgeries, verteporfin with photodynamic therapy, therapies with anti–vascular endothelial growth factor (VEGF), and injections of ranibuzamab and bevacizumab.[13] Although not an ophthalmologic emergency, patients with suspected macular degeneration should receive follow-up with ophthalmology.

Primary open-angle glaucoma

Glaucoma comprises several causes of optic-nerve damage and loss of visual field. Primary open-angle glaucoma is a chronic, slowly progressing disease process and is usually unrecognized until late in the disease process when vision is significantly diminished. Common risk factors include increasing age, family history, hypertension, diabetes, and high myopia. Symptoms are typically bilateral but occasionally may affect only one eye. Examination findings include optic disc cupping, loss of visual field, and elevated intraocular pressures. Treatment by an ophthalmologist generally includes medications to lower intraocular pressure.

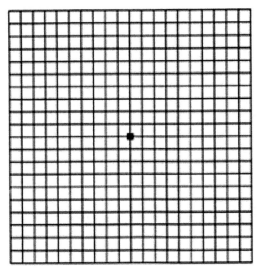

Fig. 1. Normal Amsler grid.

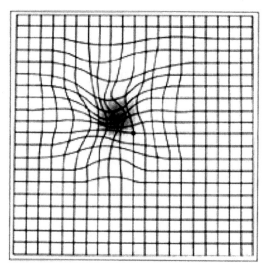

Fig. 2. Amsler grid of a patient with age-related macular degeneration.

Presbyopia

Presbyopia is the painless, bilateral, progressively diminishing ability to focus on near objects, generally considered part of the normal course of aging. Typical treatment includes corrective lenses, although surgical options now exist and can be discussed with an ophthalmologist.

Unilateral Vision Changes

Unilateral vision changes, best detected by checking separately the visual acuity of each eye, are generally the result of a primary ophthalmic cause. Disorders of the ocular media include abnormality of the cornea, lens, or vitreous. These structures require transparency in order for light to reach the retina photoreceptors. An examiner may closely observe corneal and lens disorders with a slit lamp, and subtle findings may require referral to an ophthalmologist for diagnosis.

Corneal causes that acutely affect vision usually lead to opacity or edema of the cornea. In the acute setting, most corneal changes present with pain; however, decreased cornea sensitivity resulting from herpes simplex keratitis or diabetes may mask this symptom. Severe dry eyes can be visually significant. The vision with dry eyes usually fluctuates and improves with blinking. Underlying corneal dystrophies such as Fuch dystrophy is usually worse in the morning and improves during the day.[14] The most common cause in the lens is a cataract. Macular disease classically produces painless, central loss of visual acuity or field, and patients may describe seeing distorted images (metamorphopsia). Macula edema is a common occurrence in the elderly. Diabetic macular edema is caused by leaking microaneurysms in diabetic retinopathy. Irvine-Gass syndrome is macular edema associated with cataract surgery, and usually presents in the first months after a cataract operation.[15] Less common acutely presenting diseases of the macula in the elderly include central serous retinopathy, vitreomacular traction, macular hole, and epiretinal membrane.

Retinal disorders may present with flashes of light or curtain-like loss of vision. Some of the common diseases of the retina include retinal detachment, branch or central retinal artery occlusion, branch or central retinal vein occlusion, and amaurosis fugax. Diseases of the optic nerve may affect visual acuity as well as visual-field abnormalities, and classically present with an afferent pupillary defect.

Painless disorders
Posterior vitreous detachment A posterior vitreous detachment (PVD) represents a separation of the vitreous humor from the retina. As a person ages, the vitreous undergoes liquefaction and shrinkage and ultimately separates from the retina. Patients may describe seeing black spots in the vision, floaters, flashes of light, or "cobwebs." PVD affects 24% of adults aged 50 to 59 years of age and increases to a prevalence of 87% among adults older than 80.[16] It is a relatively benign, although bothersome, condition in most patients. However, a PVD may lead to a retinal tear or detachment in a subset of patients, and a dilated fundus examination by an ophthalmologist is recommended at the time of onset of symptoms for any patient presenting with acute onset of flashes and floaters. In one study, 3.4% of patients diagnosed with an uncomplicated PVD developed a retinal tear within 6 weeks from initial presentation.[17] This finding underscores the importance of early referral to an ophthalmologist, as well as continued evaluation.

Vitreous hemorrhage Vitreous hemorrhage has a reported incidence of 7 cases per 100,000.[18] The etiology of vitreous hemorrhage includes leakage of blood from abnormal vessels (such as in diabetic retinopathy, sickle cell retinopathy, or neovascularization from a branch or central retinal vein occlusion), rupture of normal retinal vessels (as in a retinal tear or detachment, PVD, or in trauma), or extravasation of blood into the vitreous from an adjacent source (such as in wet AMD).[19] Patients see the blood and may describe it as floaters, hazy vision or even loss of vision, or a red hue to the vision. A patient's history may reveal this diagnosis; on fundus examination, depending on the amount of hemorrhage, the fundus may be partially or completely obscured. Ultrasonography of the eye is often helpful when the fundus view is obscured partially or completely by blood, and can be used to confirm the diagnosis as well as to rule out other causes, such as a retinal detachment.[20,21] Management of a vitreous hemorrhage depends on the cause of the bleed and may include conservative techniques, including elevating the head of the bed while sleeping and avoiding strenuous activity to allow the blood to settle and eventually clear. Surgical techniques such as vitrectomy may be necessary to physically remove the blood.[22] Referral to an ophthalmologist is important in helping to guide therapy (**Box 4**).

Retinal detachment A retinal detachment, or separation of the retina from the underlying ocular tissues, may occur in any age group but occurs most commonly in the elderly population. The 3 different types of retinal detachment, namely rhegmatogenous, exudative, and tractional, have differing etiology but all present similarly. A history of trauma, high myopia, diabetic retinopathy, or previous ocular surgery (including cataract surgery) places a patient at increased risk for developing a detachment.[23] The symptoms of a retinal detachment may initially include flashes of light (photopsias) caused by tractional stimulation of photoreceptors, and floaters caused by changes in the vitreous in the eye.[17] A patient may also report a change in or loss of visual acuity that often is described as the sense of a veil or curtain coming over the vision. Another common symptom described is a shadow or blackening of the vision that starts at the periphery and may move centrally. On examination, the visual acuity may be diminished; an APD is classically absent, but may be present in cases of large detachments, and confrontation visual fields in the affected eye may be abnormal. The fundus view, most easily seen through a dilated pupil, may reveal a billowing detached retina. The most reliable symptom associated with a retinal detachment is subjective

---

Box 4
Differential diagnosis of acute onset of flashes and/or floaters

Ocular Causes

Flashes and/or floaters

    PVD

    Retinal tear/retinal detachment

    Posterior uveitis

Floaters

    Vitreous hemorrhage

Flashes

    Rapid eye movements

    Wet age-related macular degeneration

Nonocular Causes

Migraine

Occipital lobe disorders

Postural hypotension

Data from Hollands H, Johnson D, Brox AC, et al. Acute onset flashes and floaters—is this patient at risk for retinal detachment? JAMA 2009;302(20):2243–9.

---

change in vision. Vitreous hemorrhage on slit-lamp examination is the best-studied finding.[17] A detachment may also be apparent on B-scan or ultrasonography.[20,21]

Management of a retinal detachment involves immediate referral to an ophthalmologist for repair, and often requires various surgical techniques.[23] Although a referral should be immediate, the timing of repair depends on the type of detachment as well as the attachment status of the macula, as macular-on retinal detachments have greater immediacy for repair.[24]

Amaurosis fugax Amaurosis fugax, or transient monocular loss of vision caused by ischemia or vascular insufficiency, is classically described as a curtain or shade coming over the vision of one eye. It is sudden, painless, and temporary, often lasting less than 30 minutes, and is followed by the complete recovery of normal vision. It may be caused by emboli, often from the carotid circulation or heart, that lodge and occlude blood flow to the optic nerve or retina, or hypoperfusion to the retinal circulation, such as that seen in atherosclerotic disease or in the ocular ischemic syndrome. It may also be secondary to a vasculitis, such as giant cell arteritis (GCA). Other causes of amaurosis fugax include hypercoagulable and hyperviscosity states, most commonly seen in young patients, as well as vasospasm such as seen in cases of migraine.[25]

Examination of the patient with amaurosis fugax may reveal a normal ophthalmologic status, especially if the vision has recovered back to baseline. A careful examination of the fundus should be performed as well as an evaluation for emboli in the retinal circulation. Workup may involve a full medical examination, including: cardiac and carotid auscultation; laboratory work to evaluate for diabetes, hyperlipidemia, and polycythemia; erythrocyte sedimentation rate (ESR), C-reactive protein (CRP), and platelet count to screen for GCA; carotid artery evaluation to rule out carotid stenosis; and cardiac evaluation with an echocardiogram to rule out cardiac disease. Treatment consists of management of the underlying etiology.[26]

Branch/central retinal artery occlusion A retinal artery occlusion typically presents as an acute, painless loss of vision over seconds in the affected eye. The patient's history may reveal a previous transient loss of vision or amaurosis fugax. A branch retinal artery occlusion will often present as a peripheral or segmental loss of vision, whereas a central retinal artery occlusion may present as complete loss of vision. On examination, visual acuity will be dramatically decreased, usually with an initial visual acuity of counting fingers or worse.[27] An afferent pupillary defect may be present, and confrontation visual fields may be decreased or may not be possible depending on the extent of loss of vision. On fundus examination a normal appearance of the retina initially may be seen, or occasionally the examiner may visualize attenuated retinal arterioles or an embolus. Within several hours of the occlusion, edema causes dramatic whitening of the retina in the posterior pole with fovea sparing, termed the "cherry-red spot." This phenomenon occurs because of preserved perfusion by the choroidal circulation. Narrowing of the retinal arterioles and segmentation of the blood in the retinal arteriole columns ("box-carring") may be appreciated. The etiology of a retinal artery occlusion and amaurosis fugax is similar and therefore the diagnostic evaluation is the same as that previously described. No treatment modality has been proved to be effective in the treatment of retinal artery occlusions.[28] There have been isolated reports of visual improvement with immediate ocular massage, anterior chamber paracentesis, intraocular pressure reduction, or with hyperventilation into a paper bag if instituted immediately after the occlusive event, but larger studies are warranted to verify the effectiveness of any of these treatments.[29] Thrombolytic therapy has been attempted in the treatment of central retinal artery occlusion, although no randomized controlled trial looking at this therapy has been completed to date.[30]

Branch/central retinal vein occlusion Similar to a retinal artery occlusion, a retinal vein occlusion presents with sudden, painless unilateral loss of vision. Peripheral or segmental loss of vision is more common with a branch retinal vein occlusion, whereas the visual disturbance may be more severe in the case of a central retinal vein occlusion. On examination, visual acuity may be reduced, an afferent pupillary defect is often absent, and confrontation visual fields may be abnormal. The diagnosis is ultimately made by a fundus examination. The fundus will have diffuse, tortuous, and engorged retinal veins and retinal hemorrhages. In a branch retinal vein occlusion, the retinal hemorrhages will be present in a sector of the retina along the involved retinal vein, whereas in a central retinal vein occlusion all quadrants of the retina will be affected. Cotton-wool spots and optic disc edema may or may not be visualized on examination. The cause of a retinal vein occlusion is most commonly atherosclerosis of the adjacent retinal artery, as both the vein and artery are contained within the same sheath. The artery compresses the retinal vein at a crossing point and this secondarily induces thrombosis in the lumen of the vein, leading to a vein occlusion. Hypertension, glaucoma, hypercoagulable states, vasculitis, and certain medications such as oral contraceptive pills have been associated with retinal vein occlusions. Medical evaluation is similar to that recommended for amaurosis fugax and retinal artery occlusions, and should include an evaluation of cardiovascular disease and hypercoagulable diseases. There is no effective treatment for a retinal vein occlusion; however, early referral to an ophthalmologist should be made to monitor for serious neovascular complications that would require urgent treatment.[31]

There are many other causes of retinal disease including rod or cone retinal dystrophies, vitamin deficiencies, and even paraneoplastic syndromes, including cancer-associated retinopathy and melanoma-associated retinopathy. These diseases are rare, require clinical workup by the ophthalmic specialist for diagnosis, and often have no treatment. If a retinal or macular disease is diagnosed or suspected, referral to the ophthalmologist and possibly a retinal specialist is warranted.

Anterior ischemic optic neuropathy Anterior ischemic optic neuropathy (AION) is caused by ischemia to the optic nerve and is the most common cause of acute optic neuropathy in patients older than 50 years. It may be classified as either arteritic (AAION), when the optic neuropathy is associated with Giant Cell Arteritis (GCA), or nonarteritic (NAION), which has a different mechanism. The clinical presentation often differs between these 2 conditions, and it is important to use the history, ophthalmologic examination, and laboratory evaluation to distinguish between them, as treatment differs greatly.[32]

Arteritic anterior ischemic optic neuropathy (AAION), caused by GCA, also termed temporal arteritis or cranial arteritis, is typically found in patients older than 60 years, with women more commonly affected than men. This disease is characterized by inflammation and thrombosis of the short posterior ciliary arteries that supply the optic nerve head. In addition to loss of vision, which may be rapid, systemic symptoms can often be elicited from patients and include headache (usually dull and in the temporal region), scalp tenderness (especially when brushing hair), and jaw claudication. The symptom most specific for AAION is jaw claudication.[33] A history of weakness, fatigue, weight loss, anorexia, fevers, and muscle aches may be present; however, up to 20% of patients with GCA will have no systemic symptoms.

When the patient presents with vision complaints, the clinical examination often reveals severe loss of vision (<20/200 in 60% of cases) and an APD unless the disease is bilateral. Loss of visual field is variable, with altitudinal or arcuate defects being the most common. On fundus examination of the affected eye, the examiner may visualize optic disc edema with pallor as well as signs of retinal ischemia (cotton-wool spots). When GCA is suspected immediate therapy is necessary, as loss of vision can quickly progress and the opposite eye may also become affected. An ESR, CRP, and complete blood count should be ordered, and concerning results include an elevated ESR and CRP as well as a low platelet count.

When GCA is suspected, immediate corticosteroid therapy must be initiated, and unilateral or bilateral temporal artery biopsy is required to confirm the diagnosis. A biopsy may be postponed until after steroids are started, and will not alter the pathology results. Several studies have shown no difference in outcomes for patients initially treated with intravenous steroids compared with those initially treated with oral prednisone.[34] If loss of vision has already occurred, it often does not improve with steroids, and the major focus of treatment is to prevent loss of vision in the fellow eye.[35] Even with prompt initiation of steroids, some patients unfortunately go on to have bilateral loss of vision. Tapering of steroids must be done very slowly, as the risk of recurrence increases once steroids are stopped. There are many side effects of long-term corticosteroid use, and all patients on steroids should be comanaged by both an ophthalmologist and their primary care physician.

Nonarteritic anterior ischemic optic neuropathy (NAION) most commonly occurs in patients older than 55 years, with men and women affected equally. The majority of patients have underlying systemic vascular disease. The pathology of this disease is not completely understood, but it is thought that there is compromise to the microcirculation of the optic disc supplied by the short posterior ciliary arteries. NAION occurs primarily in patients with a disc at risk, which is defined as an optic nerve with a very small central cup, less than one-third of the diameter of the nerve, thought to cause structural crowding of the disc. Other risk factors for NAION include hypertension, diabetes, hypercholesterolemia, nocturnal systemic hypotension, obstructive sleep apnea, and anemia. Certain medications such as erectile-dysfunction drugs and amio-darone have also been associated with NAION.

Patients typically present complaining of unilateral loss of vision or visual-field defects. Pain is usually not reported, but there may be some pain with eye movement. Vision loss in NAION is typically less severe than in AION. An APD will be present if the disease is unilateral. Loss of altitudinal or arcuate visual field is most common, although any field defect may be seen. On fundus examination the optic nerve may initially appear swollen and hyperemic (with increased color secondary to increased blood flow), and hemorrhages around the nerve may be seen. The hyperemic appear-ance of the optic nerve in NAION distinguishes this disease process from AION, whereby pale swelling is more frequently seen.[36]

There is no proven therapy for NAION, although many different treatments have been attempted including anticoagulation, fenestration of the optic nerve sheath, intravitreal injection of anti-VEGF agents, vitrectomy, optic neurotomy, hyperbaric oxygen, and others. Corticosteroid use for this condition is very controversial, and although several retrospective and prospective studies have found a potential benefit, no randomized controlled trial has yet been performed.[37,38] All patients who experi-ence an NAION should be evaluated for vascular risk factors, as they are also at risk for cerebrovascular and cardiovascular disease. About 40% of patients with NAION will have a spontaneous improvement in vision and about 15% to 25% of patients will suffer an NAION in the contralateral eye over a 5-year period.[36]

Other causes of optic neuropathy Although the most common causes of an acute optic neuropathy in the elderly population are of vascular origin, there are several other causes. Glaucoma, inflammatory diseases, compressive and infiltrative lesions, trauma, congenital causes, and toxic/metabolic etiology have all been described in detail, and many cause acute or chronic loss of vision. If any of these causes are sus-pected, an appropriate workup including laboratory tests and imaging studies should be performed (**Box 5**).

Box 5
Differential diagnosis of monocular loss of vision

Condition	Type
Optic neuritis	Idiopathic, multiple sclerosis
Ischemic optic neuropathy	AION, NAION
Inflammatory optic neuropathy	Sarcoid, systemic lupus erythematosus, Sjögren syndrome
Infectious optic neuropathy	Paranasal sinusitis, cat-scratch disease, syphilis, Lyme disease, toxoplasmosis, cytomegalovirus, cryptococcus
Compression	Paranasal mucocele, meningioma, bony compression, enlarged extraocular muscles, aneurysm
Neoplasm	Optic nerve glioma, optic nerve glioblastoma multiforme, lymphoma, leukemia, carcinomatous meningitis, metastasis
Hereditary	Leber hereditary optic neuropathy
Glaucomatous	Chronic glaucoma, acute-angle closure glaucoma
Retinal	Chronic serous chorioretinopathy, retinal artery occlusion, retinal vein occlusion, acute idiopathic blind-spot enlargement syndrome

Data from Prasad S, Volpe NJ, Balcer LJ. Approach to optic neuropathies: clinical update. Neurologist 2010;16(1):23–34.

Painful disorders

A painful, red eye is one of the most common ophthalmic complaints presented to the primary physician and emergency department.[39] There are many causes of a red eye, but only those most common or eye-threatening that may cause a decrease in visual acuity are addressed here.

Corneal abrasion/infiltrate/ulcer Corneal pathology includes abrasions, infiltrates, ulcers, or other infections. Patients may complain of pain, photophobia, and blurry vision and may have a history of trauma, contact-lens use, or have similar symptoms in the past. The visual acuity may be decreased if the abnormality lies within the visual axis. A slit-lamp examination should be performed or the patient should be referred to an ophthalmologist for further examination. Epithelial corneal defects will take up fluorescein dye and stain a yellow-green color when visualized under blue light. Whereas both abrasions and ulcers will stain with fluorescein, ulcers appear opaque and are also visualized under white light. The slit lamp is also used to examine the depth and clarity of the anterior chamber. Normally the anterior chamber is clear of any cellular material.

Simple abrasions or epithelial defects should be treated with topical erythromycin ophthalmic ointment (0.5% solution) and reevaluated 3 to 5 days later to ensure proper healing. Patients with a history of contact-lens use should be covered against *Pseudomonas* (eg, fluoroquinolone) and instructed not to wear their contacts until complete resolution. Corneal ulcers or infiltrates should be referred within 24 hours to an ophthalmologist, as these patients often need to have the infiltrates cultured, be started on fortified antibiotic drops, and reassessed daily.[40]

Conjunctivitis/iritis/uveitis Conjunctivitis is any inflammatory process involving the conjunctiva and often is caused by viral, bacterial, chemical, and allergic factors. Visual acuity remains intact, although patients may complain of blurry vision if there is significant associated discharge from the eye. By comparison, patients with iritis or uveitis generally have decreased visual acuity and profound photophobia, and have cells or flare apparent when the anterior chamber is visualized using a slit lamp. Patients deemed to have some degree of uveitis should be referred to an ophthalmologist for determination of the extent and type of inflammation and subsequent appropriate management. Topical corticosteroids are the mainstay of treatment, and cycloplegic agents are used for relief of pain and photophobia.

Endophthalmitis Recent ocular surgery carries a small but significant risk of endophthalmitis. This deep infection of the eye is a dreaded complication that occurs in 0.1% to 0.77% of patients following cornea, cataract, or lens surgeries.[41] Endophthalmitis also can be a rare complication of bacterial keratitis or ulceration, penetrating ocular trauma, or fungal infections. Patients may present with periorbital swelling, pain, eye redness, and decreased visual acuity. Other notable findings include a hypopion, purulent drainage, reduced or absent red reflex, corneal edema and infection, and fever. Emergent referral to an ophthalmologist is necessary for evaluation and treatment of the underlying cause.

Acute-angle closure glaucoma Acute-angle closure glaucoma typically presents with a dull, boring periocular pain, ipsilateral headache, nausea, vomiting, and blurry vision, and the patient may report seeing halos around lights. These complaints may appear systemic in origin, and thus it is important to maintain a high index of suspicion for this diagnosis. Clinical signs of acute-angle closure include a red eye, corneal edema, a high intraocular pressure (as measured by tonopen or by applanation tonometry), and a mid-dilated pupil.[42] As the glaucoma progresses, the pupil may remain fixed in the mid-dilated position.

Although initial management of acute angle closure may include medications to lower the intraocular pressure, the ultimate treatment is laser peripheral iridotomy. Rarely additional surgical procedures are necessary.[43] High pressures can rapidly damage the optic nerve and limit visual potential, so immediate the consultation of the ophthalmologist is critical for the best visual outcome.

Optic neuritis Optic neuritis or inflammation of the optic nerve typically occurs in younger patients and most often in females (77%). However, atypical cases may be seen in the elderly, and it has been shown that adult-onset optic neuritis behaves similarly.[44] Optic neuritis typically presents as a loss of vision in one eye over hours to days. Classically this loss of vision is accompanied by pain with eye movements, but may also be associated with a dull retroorbital ache. Visual acuity is variably reduced in the affected eye, and an APD may be present. Confrontation visual fields are often abnormal. Depending on the portion of the optic nerve affected by the inflammatory process, the nerve may or may not appear normal on fundoscopic examination. Color-vision testing may be abnormal.

Evaluation of suspected optic neuritis includes additional laboratory testing and magnetic resonance (MR) imaging of the brain and orbits, with and without contrast, to better identify optic nerve inflammation. Management of optic neuritis includes a hospital admission and intravenous steroids for 3 days followed by a gradual taper of oral steroids. The addition of intravenous steroids encourages faster visual recovery in affected patients by 1 to 2 weeks. Oral steroid treatment alone has also been associated with an increased recurrence rate of optic neuritis.[45,46]

Cavernous sinus thrombosis A cavernous sinus thrombosis, or the formation of a blood clot within the cavernous sinus, may present with ocular symptoms. A patient may present with blurred vision, ocular pain and redness, diplopia, or proptosis, in addition to generalized systemic symptoms including fever, headache, nausea, vomiting, and somnolence. Ocular signs may include eyelid and conjunctival edema, tearing, ptosis, proptosis, and restriction of extraocular movements. A sixth-nerve palsy is the most frequent early neurologic manifestation of cavernous sinus thrombosis. Symptoms are typically unilateral at onset, although they may become bilateral within hours.[47]

Examination may demonstrate decreased visual acuity, and an APD may be present. Confrontation visual fields may be abnormal, and optic nerve elevation may be seen on fundus examination. When suspected, imaging should be obtained. Computed tomography may reveal the diagnosis, although MR venography has been shown to be a more sensitive imaging modality. Both septic and aseptic forms of cavernous sinus syndrome have been described, so blood cultures should be obtained. Treatment includes antibiotics, anticoagulants, corticosteroids and, in some cases, surgery. Early involvement of the ophthalmologist as well as the neurosurgeon and otolaryngologist or oral-maxillofacial surgeon is paramount.[48]

Bilateral Vision Changes

Painless disorders

Patients complaining of bilateral painless loss of vision often have disease processes that originate outside of the eye. Common causes include cerebral stroke, vertebral basilar insufficiency, migraine, compressive mass lesions, and metabolic or toxic syndromes.

Vision loss originating from the optic chiasm is often due to a mass lesion. A bitemporal hemianopia is the classic visual-field abnormality observed, resulting from the orientation of nasal and temporal retinal fibers at the chiasm. Depending on the location of a lesion, the anterior, mid, or posterior chiasm may be affected. Visual acuity and visual-field abnormalities between these causes may be subtle and often only apparent with the use of formal visual-field testing. Lesions that affect the optic chiasm may result in an APD if one optic nerve is more significantly affected, and the nerve may appear pale on fundus examination.

The most common lesions that involve the optic chiasm include pituitary adenomas, meningiomas, craniopharyngiomas, and internal carotid artery aneurysms. In addition, inflammatory disorders, such as multiple sclerosis and sarcoidosis, may cause a similar clinical presentation. Neuroimaging may be used to differentiate between these causes, and appropriate involvement of a neurologist, endocrinologist, and neurosurgeon is appropriate once a diagnosis is suspected or confirmed.[49]

Beyond the optic chiasm, nerve fibers pass through the optic tract, lateral geniculate body, and temporal, parietal, and occipital lobe radiations. Damage to any of these structures may result in a variation of a homonymous defect of the visual field that respects the vertical midline. The most common causes are strokes, tumors, and trauma. A homonymous defect of the visual field is found in 8% of patients after a stroke.[50] Damage to bilateral occipital lobes results in cortical blindness, which is distinguished from total blindness caused by bilateral prechiasmal or chiasmal lesions, based on normal pupillary responses and optic nerve appearance. Neuroimaging is warranted if this diagnosis is suspected.

Painful disorders

Patients with painful bilateral vision changes most commonly have an ocular cause for their symptoms. Chemical exposure, photokeratitis from ultraviolet light exposure, and damage from direct sunlight exposure are in the differential diagnosis, and are often readily apparent from the patient's history. A patient's visual acuity may be variable, but pupillary response and confrontation visual fields should all be normal. A pupillary response may be abnormal if the patient has coexisting optic nerve disease. A slit-lamp examination should be performed, which often reveals damage to the cornea or other anterior ocular structures. Treatment depends on the underlying etiology and generally includes frequent lubrication to the ocular surface with or without the use of topical antibiotics or steroids.

SUMMARY

Acute vision changes are common in the elderly population. Even small changes in visual perception will prompt a visit to the emergency room or physician office. The ability to recognize emergency situations from exacerbation of chronic conditions can be challenging. Prompt evaluation and appropriate referral may prevent significant morbidity and mortality.

REFERENCES

1. Ganley JP, Roberts J. Eye conditions and related need for medical care among persons 1-74 years of age, United States, 1971-72. Vital Health Stat 11 1978;(212):i–v No 228. DHHS Pub. No (PHS)83-1678.
2. Shmuely-Dulitzki Y, Rovner BW. Screening for depression in older persons with low vision. Somatic eye symptoms and the Geriatric Depression Scale. Am J Geriatr Psychiatry 1997;5:216–20.

3. Rein DB, Zhang P, Wirth KE, et al. The economic burden of major adult visual disorders in the United States. Arch Ophthalmol 2006;124:1754–60.
4. Nawar EW, Niska RW, Xu J. National hospital ambulatory medical care survey: 2005 emergency department summary. Adv Data 2007;(386):1–32.
5. Ezra DG, Mellington F, Cugnoni H, et al. Reliability of ophthalmic accident and emergency referrals: a new role for the emergency nurse practitioner? Emerg Med J 2005;22(10):696–9.
6. Nentwich L, Ulrich AS. High-risk chief complaints II: disorders of the head and neck. Emerg Med Clin North Am 2009 Nov;27(4):713–46, x.
7. Goold L, Durkin S, Crompton J. Sudden loss of vision—history and examination. Aust Fam Physician 2009;38(10):764–7.
8. Kawasaki A. Physiology, assessment and disorders of the pupil. Curr Opin Ophthalmol 1999;10(6):394–400.
9. Budhram G. Acute glaucoma after dilated eye exam in a patient with hyphema, retinal detachment, and vitreous hemorrhage. Acad Emerg Med 2009;(16):87–8.
10. Roberts JR, Hedges JR, editors. Clinical procedures in emergency medicine. 5th edition 2009;1165–9.
11. Klein R, Klein BE, Linton KL. Prevalence of age-related maculopathy: the Beaver Dam Eye Study. Ophthalmology 1992;(99):933–43.
12. Gottlieb JL. Age-related macular degeneration. JAMA 2002;288(18):2233–6.
13. Comparison of Age-related Macular Degeneration Treatments Trials (CATT) Research Group. Ranibuzamab and bevacizumab for treatment of neovascular age-related macular degeneration: two-year results. Ophthalmology 2012;119(7):1388–98.
14. Adamis AP. Fuchs' endothelial dystrophy of the cornea. Surv Ophthalmol 1993; 38(2):149–68.
15. Ho TT, Kaiser R, Benson WE. Retinal complications of cataract surgery. Compr Ophthalmol Update 2006;7(1):1–10.
16. Hikichi T, Hirokawa H, Kado M, et al. Comparison of the prevalence of posterior vitreous detachment in whites and Japanese. Ophthalmic Surg 1995;26(1):39–43.
17. Hollands H, Johnson D, Brox AC, et al. Acute onset flashes and floaters—is this patient at risk for retinal detachment? JAMA 2009;302(20):2243–9.
18. Spraul CW, Grossniklaus HE. Vitreous hemorrhage. Surv Ophthalmol 1997;42(1): 3–39.
19. Goff MJ, McDonald HR, Johnson RN, et al. Causes and treatment of vitreous hemorrhage. Compr Ophthalmol Update 2006;7(3):97–111.
20. Yoonessi R, Hussain A, Jang TB. Bedside ocular ultrasound for the detection of retinal detachment in the emergency department. Acad Emerg Med 2010;17(9): 913–7.
21. Shinar Z, Chan L, Orlinsky M. Use of ocular ultrasound for the evaluation of retinal detachment. J Emerg Med 2011;40(1):53–7.
22. Manuchehri K, Kirkby G. Vitreous haemorrhage in elderly patients: management and prevention. Drugs Aging 2003;20(9):655–61.
23. Gariano RF, Kim CH. Evaluation and management of suspected retinal detachment. Am Fam Physician 2004;69(7):1691–8.
24. Hassan TS, Sarrafizadeh R, Ruby AJ, et al. The effect of duration of macular detachment on results after the scleral buckle repair of primary, macula-off retinal detachments. Ophthalmology 2002;109(1):146–52.
25. Biousse V, Trobe JD. Transient monocular visual loss. Am J Ophthalmol 2005; 140(4):717–21.
26. Current management of amaurosis fugax. The Amaurosis Fugax Study Group. Stroke 1990;21(2):201–8.

27. Augsburger JJ, Magargal LE. Visual prognosis following treatment of acute central retinal artery obstruction. Br J Ophthalmol 1980;64:913–7.
28. Beatty S, Au Eong KG. Acute occlusion of the retinal arteries: current concepts and recent advances in diagnosis and management. J Accid Emerg Med 2000;17(5):324–9.
29. Rumelt S, Dorenboim Y, Rehany U. Aggressive systematic treatment for central retinal artery occlusion. Am J Ophthalmol 1999;128(6):733–8.
30. Hazin R, Dixon JA, Bhatti MT. Thrombolytic therapy in central retinal artery occlusion: cutting edge therapy, standard of care therapy, or impractical therapy? Curr Opin Ophthalmol 2009;20:210–8.
31. Marcucci R, Sofi F, Grifoni E, et al. Retinal vein occlusions: a review for the internist. Intern Emerg Med 2011;6(4):307–14.
32. Hayreh SS. Management of ischemic optic neuropathies. Indian J Ophthalmol 2011;59(2):123–36.
33. Hayreh SS, Podhajsky PA, Raman R, et al. Giant cell arteritis: validity and reliability of various diagnostic criteria. Am J Ophthalmol 1997;123(3):285–96.
34. Hayreh S, Zimmerman B. Visual deterioration in giant cell arteritis patients while on high doses of corticosteroid therapy. Ophthalmology 2003;110(6):1204–15.
35. Danesh-Meyer H, Savino PJ, Gamble GG. Poor prognosis of visual outcome after visual loss from giant cell arteritis. Ophthalmology 2005;112(6):1098–103.
36. Miller NR. Current concepts in the diagnosis, pathogenesis, and management of nonarteritic anterior ischemic optic neuropathy. J Neuroophthalmol 2011;31:e1–3.
37. Lee AG, Biousse V. Should steroids be offered to patients with nonarteritic anterior ischemic optic neuropathy? J Neuroophthalmol 2010;30:193–8.
38. Hayreh SS, Zimmerman MB. Non-arteritic anterior ischemic optic neuropathy: role of systemic corticosteroid therapy. Graefes Arch Clin Exp Ophthalmol 2008;246:1029–46.
39. Cronau H, Kankanala RR, Mauger T. Diagnosis and management of red eye in primary care. Am Fam Physician 2010;81(2):137–44.
40. Wirbelauer C. Management of the red eye for the primary care physician. Am J Med 2006;119(4):302–6.
41. Donahue SP, Khoury JM, Kowalski RP. Common ocular infections. A prescriber's guide. Drugs 1996;52(4):526–40.
42. Dargin JM, Lowenstein RA. The painful eye. Emerg Med Clin North Am 2008; 26(1):199–216, viii.
43. Chew P, Sng C, Aquino MC, et al. Surgical treatment of angle-closure glaucoma. Dev Ophthalmol 2012;50:137–45.
44. Jacobson DM, Thompson HS, Corbett JJ. Optic neuritis in the elderly: prognosis for visual recovery and long-term follow-up. Neurology 1988;38(12):1834–7.
45. Beck RW, Cleary PA, Anderson MM Jr, et al. A randomized, controlled trial of corticosteroids in the treatment of acute optic neuritis. The optic neuritis study group. N Engl J Med 1992;326(9):581–8.
46. Beck RW, Cleary PA, Trobe JD, et al. The effect of corticosteroids for acute optic neuritis on the subsequent development of multiple sclerosis. The optic neuritis study group. N Engl J Med 1993;329(24):1764–9.
47. Ebright JR, Pace MT, Niazi AF. Septic thrombosis of the cavernous sinuses. Arch Intern Med 2001;161(22):2671–6.
48. Desa V, Green R. Cavernous sinus thrombosis: current therapy. J Oral Maxillofac Surg 2012;70(9):2085–91.
49. Foroozan R. Chiasmal syndromes. Curr Opin Ophthalmol 2003;14(6):325–31.
50. Fraser JA, Newman NJ, Biousse V. Disorders of the optic tract, radiation, and occipital lobe. Handb Clin Neurol 2011;102:205–21.

Geriatric Dizziness

Evolving Diagnostic and Therapeutic Approaches for the Emergency Department

Alexander X. Lo, MD, PhD[a],*, Caroline N. Harada, MD[b,c]

KEYWORDS

- Dizziness • Geriatrics • Vertigo • Stroke

KEY POINTS

- Dizziness is a common but challenging complaint in the elderly because it is often difficult to describe and encompasses a broad differential diagnosis from the life threatening to the relatively benign.
- Dizziness in the elderly patient must be approached as a syndrome, not a discrete medical diagnosis.
- The history is often critical to determining the most likely cause of dizziness.
- Common tests in the evaluation of dizziness, including magnetic resonance imaging, have suboptimal sensitivity and specificity, and an overall lack in empiric validation.
- The community or clinic physician evaluating a geriatric patient complaining of dizziness that is not clearly chronic or does not have a known benign cause, such as benign paroxysmal positional vertigo, should immediately refer the patient to the emergency department to rule out serious causes, such as a stroke.
- Even with comprehensive diagnostic testing, the true cause may still be elusive.
- Disposition decisions are not straightforward. The risk of discharging a patient with an unclear cause of dizziness must be weighed against the adverse effects of hospital admissions.

INTRODUCTION

Dizziness is a common,[1,2] but challenging complaint in the elderly because descriptions of symptoms are often vague and require a broad differential diagnosis.[3,4] Previously believed to represent a discrete diagnosis related to specific medical conditions,

Supported by a grant from the John Hartford Foundation.
[a] Department of Emergency Medicine, University of Alabama Birmingham, OHB 251, 619 19th Street South, Birmingham, AL 35249-7013, USA; [b] Birmingham Veterans Affairs Medical Center, 700 19th Street South, Birmingham, AL 35233, USA; [c] Department of Medicine, Division of Gerontology, Geriatrics and Palliative Care, University of Alabama Birmingham, CH-19-201, 1720 2nd Avenue South, Birmingham, AL 35294, USA
* Corresponding author.
E-mail address: alexanderlo@uabmc.edu

dizziness is now understood to be a geriatric syndrome, caused and defined by multiple underlying factors,[5,6] and is recognized for its complexity. Although the diagnosis and management of dizziness have been investigated in many studies, experts on the condition have nonetheless highlighted the limited evidence.[5,7,8] Most patients with dizziness have a benign condition; however, a small number (<5%) harbor a serious and potentially life-threatening cause.[9] Posterior circulation stroke is perhaps the most challenging cause, because patients can have symptoms that are identical to peripheral vertigo. National trends show a steady increase in computed tomography (CT) and magnetic resonance imaging (MRI) studies for patients with dizziness in the emergency department (ED),[2] yet this practice is not uniform.[9] The key issue is how to identify the serious causes of dizziness while being cost-efficient and avoiding unnecessary diagnostic tests.

EPIDEMIOLOGY

A 2012 review using the National Health Interview Survey, which is a national database, reported that 19.6% of people aged 65 years and older had dizziness or balance problems in the previous year.[10] This estimate is comparable with the quoted prevalence range of 21% to 29% in other community-based and population-based surveys of elderly persons in the United States[6,11] and the United Kingdom.[12] Data on the incidence of dizziness is lacking, particularly in elderly persons, although a Dutch population survey estimated an incidence rate of 47.1 per 1000 person-years across all ages.[13]

In the United States, dizziness accounts for 2.6 million (or 3.3%) of ED visits per year. The rate of visits increases with age and is higher among women.[1] It is unclear what particular features of dizziness prompt these patients to seek care in the ED as opposed to their primary care provider.

TEMPORAL CHARACTERISTICS OF DIZZINESS

Dizziness tends to be episodic; fewer than 5% of patients with dizziness report having continuous symptoms.[6,14] Estimates of the frequency of symptoms have varied across different study populations. A community survey found 35% reported having dizziness daily, 14% weekly, and 51% monthly.[6]

THE UNDERLYING CAUSE OF DIZZINESS

The causes of dizziness in the older adult are many and varied (**Fig. 1**). Studies have varied on the distribution of underlying causes for dizziness The discrepancy stems from the differences between study populations (eg, community vs clinic patients, all ages vs elderly), sampling methods (eg, random sample vs volunteers), case definition (eg, stroke vs central vertigo) and diagnostic criteria (eg, physician impression vs ICD-9 diagnostic codes). In a study of the National Hospital Ambulatory Medical Care Survey (NHAMCS) 1993 to 2005 sample, Newman-Toker and colleagues[1] found 15% of all patients with dizziness had predefined dangerous diagnoses, including 4% with stroke. Otovestibular causes accounted for 32.9%, mental disorders 7.2%, and among specifically coded cardiovascular diseases, arrhythmia (3.2%) was coded more often than angina (0.9%) or myocardial infarction (0.8%). Diagnoses were based on ICD-9 codes, but 22.1% of cases received only a symptom diagnosis without a diagnosis of the cause (eg, dizziness).

Outpatient clinic surveys have reported that as much as 6% of dizziness is due to stroke,[5] but the reported proportion of stroke and cardiovascular diseases was as high as 15% in 1 small ED series.[15] The risk of serious diagnoses increases with age.

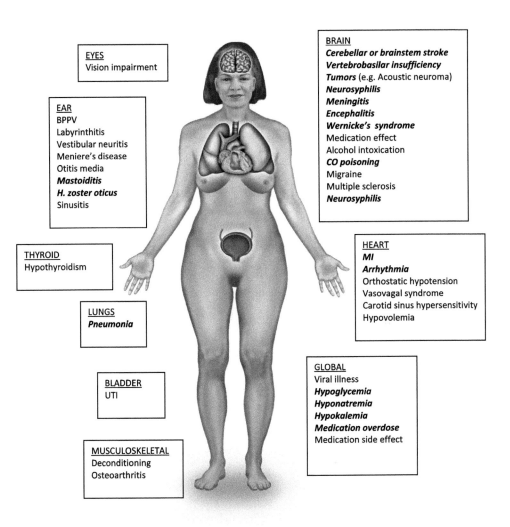

Fig. 1. Underlying causes of dizziness in the elderly. Conditions requiring rapid diagnosis in the ED are shown in bold italic type.

In the national ED sample reported by Newman-Toker and colleagues,[1] the risk was higher in the elderly, with 21% of dangerous diagnoses in persons 50 years and older, compared with 9% in those less than 50 years. A psychiatric cause of dizziness, often considered a diagnosis of exclusion, is also less likely in older patients, whereas more serious underlying causes are more likely.[1,16] Even though the proportion of dizziness due to stroke is small, data from a small series found a remarkably high mortality rate of 40% from cerebellar strokes presenting as dizziness,[17] supporting the argument in favor of using costly resources to rule out strokes in the dizzy elderly patient.

RISK FACTORS FOR DIZZINESS

Aside from increasing age and female gender, several clinical characteristics have been independently associated with dizziness as shown in **Table 1**. These data were derived from multivariate analyses of 3 population-based studies from the United

Table 1
Patient and clinical characteristics associated with dizziness

Characteristic		Tinetti et al,[6] 2000 (US) OR	95% CI	Stevens et al,[12] 2008 (UK) OR	95% CI	Maarsingh et al,[13] 2010 (The Netherlands) OR	95% CI
Female		NR		1.81	1.38–2.38	NR	
Living alone		NR		NR		1.3	1.2–1.4
Education[a]		NR		NR		1.2	1.1–1.3
≥5 medications		1.3	1.01–1.68	NR		NR	
Depression		1.36	1.02–1.8	2.17	1.56–3.01	NR	
Anxiety		1.69	1.24–2.30	NR		NR	
Poor hearing		1.27	0.99–1.63	1.81	1.35–2.43	NR	
Poor vision		NR		1.72	1.23–2.39	NR	
Any cerebrovascular disease		NR		NR		1.3	1.1–1.5
Any cardiovascular disease		NR		1.34	0.91–1.96	NR	
Past myocardial infarction		1.31	1.00–1.71	NR		NR	
Hypertension		NR		NR		1.2	1.1–1.3
Abnormal heart rhythm		NR		1.85	1.23–2.77	NR	
Grip strength	Third vs first quintile	NR		0.67	0.46–0.98	NR	
	Fourth vs first quintile	NR		0.41	0.25–0.68	NR	
	Fifth vs first quintile	NR		0.58	0.32–1.00	NR	

Abbreviation: NR, not reported.
[a] Education compared elementary versus college/university.

States,[6] the United Kingdom,[12] and the Netherlands.[13] Tinetti and colleagues[6] also reported a dose-response relationship involving these characteristics, whereby the prevalence of dizziness increased with increasing number of characteristics present, from 10% in persons with none to 68% in persons with 5 or more, supporting the hypothesis that dizziness in the elderly has a multifactorial cause. The lack of robust prospective data prohibits the establishment of a true cause and effect relationship.[18]

IMPACT OF DIZZINESS

The most obvious impact of dizziness in the elderly is a fall. Dizziness increases the risk of falls in the elderly,[19–21] with approximately half of patients with vestibular disease reporting a fall, and half of that group reporting more than 1 fall in the past year.[21] Accidental falls have been reported to increase the risk of head injury in the elderly,[22] and the elderly are at increased risk of mortality from a traumatic head injury compared with younger people.[23]

Even in the absence of a fall or trauma, dizziness alone negatively affects function and quality of life in the elderly. The adverse effects of dizziness include increased anxiety, decline in function, fear of falling, limitations of activities in everyday life, along with an indirect substantial health care cost.[18,24,25] Two separate population-based studies have found that between 50% and 60% of patients with dizziness reported moderate to severe limitations on everyday life.[24,25]

The economic impact of dizziness is also worth considering. Patients presenting to the ED with dizziness, compared with those without, were higher users of health care resources because they were more likely to arrive by ambulance, undergo CT or MRI imaging studies, stay longer in the ED, and be admitted to the hospital.[1]

THE DIAGNOSTIC APPROACH TO THE PATIENT WITH DIZZINESS
Overview

The challenge for the ED physician taking care of a dizzy elderly patient is to rule out potentially life-threatening causes of dizziness, identify the cause of dizziness (to the extent possible), and design a management plan. Overlap exists in the presentation of benign and dangerous dizziness, and seemingly benign features, such as isolated dizziness, can mask a potentially life-threatening cause, although this is rare (<1%).[26,27]

A detailed list of recommended history, physical examination, laboratory tests and imaging studies, and their rationales are provided in **Table 2**, and more elaborate discussions on their respective usefulness or accuracy are discussed in the following sections. The discussions address the global complaint of dizziness in the ED, beyond vertigo alone. The application of history and physical examination components to differentiate peripheral versus central vertigo is also discussed.

History

Dizziness is a self-reported subjective symptom that is vulnerable to different interpretations by both patients and physicians.[5,28,29] The symptom parameters introduced by Drachman and Hart[30] have helped to establish some consistency in its definition by categorizing dizziness into vertigo, presyncopal lightheadedness, disequilibrium, and other dizziness (**Table 3**).

Although the dizziness subtypes of Drachman and Hart can be very helpful, as many as 56% of patients described symptoms that fit into multiple rather than individual discrete subtypes.[6,31] This was especially true for older adults. Tinetti and colleagues[6] reported 59% with loss of balance, 33% with vertigo, 42% with presyncope, and 17% with other sensations, in addition to at least 1 of the other subtypes. One study with more than 300 patients reported that more than half of patients were vague, inconsistent, or contradictory in describing their symptoms.[28] In addition, a population-based study of ED patients found that a report of vertigo, compared with other dizziness symptom subtypes, could not differentiate the presence or absence of stroke.[26] In contrast, another study reported that a description of dizziness as vertigo accurately predicted an underlying peripheral vestibular disease with a sensitivity as high as 87%.[32]

Specific historical features, including frequency, tempo, onset, triggers, and associated symptoms of dizziness have been found to be useful in distinguishing between peripheral and central causes of vertigo (**Table 4**).[4,7,33] A systematic review by Tarnutzer and colleagues[7] explored the accuracy of various clinical history elements to discriminate between peripheral and central vertigo. They found that multiple prodromal dizziness episodes, age more than 50 years, and a normal result for the head impulse test were strong predictors of stroke, whereas the absence of dangerous signs in the head impulse-nystagmus-test of skew (HINTS) battery of tests (**Table 5**) was a very strong (negative likelihood ratio of 0.02) predictor of vestibular neuritis. HINTS is discussed below in Physical Examination section.

A retrospective analysis of 907 consecutive patients presenting to a university ED with dizziness incorporated the application of the ABCD2 scoring system for transient ischemic attack (TIA). This study determined a potential usefulness for the ABCD2 score as a stroke screen in patients with dizziness.[34] The ABCD2 TIA score incorporates Age, Blood pressure, Clinical features, Duration and Diabetes to predict the risk of stroke after a TIA.[35,36] Critics have challenged its usefulness based on the relatively small proportion of patients with confirmatory neuroimaging (35%), the biased referral

Table 2
Diagnostic approach to the dizzy elderly patient

Symptoms and Characteristics	Rationale
History of Present Illness	
Description of dizziness	Clarify what the patient means by dizziness
Is dizziness recurrent or new?	New onset dizziness requires broader differential and attention to serious causes
Dizziness onset and severity	Marginal discriminator between peripheral or central cause
Dizziness frequency, tempo, and duration	BPPV is episodic; neuritis rarely involves >1 episode
Neurologic symptoms	Other neurologic symptoms may indicate need for stroke evaluation
Weakness	Focal numbness suggests stroke
Numbness	Focal weakness suggests stroke
Gait or balance problem	Problem with gait or station suggests stroke
Cardiac symptoms	Serves to indicate possible cardiac cause
Chest pains	Evaluate for acute coronary syndrome, rule out myocardial infarction
Palpitations	Suggests ruling out arrhythmia
Dyspnea, orthopnea	Suggests ruling out other cardiac process
Recent bleeding (menses, gastrointestinal bleed)	Indicates hypovolemia from bleeding
Head trauma	Rule out traumatic intracranial injury (eg, intracranial hemorrhage)
Past Medical/Medication/Social History	
Medical history	Focus on potential triggers or underlying cause of dizziness
Vestibular diseases	History of BPPV, labyrinthitis, neuritis, or Meniere's disease can clarify current symptoms
Stroke	Previous stroke increases risk of stroke
Cardiac disease	Cardiac disease indicates workup for cardiac causes (myocardial infarction, arrhythmia)
Cancer	History of cancer increases the risk of brain metastases
Human immunodeficiency virus (HIV)	History of HIV increases the risk of brain lesions; eg, toxoplasmosis
Psychiatric disorders	Depression and anxiety are associated with complaint of dizziness
Medication history	New medications or dosage changes may indicate medication side effect
Alcohol use	Alcohol intoxication or Wernicke disease may explain dizziness
Physical Examination	
Vital signs	Bradycardia or hypotension may point to underlying cause
Orthostatics	Rule out orthostatic hypotension as cause of dizziness

(continued on next page)

Table 2 (continued)	
Symptoms and Characteristics	**Rationale**
Head, eyes, ears, nose, and throat	
Ear examination	Rule out otitis media, mastoiditis; test hearing
Vestibular examination	Dix-Hallpike for BPPV or other tests of vestibular dizziness (see text)
Neurologic examination	
Eye examination	Evaluate for nystagmus (see **Table 4**) or vision changes (may suggest stroke)
Speech/language	Dysarthria or aphasia suggests stroke
Motor examination	Focal weakness suggests stroke; global weakness suggests deconditioning
Sensory examination	Focal sensory deficit suggests stroke
Cerebellar	Cerebellar signs (dysmetria, ataxia) suggests posterior stroke
Cardiac examination	Evaluate for arrhythmia, diaphoresis, signs of tamponade, and so forth
Respiratory examination	Pneumonia may cause dizziness
Remainder of general examination	Helps with broad differential for dizziness
Laboratory Tests	
Complete blood count	Infection, severe anemia
Electrolyte panel	Hyponatremia, hypokalemia, dehydration, or gastrointestinal bleed (blood urea nitrogen)
Cardiac panel if indicated	Cardiac ischemia
Thyroid panel	Hypothyroidism
Urinalysis	Urinary tract infection, dehydration
Urine drug screen	Medication effect (opioids, benzodiazepines)
Radiologic and Other Studies	
Electrocardiograph	Rule out arrythmia or myocardial infarction
Chest radiograph	Pneumonia
CT scan (head)	Rule out acute intracranial hemorrhage or space-occupying lesions
MRI (brain)	Evaluate for ischemic stroke in cerebellum or brainstem, or other lesions

Adapted from Refs.[4,7,39,43]

of a tertiary patient population with greater likelihood of dizziness with serious (cerebrovascular) causes, the reliance on chart review, and the modest calculated sensitivity (86%) and specificity (58%).[37] Nonetheless, the lack of an alternative decision aid and wide practice variability merit further investigation of the usefulness of this instrument as a screening tool for dizziness related to stroke. Inclusion of older patients in future studies is critical.

Medication History

As many as 1 in 4 cases of dizziness have been attributed to medications.[10,38] Different classes of commonly prescribed medications can exert effects via multiple

Table 3
Dizziness subtypes

Subtype	Description or Terms Used	Prevalence (%)		
		Tinetti et al, 2000[6]	Lin and Bhattacharyya, 2012[10]	Colledge, 1994[104]
Vertigo	Spinning, sensation of movement	33	30	32
Disequilibrium	Off balance, unsteadiness, sensation of falling when walking	59	68	42
Presyncopal lightheadedness	Near faint, almost passing out	42	30	39
Nonspecific or other		17	NR	NR

Abbreviation: NR, not reported.
Adapted from Refs.[6,10,30,104]

Table 4
Differentiating between peripheral and central vertigo

	Peripheral Vertigo			Central Vertigo	
	Labyrinthitis/ Vestibular Neuritis	BPPV	Meniere's Disease	Stroke/TIA	Migraine
Tempo	Acute (<3 d)	Episodic Lasts seconds	Episodic Lasts hours	Constant (stroke) Hours/minutes (TIA)	Episodic Minutes to days
Clues from history	Unlikely if >1 episode Spontaneous Worsened by head movement Auditory symptoms if labrynthitis	Triggered by change in position, eg, lying down or turning in bed	Unilateral tinnitus Hearing loss Sense of ear fullness	Spontaneous Continuous	Precipitated by movement
Dix-Hallpike or supine roll	Negative	Positive	Negative	Negative	Negative
Spontaneous nystagmus	Horizontal	Horizontal	Horizontal if present	Purely vertical Purely torsional Gaze-evoked and bidirectional	May be present Direction varies
Head thrust	Positive	Normal	Normal	Normal	May be positive
Gait	Wide-based Slow, cautious	Normal	Unknown	Often impaired	Normal
Romberg	Negative	Negative	Negative	Positive if cerebellar lesion	Negative

Adapted from Tusa RJ, Gore R. Dizziness and vertigo: emergencies and management. Neurol Clin 2012;30(1):61–74. vii–viii; Kerber KA. Vertigo and dizziness in the emergency department. Emerg Med Clin North Am 2009;27(1):39–50. viii.

Table 5 Accuracy of HINTS				
Test	**Sensitivity (%)**	**Specificity (%)**	**NLR**	**PLR**
Head impulse test	85	95	0.16	18.39
Gaze-evoked nystagmus	38	92	0.68	4.51
Test of skew	30	98	0.71	19.66
HINTS	98	85	0.02	NR

Abbreviations: NLR, negative likelihood ratio; PLR, positive likelihood ratio.
Data from Tarnutzer AA, Berkowitz AL, Robinson KA, et al. Does my dizzy patient have a stroke? A systematic review of bedside diagnosis in acute vestibular syndrome. CMAJ 2011;183(9):E571–92.

pathways (**Table 6**). Many psychiatric and antiepileptic medications cause dizziness through effects on the central nervous system. Cardiac medications, especially antihypertensive medications such as beta-blockers and calcium channel blockers, have been independently associated with dizziness[6] and can cause a drop in blood pressure, leading to a presyncopal type of dizziness. Diuretics can theoretically cause sufficient hypovolemia to cause dizziness. Any ototoxic drug, such as aminoglycosidic antibiotics, can cause dizziness through otovestibular effects.[39,40] When inquiring about medications, it is important to identify new medications or new dosages of usual medications that may have preceded the current episode of dizziness.

Physical Examination

Whether the patient is seen in a general practice clinic or the ED, a thorough examination is recommended, with special attention paid to the otolaryngologic and neurologic examinations. The physical examination serves the dual purpose of confirming a benign vestibular cause of dizziness if present, while simultaneously screening for signs and symptoms that could signal a possible underlying neurologic or cardiac cause that is more serious.

Table 6 Medications that may cause dizziness	
Hypothesized Mechanism	**Medication Category**
Central nervous system	Anticonvulsants Antidepressants Antipsychotics Anxiolytic/sedative Mood stabilizers
Cardiogenic	Antihypertensive agents Nitrates Cardiac glycosides
Metabolic	Diuretics Insulin Oral hypoglycemic agents
Ototoxicity	Aminoglycoside antimicrobial agents Chemotherapeutic agents (vincristine)

Adapted from Chawla N, Olshaker JS. Diagnosis and management of dizziness and vertigo. Med Clin North Am 2006;90(2):291–304; Tinetti ME, Williams CS, Gill TM. Dizziness among older adults: a possible geriatric syndrome. Ann Intern Med 2000;132(5):337–44.

Classic teaching suggests several physical examination maneuvers that can be used to distinguish peripheral from central vertigo.[4] A summary of physical examination findings that can help distinguish peripheral from central vertigo[4,7,33,41–44] is provided in **Table 4**. The Dix-Hallpike[45] (or Nylan-Barany) test (see **Fig. 2**) has been the main confirmatory examination for benign paroxysmal positional vertigo (BPPV) for years, but 1 review found only modest to moderate sensitivity (59%–87%).[43] The Side-Lying maneuver has been recommended as an alternative maneuver for patients unable to participate in the Dix-Hallpike, but had a sensitivity of only 65%.[43] These estimates were derived from samples of fewer than 30 patients and the gold standard against which these maneuvers are measured is usually clinical judgment, which is arguably subjective.[46] Although the Dix-Hallpike maneuver is sensitive for posterior semicircular canal BPPV, 10% of BPPV affects the horizontal semicircular canal; the Supine Roll test can be used in these cases,[47] but sensitivity and specificity for this test have not been determined. A description of the Supine Roll test is available online at http://www.mayoclinicproceedings.org.

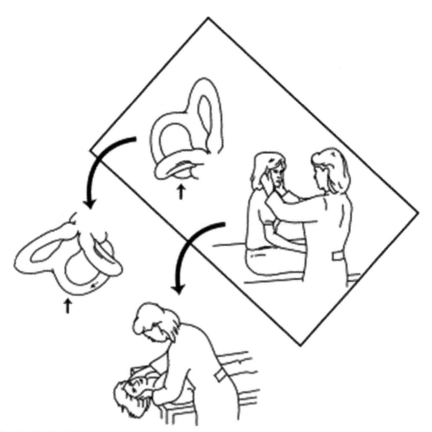

Fig. 2. Dix-Hallpike maneuver. (1) The patient sits upright while the examinee rotates the patient's head 45° to one side. (2) With eyes open, the patient lies back with head hanging slightly below the level of the examination table while the examiner observes for nystagmus and inquires about subjective vertigo. Latency, duration, and direction of nystagmus should be noted. (3) If negative, repeat the maneuver with patient's head rotated to the opposite side. (*From* Tusa RJ. Vertigo. Neurol Clin 2001;19:39; with permission.)

Recent studies have proposed a specific battery of tests termed HINTS (horizontal head impulse test, nystagmus and test of skew) that can be performed at the bedside and with 100% sensitivity and 96% specificity, based on 101 patients identified from an academic hospital ED and inpatient stroke service.[48] Results did not separate ED patients from the stroke service. The accuracy of HINTS and its component tests from a systematic review are shown in **Table 5**. HINTS awaits further validation studies in other patient populations, especially the elderly, before it proves to be an effective prediction rule.[7] A video demonstration of the HINTS battery of tests is available online at http://stroke.ahajournals.org/content/suppl/2009/10/01/STROKEAHA.109.551234.DC1.html.

In a review of the accuracy of dizziness tests involving 26 studies, Dros and colleagues[43] found that none was conducted exclusively in elderly patients; only 1 study reported a median age greater than 65 years (79 years, range 33–90 years) and the remainder of the studies that reported age had a mean age ranging from 47 to 64 years.[49]

Laboratory Tests

Laboratory studies help to rule out metabolic, toxicologic, infectious, and cardiac causes of dizziness. Complete blood counts and basic metabolic panels should, if possible, be interpreted in the context of prior results, as certain chronic abnormalities (eg, anemia, kidney disease) may be more common in the elderly. When a cardiac cause is suspected, clinicians are encouraged to lower their threshold for ordering cardiac enzymes, as acute coronary syndromes can be subtle in the elderly.[50]

Radiologic Studies

CT and MRI studies of the brain are often recommended to investigate serious causes of dizziness. There are currently no guidelines and little evidence to clarify the role of brain imaging studies in dizziness. There is large variation in the use of brain imaging for ED patients with dizziness although increased imaging rates did not translate into higher rates of stroke diagnoses.[9] Given the increasing rates of CT scans in the ED,[51] it is not surprising that a recent study on the efficiency of brain CT scans for patients presenting to the ED with dizziness found that only 6% of all CT scans identified a central nervous system cause, such as a stroke or intracranial mass.[26]

CT scans of the head are used primarily to evaluate for acute intracranial bleeds, skeletal injuries, anatomic changes (hydrocephalus, midline shift, cerebral atrophy), or space-occupying lesions. The sensitivity of CT scans in diagnosing acute ischemic strokes is poor (16%).[7] Diffusion-weighted MRI is more sensitive, especially for pathology in the posterior circulation but is far from perfect, with only 83% sensitivity overall and 80% in the first 24 hours.[7,52]

Among northern California hospitals, there was a 1.5-fold difference in the use of head CT and a 6.4-fold difference in the use of brain MRI for patients with dizziness in the ED, even after adjusting for site differences. Higher use of CT and MRI did not translate into an increase in stroke diagnosis.[9]

In a retrospective study of ED patients with vertigo or dizziness based on ICD-9 codes who underwent a head CT scan, only 2.2% (10/448) of initial head CT scans had a positive finding, and of those, only 7 of the 10 represented an acute process. Of the 448 initial studies, 87 received a follow-up MRI within an unspecified time period, but MRI changed the CT diagnosis from a false-negative to a true-positive process in 16% of cases and acutely in 8% of cases. The investigators concluded that CT had a low diagnostic yield, and from a cost standpoint, represented only $1 of usefulness for every $63.81 of CT expenditure, although the potential cost savings associated with hospitalization and overall costs of a misdiagnosed case were not included in the analysis.[53] Another study found a 0% diagnostic yield for stroke or other intracranial abnormalities from head CT of 344 ED patients and concluded that head CT studies were not cost-effective for the evaluation of dizziness.[54]

TREATMENT OF DIZZINESS
Pharmacologic Therapies for Vertigo Symptoms

There are 2 categories of pharmacologic therapies for dizziness (**Table 7**): those that offer symptom relief and those that are disease specific. Symptom relief medications are known as vestibular suppressants, which can be used to reduce the sensation of movement in vertigo and, in some cases, the associated motion sickness symptoms (usually nausea, vomiting, or diarrhea).

Unfortunately there are few high-quality studies confirming the efficacy of these medications. Meclizine is the most commonly used medication for vestibular

Table 7
Vestibular suppressants

Medication (Examples in Parentheses)	Proposed Mechanism	Considerations for Use in Older Adults
Antihistamines (meclizine, diphenhydramine, dimenhydrinate)	Suppress histamine activity in brain vomiting center, also block acetylcholinergic activity	On the Beers list[55] of potentially inappropriate medications for older adults due to concern for anticholinergic side effects[a]
Benzodiazepines (diazepam, lorazepam)	Enhance inhibitory effect of γ-aminobutyric acid in vestibular system	On the Beers list of potentially inappropriate medications for older adults due to concern for cognitive impairment, falls, fractures, and motor vehicle accidents
Calcium channel antagonists (flunarizine, cinnarizine)	Directly suppress vestibular activity, also some central anticholinergic and/or antihistaminic activity	Not available in United States Similar adverse effects to antihistamines
Metoclopramide	Blocks dopamine activity in brain's chemoreceptor trigger zone	On the Beers list of potentially inappropriate medications for older adults due to extrapyramidal side effects
Phenothiazines (prochlorperazine, promethazine)	Block various neurotransmitter (dopamine, histamine, acetylcholine) activity in brain	On the Beers list of potentially inappropriate medications for older adults due to concern for anticholinergic side effects[a]
Anticholinergics (scopolamine)	Block acetylcholinergic activity in vestibular nucleus of brain	On the Beers list of potentially inappropriate medications for older adults due to concern for anticholinergic side effects[a]

[a] Anticholinergic side effects include confusion, dry mouth, constipation, blurry vision, and urinary retention.
Data from American Geriatrics Society Beers Criteria Update Expert Panel. American Geriatrics Society updated Beers Criteria for potentially inappropriate medication use in older adults. J Am Geriatr Soc 2012;60(4):616–31; Hain TC, Uddin M. Pharmacologic treatment of vertigo. CNS Drugs 2003;17(2):85–100; and Rudolph JL, Salow MJ, Angelini MC, et al. The anticholinergic risk scale and anticholinergic adverse effects in older persons. Arch Intern Med 2008;168(5):508–13.

diagnoses in the United States.[56] A literature search revealed only 2 randomized controlled trials of meclizine for symptoms of vertigo. One randomized, double-blind, placebo-controlled study of 12 subjects reported that meclizine was no better than placebo for reducing vertigo symptoms on the first day of treatment, although it was superior to placebo by the seventh day.[57] Another study of 40 subjects demonstrated that meclizine was equivalent to thiethylperazine in reducing symptoms of vertigo.[58]

Vestibular suppressants are not appropriate for BPPV and should not be used indiscriminately for all types of vertigo.[47,59] One study of ED management of vestibular diagnoses throughout the United States demonstrated the widespread inappropriate use of meclizine (which was prescribed in 59% of cases of BPPV). They noted that physicians were prescribing vestibular suppressants for the diagnosis of dizziness without tailoring therapy to address the specific cause of the dizziness, such as the significant underuse of corticosteroids for vestibular neuritis.[56]

Current recommendations are that vestibular suppressants should be used for acute vertigo only and should be tapered quickly, because of concerns that these medications inhibit the brain's natural ability to compensate for vertigo over time.[33,60,61] Most medications used to treat vertigo are associated with a high risk of adverse effects for older adults (see **Table 7**), so prescribing these medications appropriately is all the more difficult in the geriatric population. One common practice that should certainly be avoided in older patients is the prescription of 2 medications simultaneously for vertigo: one to suppress the vertigo itself and another to combat associated nausea. The risk of adverse drug reactions and drug interactions in older patients increases significantly as the number of medications increases.

Bottom line: Disease-specific therapies and vestibular rehabilitation are preferred over nonspecific symptomatic treatment. All the vestibular suppressants are considered high risk for use in older adults, so they should be reserved for extreme cases when symptoms are severely limiting. In those cases, a vestibular suppressant such as meclizine can be used at the lowest possible dose for the shortest possible time. Patients should receive counseling on the risks of these medications at the time they are prescribed.

Therapies Directed at Specific Diagnoses

It is worthwhile focusing on disease-specific pharmacologic treatment of the 3 most common causes of peripheral vertigo.

BPPV

Current guidelines recommend avoiding vestibular suppressants in favor of canalith repositioning maneuvers, such as the Epley maneuver, and possibly also pursuing vestibular rehabilitation.[47,59] This recommendation is based on 2 studies[62,63] of vestibular suppressants, one of which failed to show superiority to placebo and another that showed that canalith repositioning maneuvers were superior to medication. Vestibular suppressants can be used for brief periods in patients with severe symptoms, especially if needed for patients to be able to tolerate canalith repositioning maneuvers.

The Epley maneuver (**Fig. 3**) is used to reposition canaliths in the posterior semicircular canal.[64,65] Epley reported a 100% success rate in his series of 30 patients.[65] This maneuver has been shown to be both easy to use and effective at diagnosing BPPV by general practitioners in the clinic.[66] In the ED, the Epley maneuver has been reported to be efficacious versus a sham maneuver in 1 randomized clinical trial that used a 10-point vertigo severity score. In this study, Epley-treated patients reported a median

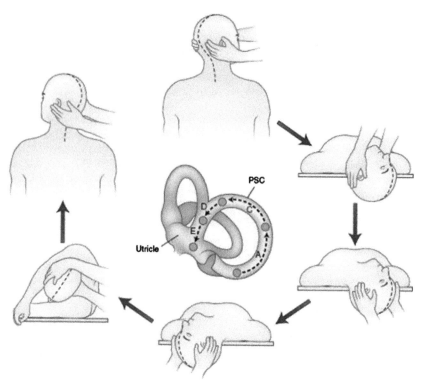

Fig. 3. Epley maneuver. (1) The patient sits upright with head turned 45° toward the affected ear. (2) Lay the patient down with head hanging slightly below the level of the examination table for 30 seconds. (3) Turn the head 90° toward the unaffected side and hold for 30 seconds. (4) Roll the patient onto his or her side to turn the head a further 90° toward the unaffected side. The head should now be almost facing the floor. Hold for 30 seconds. (5) Sit patient upright. (6) Some experts recommend keeping head upright for 24 hours after the maneuver. (*From* Rakel RE. Conn's current therapy 1995. Philadelphia: WB Saunders; 1995. p. 839; with permission.)

improvement of 6 points and sham-treated patients 1 point improvement ($P = .001$).[67] One reported complication following the Epley maneuver was the sensation of falling.[68]

Bottom line: Canalith repositioning maneuvers are first-line treatment; use of vestibular suppressants should be avoided.

Vestibular neuritis

Vestibular suppressants can be useful for symptomatic relief of vestibular neuritis when used in the first 3 days of symptoms.[69,70] In addition, corticosteroids have been demonstrated to speed up the resolution of symptoms.[61] In a prospective randomized, double-blind trial of methylprednisolone, valacyclovir, or placebo involving 141 patients with vestibular neuritis, methylprednisolone increased the recovery of vestibular function from 40% to 62% 1 year after onset of symptoms.[71] The mean age of the subjects in this study was 46 to 52 years; the oldest subject was 71 years old. Antiviral medication was not useful.[71] A subsequent prospective, randomized, controlled trial of 30 patients showed that prednisone may enhance early recovery, but the oldest subject was 72 years old and the mean age was 48 years.[72] However, a recent meta-analysis of 3 prospective, randomized, controlled trials (including the 2 studies mentioned earlier) reported that although caloric testing results were improved with corticosteroids, symptomatic recovery from acute vestibular neuritis was not, thus casting some uncertainty on the role of steroids.[73] Another important factor in the management of this condition is that, in some patients, symptoms may persist for months to years, so if after 3 days the patient still has significant symptoms, a referral for vestibular rehabilitation should be made.

Bottom line: In days 1 to 3 of symptom onset, the authors still advocate the use of steroids (prednisone 1 mg/kg initially tapered off over 20 days) in older patients in whom steroids are low risk. Vestibular suppressants can be added for symptom relief, but should be stopped after day 3. Symptoms usually resolve spontaneously even without treatment.[70]

Meniere's disease

There is little evidence to guide the management of Meniere's disease.[61] Betahistine is an antihistamine available in Europe, but a Cochrane review in 2001 concluded there was insufficient evidence to confirm efficacy for Meniere's disease.[74] Other commonly used treatments include those aimed at lowering endolymphatic pressure, such as maintaining a diet low in sodium (less than 1–2 g of salt daily) and diuretics (usually a combination of hydrochlorothiazide and triamterene). These treatments have not been rigorously evaluated for efficacy. A 2006 Cochrane review identified no articles that met their threshold for inclusion.[75] Patients who fail medical management are usually sent for surgical interventions, including endolymphatic sac decompression and intratympanic injections.[76]

Bottom line: Although there is little high-quality evidence to support any of the current treatments, a low-salt diet and diuretics are generally better tolerated by older adults than antihistamines or other vestibular suppressants. Systemic steroids can also be tried in patients who are low risk, but if symptoms are difficult to control medically, surgical interventions may be required.

Other conditions with disease-specific therapies

Vestibular migraine responds well to antimigraine therapies.[60,61,76] Psychogenic vertigo should be treated with benzodiazepines or antidepressants.[60] Episodic ataxia type 2 responds to acetazolamide and 4-aminopyridine can also be used, although this is based on several nonrandomized studies.[61]

Vestibular Rehabilitation

Several studies have shown the benefits of vestibular rehabilitation, which is a structured program of movement exercises aimed at retraining the vestibular system to decrease symptoms and permit return to normal activities.[77–81] Unfortunately, these studies tend to be small and inconsistent in the type of vestibular rehabilitation and outcomes measured. Vestibular rehabilitation is delivered by a specially trained physical or occupational therapist, however, 1 study demonstrated that nurses in a primary care clinic can be trained to administer effective vestibular rehabilitation.[77] Currently, this therapeutic option is used in only a small fraction of patients with chronic dizziness.[82] Although vestibular rehabilitation is effective for most patients, 10% to 66% of patients do not experience improvement in symptoms.[82,83] Research is needed to better define which patients are most likely to benefit from vestibular rehabilitation.[83]

Any patient can be referred for vestibular rehabilitation from the ED, but those most likely to benefit are those suffering from acute or chronic vertigo caused by peripheral vestibular dysfunction.[84] Vestibular rehabilitation is also appropriate for patients with central causes of vertigo, although complete recovery is rare.[79,84] Because of the risks associated with vestibular suppressant medications for older patients, vestibular rehabilitation is an important and underused option for treatment of vertigo. For patients unable to complete formal vestibular rehabilitation, a simple regimen of low-level physical activity has been shown to help elderly patients with chronic dizziness overcome a fear of falling and improve quality of life.[85]

OUTPATIENT AND PREHOSPITAL MANAGEMENT OF THE DIZZY PATIENT

The evaluation and management of dizziness can be challenging due to (1) the subjective nature of the patient's symptom complaint, (2) the absence of an objective and reliable measure of dizziness, and (3) the suboptimal accuracy of bedside examinations.

Therefore, the authors propose the following courses of action. If the patient has an established benign and recurrent condition, such as BPPV, and is being evaluated by the primary care provider most familiar with the patient, then the physician can take a conservative route. This course relies on an office-based evaluation and focuses on symptomatic relief. However, if the physician suspects a more serious cause, then more in-depth evaluation is required.

As cardiovascular and cerebrovascular causes are two of the more worrisome causes of dizziness,[26,86] this subset of patients with suspected serious causes should be referred to the ED.[4] The purpose of this emergent referral is to rule out a stroke or cardiac event. In preparation, a complete medical and medication history will be most helpful to the ED, especially information on allergies and use of anticoagulants. More importantly, communicating the neurologic examination in the clinic to the ED physician will help establish a baseline and determine if neurologic deficits are progressing.

Outpatient providers should avoid any delay if a stroke is suspected to optimize the time to treatment, especially if the patient might be a candidate for thrombolysis of ischemic strokes. In such situations, immediate transfer to the nearest ED by emergency medical services is recommended. The treatment window for acute thrombolysis with tissue plasminogen activator (t-PA) in acute ischemic stroke has traditionally been designated as 3 hours beginning at the onset of symptoms.[87] Subsequent treatment trials, however, have extended the treatment window to 4.5 hours; cerebrovascular reperfusion therapy for appropriate patients within this extended treatment window enhances favorable disability outcomes at 90 days (52.4% vs 45.2%; odds ratio [OR] 1.34, 95% confidence interval [CI] 1.02–1.76) at the cost of higher rates of intracranial hemorrhages (27.0% vs 17.6%; $P = .001$) but without significant difference in 90-day mortality (7.7% vs 8.4%; $P = .68$).[88]

ED MANAGEMENT

Patients whose dizziness symptoms are new or different from previous episodes are of particular concern. The priority for the ED is to rule out a dangerous cause of dizziness. In particular, an ST-segment elevation myocardial infarction (STEMI) and an acute stroke must be ruled out, as these two disease entities have a specific time window within which optimal treatment should be administered.[87–90] Screening for an acute stroke is enhanced by the use of the Cincinnati Prehospital Stroke Scale, which has been demonstrated to be reproducible and valid.[91] The process of ruling out STEMI, stroke, and other serious causes of dizziness benefits from the process of ruling in a peripheral vestibular cause.[4] A recommended ED diagnostic pathway is shown in **Fig. 4**.

Both CT and MRI are imperfect studies, and even negative results do not rule out a stroke with absolute certainty. In cases of suspected stroke with negative MRI

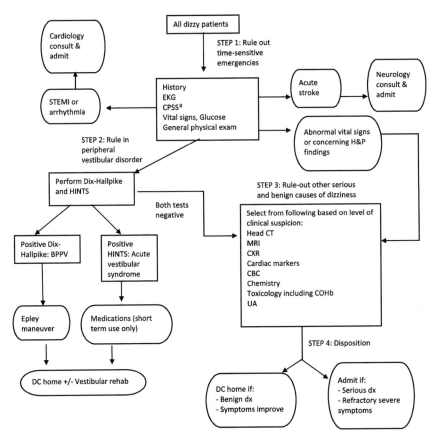

Fig. 4. A recommended pathway for the ED management of the older dizzy patient. [a] CPSS, Cincinnati Pre-Hospital Stroke Scale, a 3-item stroke scale designed for rapid screening for stroke by evaluating for facial droop, arm drift, and abnormal speech. The scale is reproducible (interclass correlation 0.92, 95% CI 0.89–0.93), with any of the 3 items having a sensitivity of 66% and a specificity of 87%. (*Data from* Kothari RU, Pancioli A, Liu T, et al. Cincinnati Prehospital Stroke Scale: reproducibility and validity. Ann Emerg Med 1999;33(4):373–8.)

studies, the ED physician should consult a neurologist and may choose to admit the patient for close observation and repeat MRI if the suspicion for stroke is strong, given the imperfect sensitivity of MRI in the acute setting.[7] In a single academic center, dizziness accounted for 16% of all neurology consultations from the ED.[92] In some cases, an otolaryngologist may also be consulted for vestibular problems refractory to conventional therapy (medications, canalith repositioning maneuvers).

CLINICAL AND MEDICOLEGAL PITFALLS

Given the complexities of diagnosing and managing dizziness in the elderly, it is reasonable to anticipate that unintentional errors may occur.

Few studies have evaluated the accuracy of physician's dizziness assessments. Royl and colleagues[93] found that among German patients presenting with vertigo to the ED, 44% of the diagnoses were incorrect, based on further evaluation by neurologists. Seven percent of patients had a more serious diagnosis mistaken as benign, and 23% were given a serious diagnosis that was later labeled benign. A Canadian study of 493 neurologic consultations from the ED for all neurologic problems found agreement between the referring ED physician and the final diagnosis by the neurologist in only 66% of cases, disagreement between ED diagnosis and final neurologist diagnosis in 17%, and disagreement between both ED diagnosis and initial neurologist diagnosis and the final neurologist diagnosis in 5%. In addition, the consulting neurologist's initial diagnosis agreed with the final neurologist diagnosis 80% of the time.[94] As many as 35% of patients presenting to the ED with dizziness that was ultimately confirmed as cerebrovascular events were initially misdiagnosed.[26]

Presently, no ED-based prediction rule exists to guide the diagnosis of stroke in patients presenting with dizziness. Data from Hong Kong showed that age 65 years or more (OR = 6.13, 95% CI 1.97–19.09), ataxia symptoms (OR = 11.39, 95% CI 2.404–53.95), focal neurologic symptoms (OR = 11.78, 95% CI 1.61–86.29), previous stroke (OR = 3.89, 95% CI 1.12–13.46), and diabetes mellitus (OR = 3.57, 95% CI 1.04–12.28) predicted central causes of dizziness.[95] Kerber and colleagues[96] found that the description of nystagmus in the ED medical records conflicted with the ED physician's diagnosis of peripheral vestibular process in 81% of cases. Using NHAMCS data, Newman-Toker and colleagues[56] concluded that there is overuse of CT and underuse of MRI in patients given a final diagnosis of BPPV or acute vestibular syndrome. These studies suggest that targeted specialized training for ED staff and trainees can be helpful in the diagnosis and management of dizziness.

Given the difficulties in identifying the true cause of an older patient's dizziness, it may be tempting to adopt a conservative approach to disposition and simply hospitalize all elderly patients presenting with dizziness. Recent data caution against this approach, as hospital admissions for older adults independently increase the risk of loss of independence, decline in function, and delirium.[97,98]

Although the geriatric patient with dizziness represents a high-risk population, an intracranial hemorrhage is unlikely.[9,27] Safe disposition can be extremely difficult, especially if the dizziness has not resolved. If available, a geriatric consultation is recommended. Alternatively, either a discussion with the patient's primary care provider or a more thorough patient assessment that includes function and home safety assessment may be helpful. However, in a busy setting, such as a high-volume ED, the latter is not practical. In such situations, admitting the patient to obtain a more comprehensive workup will prove to be the best approach. If a dizzy patient is sent home directly from the ED, it is essential to ensure that a family member or friend is available to provide 24-hour supervision until the symptoms abate or resolve.

The dizzy patient is at increased risk for falls[99] and fall-related injuries[100] and therefore must be carefully evaluated for injuries. Head trauma can result in short-term amnesia, which further complicates the history. Subtle fractures may also be less apparent on plain radiographs in the setting of significant osteopenia. If acute traumatic injuries in the setting of dizziness are suspected, a thorough trauma assessment, including primary, secondary, and tertiary surveys, may be indicated.

Any physician attempting either the Epley or horizontal head impulse test in the older patient must exercise caution and avoid forceful or jarring movements. No specific traumatic injuries involving the Epley maneuver have been reported. However, the medical literature includes several case reports of serious complications after spinal manipulation, including vertebral fracture, spinal cord injury, vertebrobasilar vascular injury, and disk herniation.[101,102] Allowing the patients to move their heads at their own pace during the HINTS test may optimize patient safety.

DISCHARGE FROM THE ED

At discharge, patients diagnosed with peripheral vestibular dizziness or in whom a life-threatening cause has been ruled out, should be provided with the following:

Referral: Patients should be referred to their primary care provider for follow-up within 1 to 2 weeks or sooner if symptoms return. Referral for vestibular rehabilitation, if available locally, can help patients with vestibular retraining.

Treatment: When indicated, a prescription for any of the medications discussed earlier should be provided. For patients with BPPV, instructions for canalith repositioning maneuvers are helpful. Videos for maneuvers are also available online at www.youtube.com.[103]

Diagnosis: An underlying cause for the dizziness should ideally be given as the diagnosis (eg, vestibular neuritis, hypoglycemia) rather than a symptom (eg, dizziness, vertigo not otherwise specified).

Return instructions: Patients should call the emergency service (9-1-1) and return to the ED for any worrisome signs or symptoms such as (1) signs of stroke (difficulty speaking, sudden loss of vision, sudden weakness, or paralysis), (2) chest pain, (3) difficulty breathing, (4) palpitations or irregular heartbeat, (5) syncope, or (6) head trauma.

FUTURE DIRECTIONS

Further research is needed to optimize the ED management of the dizzy patient. Studies are needed to better understand the epidemiology of dizziness, as well as the diagnostic accuracy of bedside tests, how best to identify patients whose dizziness is due to stroke, and which therapies are best to mitigate the symptoms of vertigo. Disease-specific therapies also need extensive investigation. Cost-effectiveness studies would be invaluable in optimizing ED management. Older adults should be a particular focus of future research, as diagnosis can be more challenging and treatment options are limited. This type of research is challenging because of the lack of consistent diagnostic criteria, the wide diversity of causes of dizziness, the rarity of some of the causes, and because symptoms often resolve spontaneously with time.

SUMMARY

As shown by the often discrepant data on geriatric dizziness, there is limited evidence to guide bedside diagnostic, therapeutic, or disposition decision making for the geriatric patient with dizziness in the ED. Sloan and Dallara[3] compared the evidence on geriatric dizziness with the story of the three blind men, each of whom described different parts of the elephant and had different impressions of what an elephant looks like. Despite such ambiguity, dizziness is a common complaint. The clinician is faced with the dilemma of choosing between taking a conservative approach by assuming a benign cause or committing costly and increasingly limited resources to pursue a relatively infrequent but potentially devastating underlying cause. It is our hope that future research will illuminate the true nature of the elephant.

REFERENCES

1. Newman-Toker DE, Hsieh YH, Camargo CA Jr, et al. Spectrum of dizziness visits to US emergency departments: cross-sectional analysis from a nationally representative sample. Mayo Clin Proc 2008;83(7):765–75.

2. Kerber KA, Meurer WJ, West BT, et al. Dizziness presentations in U.S. emergency departments, 1995-2004. Acad Emerg Med 2008;15(8):744–50.
3. Sloane PD, Dallara J. Clinical research and geriatric dizziness: the blind men and the elephant. J Am Geriatr Soc 1999;47(1):113–4.
4. Kerber KA. Vertigo and dizziness in the emergency department. Emerg Med Clin North Am 2009;27(1):39–50, viii.
5. Sloane PD, Coeytaux RR, Beck RS, et al. Dizziness: state of the science. Ann Intern Med 2001;134(9 Pt 2):823–32.
6. Tinetti ME, Williams CS, Gill TM. Dizziness among older adults: a possible geriatric syndrome. Ann Intern Med 2000;132(5):337–44.
7. Tarnutzer AA, Berkowitz AL, Robinson KA, et al. Does my dizzy patient have a stroke? A systematic review of bedside diagnosis in acute vestibular syndrome. CMAJ 2011;183(9):E571–92.
8. Kerber KA, Fendrick AM. The evidence base for the evaluation and management of dizziness. J Eval Clin Pract 2010;16(1):186–91.
9. Kim AS, Sidney S, Klingman JG, et al. Practice variation in neuroimaging to evaluate dizziness in the ED. Am J Emerg Med 2012;30(5):665–72.
10. Lin HW, Bhattacharyya N. Balance disorders in the elderly: epidemiology and functional impact. Laryngoscope 2012;122(8):1858–61.
11. Agrawal Y, Carey JP, Della Santina CC, et al. Disorders of balance and vestibular function in US adults: data from the National Health and Nutrition Examination Survey, 2001-2004. Arch Intern Med 2009;169(10):938–44.
12. Stevens KN, Lang IA, Guralnik JM, et al. Epidemiology of balance and dizziness in a national population: findings from the English longitudinal study of ageing. Age Ageing 2008;37(3):300–5.
13. Maarsingh OR, Dros J, Schellevis FG, et al. Dizziness reported by elderly patients in family practice: prevalence, incidence, and clinical characteristics. BMC Fam Pract 2010;11:2.
14. Sloane P, Blazer D, George LK. Dizziness in a community elderly population. J Am Geriatr Soc 1989;37(2):101–8.
15. Herr RD, Zun L, Mathews JJ. A directed approach to the dizzy patient. Ann Emerg Med 1989;18(6):664–72.
16. Kroenke K, Lucas CA, Rosenberg ML, et al. Causes of persistent dizziness. A prospective study of 100 patients in ambulatory care. Ann Intern Med 1992;117(11):898–904.
17. Savitz SI, Caplan LR, Edlow JA. Pitfalls in the diagnosis of cerebellar infarction. Acad Emerg Med 2007;14(1):63–8.
18. Neuhauser HK, Radtke A, von Brevern M, et al. Burden of dizziness and vertigo in the community. Arch Intern Med 2008;168(19):2118–24.
19. Pluijm SM, Smit JH, Tromp EA, et al. A risk profile for identifying community-dwelling elderly with a high risk of recurrent falling: results of a 3-year prospective study. Osteoporos Int 2006;17(3):417–25.
20. Tinetti ME. Clinical practice. Preventing falls in elderly persons. N Engl J Med 2003;348(1):42–9.
21. Herdman SJ, Blatt P, Schubert MC, et al. Falls in patients with vestibular deficits. Am J Otol 2000;21(6):847–51.
22. Gaetani P, Revay M, Sciacca S, et al. Traumatic brain injury in the elderly: considerations in a series of 103 patients older than 70. J Neurosurg Sci 2012;56(3):231–7.
23. Fortuna GR, Mueller EW, James LE, et al. The impact of preinjury antiplatelet and anticoagulant pharmacotherapy on outcomes in elderly patients with hemorrhagic brain injury. Surgery 2008;144(4):598–603 [discussion: 603–5].

24. Dros J, Maarsingh OR, Beem L, et al. Impact of dizziness on everyday life in older primary care patients: a cross-sectional study. Health Qual Life Outcomes 2011;9:44.
25. Murphy SL, Dubin JA, Gill TM. The development of fear of falling among community-living older women: predisposing factors and subsequent fall events. J Gerontol A Biol Sci Med Sci 2003;58(10):M943–7.
26. Kerber KA, Brown DL, Lisabeth LD, et al. Stroke among patients with dizziness, vertigo, and imbalance in the emergency department: a population-based study. Stroke 2006;37(10):2484–7.
27. Kerber KA, Burke JF, Brown DL, et al. Does intracerebral haemorrhage mimic benign dizziness presentations? A population based study. Emerg Med J 2012;29(1):43–6.
28. Newman-Toker DE, Cannon LM, Stofferahn ME, et al. Imprecision in patient reports of dizziness symptom quality: a cross-sectional study conducted in an acute care setting. Mayo Clin Proc 2007;82(11):1329–40.
29. Stanton VA, Hsieh YH, Camargo CA, et al. Overreliance on symptom quality in diagnosing dizziness: results of a multicenter survey of emergency physicians. Mayo Clin Proc 2007;82(11):1319–28.
30. Drachman DA, Hart CW. An approach to the dizzy patient. Neurology 1972; 22(4):323–34.
31. Sloane PD, Baloh RW. Persistent dizziness in geriatric patients. J Am Geriatr Soc 1989;37(11):1031–8.
32. Lawson J, Fitzgerald J, Birchall J, et al. Diagnosis of geriatric patients with severe dizziness. J Am Geriatr Soc 1999;47(1):12–7.
33. Tusa RJ, Gore R. Dizziness and vertigo: emergencies and management. Neurol Clin 2012;30(1):61–74, vii–viii.
34. Navi BB, Kamel H, Shah MP, et al. Application of the ABCD2 score to identify cerebrovascular causes of dizziness in the emergency department. Stroke 2012;43(6):1484–9.
35. Rothwell PM, Giles MF, Flossmann E, et al. A simple score (ABCD) to identify individuals at high early risk of stroke after transient ischaemic attack. Lancet 2005;366(9479):29–36.
36. Johnston SC, Rothwell PM, Nguyen-Huynh MN, et al. Validation and refinement of scores to predict very early stroke risk after transient ischaemic attack. Lancet 2007;369(9558):283–92.
37. Maarsingh OR, van der Wouden JC. Letter by Maarsingh and van der Wouden regarding article, "Application of the ABCD2 score to identify cerebrovascular causes of dizziness in the emergency department". Stroke 2012;43(8):e78 [author reply: e79].
38. Maarsingh OR, Dros J, Schellevis FG, et al. Causes of persistent dizziness in elderly patients in primary care. Ann Fam Med 2010;8(3):196–205.
39. Chawla N, Olshaker JS. Diagnosis and management of dizziness and vertigo. Med Clin North Am 2006;90(2):291–304.
40. Ishiyama G, Ishiyama A, Kerber K, et al. Gentamicin ototoxicity: clinical features and the effect on the human vestibulo-ocular reflex. Acta Otolaryngol 2006; 126(10):1057–61.
41. Adams ME, Heidenreich KD, Kileny PR. Audiovestibular testing in patients with Meniere's disease. Otolaryngol Clin North Am 2010;43(5):995–1009.
42. von Brevern M, Zeise D, Neuhauser H, et al. Acute migrainous vertigo: clinical and oculographic findings. Brain 2005;128(Pt 2):365–74.
43. Dros J, Maarsingh OR, van der Horst HE, et al. Tests used to evaluate dizziness in primary care. CMAJ 2010;182(13):E621–31.

44. Hotson JR, Baloh RW. Acute vestibular syndrome. N Engl J Med 1998;339(10): 680–5.

45. Dix MR, Hallpike CS. The pathology symptomatology and diagnosis of certain common disorders of the vestibular system. Proc R Soc Med 1952;45(6): 341–54.

46. Halker RB, Barrs DM, Wellik KE, et al. Establishing a diagnosis of benign paroxysmal positional vertigo through the Dix-Hallpike and side-lying maneuvers: a critically appraised topic. Neurologist 2008;14(3):201–4.

47. Bhattacharyya N, Baugh RF, Orvidas L, et al. Clinical practice guideline: benign paroxysmal positional vertigo. Otolaryngol Head Neck Surg 2008;139(5 Suppl 4):S47–81.

48. Kattah JC, Talkad AV, Wang DZ, et al. HINTS to diagnose stroke in the acute vestibular syndrome: three-step bedside oculomotor examination more sensitive than early MRI diffusion-weighted imaging. Stroke 2009;40(11):3504–10.

49. Chan TP. Is benign paroxysmal positional vertigo underdiagnosed in hospitalised patients? Hong Kong Med J 2008;14(3):198–202.

50. Canto JG, Fincher C, Kiefe CI, et al. Atypical presentations among Medicare beneficiaries with unstable angina pectoris. Am J Cardiol 2002;90(3):248–53.

51. Kocher KE, Meurer WJ, Fazel R, et al. National trends in use of computed tomography in the emergency department. Ann Emerg Med 2011;58(5): 452–462.e3.

52. Chalela JA, Kidwell CS, Nentwich LM, et al. Magnetic resonance imaging and computed tomography in emergency assessment of patients with suspected acute stroke: a prospective comparison. Lancet 2007;369(9558):293–8.

53. Lawhn-Heath C, Buckle C, Christoforidis G, et al. Utility of head CT in the evaluation of vertigo/dizziness in the emergency department. Emerg Radiol 2012. [Epub ahead of print].

54. Wasay M, Dubey N, Bakshi R. Dizziness and yield of emergency head CT scan: is it cost effective? Emerg Med J 2005;22(4):312.

55. American Geriatrics Society Beers Criteria Update Expert Panel. American Geriatrics Society updated Beers Criteria for potentially inappropriate medication use in older adults. J Am Geriatr Soc 2012;60(4):616–31.

56. Newman-Toker DE, Camargo CA Jr, Hsieh YH, et al. Disconnect between charted vestibular diagnoses and emergency department management decisions: a cross-sectional analysis from a nationally representative sample. Acad Emerg Med 2009;16(10):970–7.

57. Schmitt LG, Shaw JE. Alleviation of induced vertigo. Therapy with transdermal scopolamine and oral meclizine. Arch Otolaryngol Head Neck Surg 1986; 112(1):88–91.

58. Jungert S. Comparative investigation between thiethylperazine and meclizine in vertigo of different genesis. Acta Otorhinolaryngol Belg 1978;32(3):264–72.

59. Fife TD, Iverson DJ, Lempert T, et al. Practice parameter: therapies for benign paroxysmal positional vertigo (an evidence-based review): report of the Quality Standards Subcommittee of the American Academy of Neurology. Neurology 2008;70(22):2067–74.

60. Hain TC, Uddin M. Pharmacological treatment of vertigo. CNS Drugs 2003; 17(2):85–100.

61. Strupp M, Thurtell MJ, Shaikh AG, et al. Pharmacotherapy of vestibular and ocular motor disorders, including nystagmus. J Neurol 2011;258(7):1207–22.

62. McClure JA, Willett JM. Lorazepam and diazepam in the treatment of benign paroxysmal vertigo. J Otolaryngol 1980;9(6):472–7.

63. Salvinelli F, Trivelli M, Casale M, et al. Treatment of benign positional vertigo in the elderly: a randomized trial. Laryngoscope 2004;114(5):827–31.

64. Epley JM. New dimensions of benign paroxysmal positional vertigo. Otolaryngol Head Neck Surg (1979) 1980;88(5):599–605.

65. Epley JM. The canalith repositioning procedure: for treatment of benign paroxysmal positional vertigo. Otolaryngol Head Neck Surg 1992;107(3):399–404.

66. Cranfield S, Mackenzie I, Gabbay M. Can GPs diagnose benign paroxysmal positional vertigo and does the Epley manoeuvre work in primary care? Br J Gen Pract 2010;60(578):698–9.

67. Chang AK, Schoeman G, Hill M. A randomized clinical trial to assess the efficacy of the Epley maneuver in the treatment of acute benign positional vertigo. Acad Emerg Med 2004;11(9):918–24.

68. Uneri A. Falling sensation in patients who undergo the Epley maneuver: a retrospective study. Ear Nose Throat J 2005;84(2):82, 84–5.

69. Walker MF. Treatment of vestibular neuritis. Curr Treat Options Neurol 2009; 11(1):41–5.

70. Baloh RW. Clinical practice. Vestibular neuritis. N Engl J Med 2003;348(11): 1027–32.

71. Strupp M, Zingler VC, Arbusow V, et al. Methylprednisolone, valacyclovir, or the combination for vestibular neuritis. N Engl J Med 2004;351(4):354–61.

72. Shupak A, Issa A, Golz A, et al. Prednisone treatment for vestibular neuritis. Otol Neurotol 2008;29(3):368–74.

73. Goudakos JK, Markou KD, Franco-Vidal V, et al. Corticosteroids in the treatment of vestibular neuritis: a systematic review and meta-analysis. Otol Neurotol 2010;31(2):183–9.

74. James AL, Burton MJ. Betahistine for Meniere's disease or syndrome. Cochrane Database Syst Rev 2001;(1):CD001873.

75. Thirlwall AS, Kundu S. Diuretics for Meniere's disease or syndrome. Cochrane Database Syst Rev 2006;(3):CD003599.

76. Swartz R, Longwell P. Treatment of vertigo. Am Fam Physician 2005;71(6): 1115–22.

77. Yardley L, Donovan-Hall M, Smith HE, et al. Effectiveness of primary care-based vestibular rehabilitation for chronic dizziness. Ann Intern Med 2004;141(8): 598–605.

78. Strupp M, Arbusow V, Maag KP, et al. Vestibular exercises improve central vestibulospinal compensation after vestibular neuritis. Neurology 1998;51(3): 838–44.

79. Kammerlind AS, Hakansson JK, Skogsberg MC. Effects of balance training in elderly people with nonperipheral vertigo and unsteadiness. Clin Rehabil 2001;15(5):463–70.

80. Venosa AR, Bittar RS. Vestibular rehabilitation exercises in acute vertigo. Laryngoscope 2007;117(8):1482–7.

81. Yardley L, Barker F, Muller I, et al. Clinical and cost effectiveness of booklet based vestibular rehabilitation for chronic dizziness in primary care: single blind, parallel group, pragmatic, randomised controlled trial. BMJ 2012;344:e2237.

82. Krebs DE, Gill-Body KM, Parker SW, et al. Vestibular rehabilitation: useful but not universally so. Otolaryngol Head Neck Surg 2003;128(2):240–50.

83. Hall CD, Cox LC. The role of vestibular rehabilitation in the balance disorder patient. Otolaryngol Clin North Am 2009;42(1):161–9, xi.

84. Whitney SL, Rossi MM. Efficacy of vestibular rehabilitation. Otolaryngol Clin North Am 2000;33(3):659–72.

85. Ekwall A, Lindberg A, Magnusson M. Dizzy - why not take a walk? Low level physical activity improves quality of life among elderly with dizziness. Gerontology 2009;55(6):652–9.

86. Newman-Toker DE, Dy FJ, Stanton VA, et al. How often is dizziness from primary cardiovascular disease true vertigo? A systematic review. J Gen Intern Med 2008;23(12):2087–94.

87. Tissue plasminogen activator for acute ischemic stroke. The National Institute of Neurological Disorders and Stroke rt-PA Stroke Study Group. N Engl J Med 1995;333(24):1581–7.

88. Hacke W, Kaste M, Bluhmki E, et al. Thrombolysis with alteplase 3 to 4.5 hours after acute ischemic stroke. N Engl J Med 2008;359(13):1317–29.

89. Cannon CP, Braunwald E. Time to reperfusion: the critical modulator in thrombolysis and primary angioplasty. J Thromb Thrombolysis 1996;3(2):117–25.

90. Zijlstra F, Patel A, Jones M, et al. Clinical characteristics and outcome of patients with early (<2 h), intermediate (2-4 h) and late (>4 h) presentation treated by primary coronary angioplasty or thrombolytic therapy for acute myocardial infarction. Eur Heart J 2002;23(7):550–7.

91. Kothari RU, Pancioli A, Liu T, et al. Cincinnati Prehospital Stroke Scale: reproducibility and validity. Ann Emerg Med 1999;33(4):373–8.

92. Hansen CK, Fisher J, Joyce N, et al. Emergency department consultations for patients with neurological emergencies. Eur J Neurol 2011;18(11):1317–22.

93. Royl G, Ploner CJ, Leithner C. Dizziness in the emergency room: diagnoses and misdiagnoses. Eur Neurol 2011;66(5):256–63.

94. Moeller JJ, Kurniawan J, Gubitz GJ, et al. Diagnostic accuracy of neurological problems in the emergency department. Can J Neurol Sci 2008;35(3): 335–41.

95. Cheung CS, Mak PS, Manley KV, et al. Predictors of important neurological causes of dizziness among patients presenting to the emergency department. Emerg Med J 2010;27(7):517–21.

96. Kerber KA, Morgenstern LB, Meurer WJ, et al. Nystagmus assessments documented by emergency physicians in acute dizziness presentations: a target for decision support? Acad Emerg Med 2011;18(6):619–26.

97. Covinsky KE, Palmer RM, Fortinsky RH, et al. Loss of independence in activities of daily living in older adults hospitalized with medical illnesses: increased vulnerability with age. J Am Geriatr Soc 2003;51(4):451–8.

98. Gill TM, Allore HG, Holford TR, et al. Hospitalization, restricted activity, and the development of disability among older persons. JAMA 2004;292(17): 2115–24.

99. Tinetti ME, Speechley M, Ginter SF. Risk factors for falls among elderly persons living in the community. N Engl J Med 1988;319(26):1701–7.

100. Beckman A, Hansson EE. Fractures in people with dizziness: 5-year follow-up. J Am Geriatr Soc 2011;59(9):1767–9.

101. Stevinson C, Ernst E. Risks associated with spinal manipulation. Am J Med 2002;112(7):566–71.

102. Tamburrelli FC, Genitiempo M, Logroscino CA. Cauda equina syndrome and spine manipulation: case report and review of the literature. Eur Spine J 2011; 20(Suppl 1):S128–31.

103. Kerber KA, Burke JF, Skolarus LE, et al. A prescription for the Epley maneuver: www.youtube.com? Neurology 2012;79(4):376–80.

104. Colledge NR, Wilson JA, MacIntyre CC, et al. The prevalence and characteristics of dizziness in an elderly community. Age Ageing 1994;23(2):117–20.

Emergency Management of Palpitations in the Elderly

Epidemiology, Diagnostic Approaches, and Therapeutic Options

Namirah Jamshed[a],*, Jeffrey Dubin, MD, MBA[a],
Zayd Eldadah, MD, PhD[a],[b]

KEYWORDS

- Palpitations • Emergency department • Arrhythmias • Atrial fibrillation • Elderly

KEY POINTS

- Palpitations are a common reason for presentation to the emergency department.
- Most palpitations are benign but older people have risk factors that make them more vulnerable to cardiac arrhythmias causing palpitations.
- Ambulatory cardiac monitoring maybe useful in high-risk elderly patients with palpitations for further diagnosis.
- Atrial fibrillation is the most common type of arrhythmia in the elderly. Anticoagulation for atrial fibrillation is individualized weighing the risks of bleeding against the benefits of thromboembolic stroke prevention.

INTRODUCTION

Older people often present to the emergency department (ED) with complaints of palpitations. These palpitations are described mostly as a heightened or uncomfortable awareness of the heartbeat.[1] The prevalence of palpitations is as high as 16% in the adult outpatient setting.[2] In a study of the evaluation and outcome of adult patients with palpitations who presented to the ED, clinic, or a hospital, 43% had cardiac disease and 31% had symptoms of anxiety.[3] On further evaluation for those who specifically presented to the ED, 47% had palpitations related to a cardiac cause, 27% caused by psychiatric causes, and the rest were either miscellaneous or of unknown causes.[3]

Although palpitations may indicate the presence of a life-threatening cardiac arrhythmia, they are mostly benign. Fewer than half of the patients presenting with

The authors have no conflicts of interest to declare.
[a] MedStar Washington Hospital Center, Georgetown University School of Medicine, Washington, DC, USA; [b] Johns Hopkins University School of Medicine, Baltimore, MD, USA
* Corresponding author.
E-mail address: Namirah.Jamshed@Medstar.net

Clin Geriatr Med 29 (2013) 205–230
http://dx.doi.org/10.1016/j.cger.2012.10.003
0749-0690/13/$ – see front matter © 2013 Elsevier Inc. All rights reserved.

palpitations have a pathologic cardiac arrhythmia.[4] The relationship between palpitations and structural heart disease is not particularly robust.[5,6] Weber and Kapoor[3] found that older age, male sex, description of irregular heartbeat, history of coronary artery disease, and palpitations lasting longer than 5 minutes were independent predictors of a cardiac cause. The pretest probability of palpitations reflecting a pathologic cardiac arrhythmia in adult patients with primary cardiac disease is 39%.[4,7] Palpitations are subjective, and there is significant variability among individuals' cardiac rhythm or rate.[8] Among the elderly, palpitations caused by arrhythmias can be a significant cause of falls, physical disability, and frequent hospital admissions.[9,10] In addition, older people may be more likely to have cardiac arrhythmias as the source of their palpitations because of the effects of aging on the cardiovascular system.[11,12]

Palpitations may also be associated with noncardiac causes, such as fever, anemia, and anxiety.[13] Conversely, patients presenting with paroxysmal supraventricular tachycardia (PSVT) may mimic symptoms of panic disorder.[14] In one study, 55% of the patients diagnosed with panic disorder had unrecognized PSVT.[14] Barsky and colleagues[15] studied the prevalence of psychiatric diseases in patients with palpitations who underwent Holter monitoring and found that about 45% had at least one lifetime anxiety or depressive episode. The prevalence of anxiety and major depression was 27.6% and 20.8%, respectively. Palpitations can be debilitating even when benign. Another study showed 84% of the patients who initially presented with palpitations had recurrence.[16] Patients with palpitations had a higher prevalence of panic disorders, other psychological symptoms, and somatization. Functional impairment in patients with recurrent palpitations is also a significant issue. A 10-item screening instrument was designed to distinguish patients whose palpitations are more likely to result from panic disorder and in whom monitoring might be avoided, but this decision tool requires further validation and has not been tested in the ED setting.[17] Many patients with palpitations may indeed have an underlying psychiatric disorder, but it is important to carefully explore all other differentials before making a final diagnosis, especially in the elderly population.

QUALITY OF LIFE

Palpitations can impair quality of life. Weber and Kapoor[3] noted that 77% of patients with palpitations experienced a recurrence. One-third of the patients reported that they had difficulty performing house chores, 19% complained of decreased working ability, and 12% of those who worked had to take time off. However, the mean of patients in this population was 46. Barsky and colleagues[16] confirmed these finding in a subsequent prospective study on 145 adult patients with palpitations. Investigators followed these patients for 6 months and compared them with a group that had no symptoms. The results indicated that patients who presented with palpitations remained symptomatic and had functional impairment over time. In addition, they had a higher incidence of panic attacks and psychological symptoms.[16] For older patients with palpitations, this can become an additional chronic problem negatively affecting their quality of life.

DEFINITION

Palpitations are an abnormal awareness of the heartbeat. They are frequently described as fluttering, skipping, pounding, or racing sensations. They may also be described by patients as disagreeable sensations of pulsation or movement in the chest and/or adjacent areas.[18,19] The term is often used to describe patients' subjective perception of a cardiac nature, which may or may not be associated with a cardiac arrhythmia. Because palpitations may be associated with a large number of conditions and causes, they do not have strict clinical correlations. Subjective palpitations may be perfectly normal if experienced during or after vigorous physical activity or emotional stress. These palpitations are typically physiologic and are an expected response to a discrete stimulus or stimuli. Palpitations outside of this norm are pathologic and considered abnormal.[13,19–22]

THE AGING HEART

Aging is associated with cellular and structural changes of the cardiovascular system. There is a reduction of pacemaker cells within the sinoatrial node and degenerative changes in the conduction system.[23] Evidence exists that these changes make the older host more susceptible to cardiac disease. Principal changes include increased stiffness of central elastic arteries,[24] impaired left ventricular filing, increased afterload, and prolonged availability of intracellular calcium. In addition, the elderly exhibit decreased responsiveness to beta-adrenergic receptor stimulation, which limits the increase in heart rate and contractility in response to exercise. Aging is also associated with atrial dilatation, which may increase the risk of atrial fibrillation (AF) and other arrhythmias.[11] **Fig. 1** illustrates the clinical consequences of these changes with aging.[25] All of these changes in the aging heart make it more vulnerable to cardiac arrhythmias as a cause of palpitations.

PATHOPHYSIOLOGY OF CARDIAC ARRHYTHMIAS

Multiple mechanisms can cause palpitations. These palpitations can range from irregular, slow or too rapid contractions of the heart, intense or anomalous contractions of

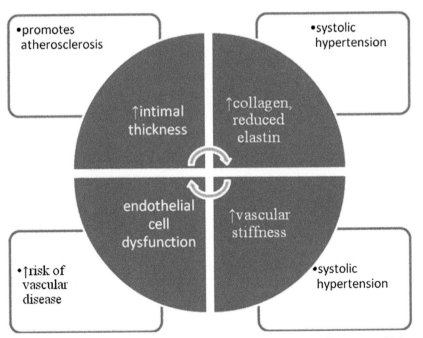

Fig. 1. Age-related changes in the vasculature. (*Data from* Tallis R, Fillit HM. Brocklehurst's textbook of geriatric medicine and gerontology. 6th edition. Philadelphia: Churchill Livingstone; 2003.)

the heart, and/or heterogeneity in the subjective perception of a heartbeat.[26] Cardiac arrhythmias usually result from abnormalities in impulse formation, impulse conduction, or a combination of these mechanisms. Slowed or rapid firing of the sinoatrial (SA) node may result in either sinus bradycardia or sinus tachycardia, respectively. Impulses that originate in the sinus node or elsewhere in the atrium are termed supraventricular and depolarize both atria en route to the atrioventricular (AV) node. The impulse is delayed and processed there before being perpetuated to the His-Purkinje system, which leads to ventricular depolarization. Ventricular activation is normally completed within 120 milliseconds. Ectopic atrial rhythms may originate from any site outside the SA node and can develop as a result of electrolyte disturbances, ischemia, and excessive myocardial fiber stretch as with aging, drugs, and contact with toxins.[27] An impulse that is generated at an ectopic ventricular site, however, cannot reach the Purkinje fibers as rapidly as a normal impulse, and ventricular activation is delayed. The QRS complex from an ectopic ventricular focus is, therefore, wider, signifying aberrant ventricular conduction. Arrhythmias that derive from a supraventricular source typically manifest with a narrow QRS complex. The width of the QRS complex generally can be used to distinguish supraventricular from ventricular arrhythmias. A rapid ventricular rate with a narrow QRS complex indicates an atrial origin.[19] It is useful to identify the presence of atrial activity (P waves) when ventricular rates are rapid. The absence of P waves with an irregular rate suggests AF. A wide QRS complex with tachycardia suggests possible ventricular tachycardia (VT) (vs supraventricular tachycardia [SVT] with aberrant conduction).[28]

EPIDEMIOLOGY OF PALPITATIONS

The variability of the definition of palpitations makes it difficult to make an accurate quantification of the prevalence. There is evidence, however, that palpitations are a common symptom in the general population and in those suffering from heart disease and hypertension.[13] Many older patients have both hypertension and heart disease and, therefore, are more prone to palpitations, which often necessitate a cardiac evaluation. Palpitations are a common presenting symptom to the general practitioner and, after chest pain, a leading cause of cardiology evaluation.[29,30] A study from Netherlands looked at the common reasons for cardiology consultation from noncardiac departments in patients with mean age of 70 years. The most common reasons for the consultation were, suspected heart failure (20%), suspected infective endocarditis (15%), suspected rhythm problems (14%) and suspected acute coronary syndrome (13%).[31] The study concluded that consultation is mostly needed for elderly people with a high prevalence of cardiac disease and high in-house mortality.

Many patients presenting with palpitations may have no underlying cardiac arrhythmia that requires further management. Others, however, have clinically significant arrhythmias. Weber and Kapoor[3] looked at 190 patients who presented with complaints of palpitations to a university medical center. Forty-one percent of these patients had underlying arrhythmias, of which 16% had AF or atrial flutter, 10% had SVT, and 2% had VT. Three percent had structural disease as a cause of their symptom, 31% had a psychosomatic cause, and 4% had systemic causes. Medication and illicit drugs were responsible for about 6% of the underlying cause. Independent risk factors for a cardiac cause included male sex, irregular heartbeat complaints, history of heart disease, and duration of symptoms for more than 5 minutes. In general, older patients and men are more likely to suffer from palpitations because of an underlying arrhythmia when compared with younger and female patients.[3,4,7,32,33]

CAUSE

The cause of palpitations may be divided into cardiac and noncardiac. **Fig. 2** gives an outline of these causes.[34] Older people are often on multiple medications because of comorbid conditions. Drugs that can cause sinus tachycardia include sympathomimetics, anticholinergics, vasodilators, and hydralazine.[35] Abrupt cessations of beta-blockers or new therapy with beta-blockers can both lead patients to complain of palpitations. The latter may occur because of the perception during increased stroke volume and lower heart rate. Other recreational drugs, such as caffeine and nicotine, or illicit drugs can cause sympathetic stimulation and sinus tachycardia leading to the feeling of palpitations even if there is no underlying heart disease.[36,37]

PRESENTATION OF DISEASE

Palpitations occurring in the setting of presyncope, dizziness, or syncope suggests cardiac arrhythmia. A minority of patients may have palpitations during a routine physical examination. It is challenging to document a cardiac rhythm during symptoms. Event monitoring may facilitate this, but the yield depends on the frequency and duration of symptoms. Older patients with an arrhythmia may present with atypical signs and symptoms, such as falls, worsening heart failure, worsening or new angina, delirium, fatigue, or dizzy spells.[10,38] Palpitations can frequently have multiple underlying causes. To be able to attribute them to a cardiac arrhythmia, a rhythm recording is essential; however, obtaining one can be challenging.

DIAGNOSIS AND HISTORICAL CLUES

Patients' age is an important factor to consider when evaluating palpitations. Tachyarrhythmia that may present as palpitations, such as AF, atrial flutter, or atrial tachycardia and VT, are more common in the elderly and are associated with structural heart disease.[32] On the other hand, bradyarrhythmias rarely present with palpitations.[34] A prior history of cardiac disease increases the risk of more serious cardiac

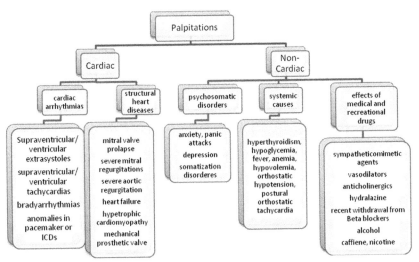

Fig. 2. Cardiac and noncardiac causes of palpitations. ICDs, implantable cardioverter defibrillators.

arrhythmias.[3] A history of panic disorders should also be recorded.[39] It is important to note, however, that patients can have both a psychosomatic disorder and cardiac arrhythmias.[17,20] Family history may not be as important as in younger patients, but a family history of arrhythmogenic right ventricular dysplasia or AF may be helpful in older patients.[40,41]

If possible, patients should be asked to tap out their palpitation. An irregular heartbeat would suggest AF. Patients with polyuria and palpitations may have an SVT caused by the increased atrial pressures stimulating the production of natriuretic peptides.[42] Visible movements of patients' clothes during palpitations, shirt flapping, and fast pounding sensation in the neck may signify AV nodal reentrant tachycardia (AVNRT). This tachycardia occurs when the contraction of the atria against closed valves produces increased right atrial pressures and reflux into the superior vena cava.[43,44] Ventricular arrhythmias are associated with presyncope or syncope.[20] Sinus tachycardia can occur in the setting of panic disorder or hyperthyroidism. In addition, before attributing palpitations to a psychiatric diagnosis, it is important to exclude all other clinically significant causes.[14] **Table 1** outlines further symptom presentation and possible associated cardiac arrhythmias based on history.[34,45]

CARDIAC ARRHYTHMIAS AS A CAUSE OF PALPITATIONS

History and physical examination often aid us in coming to a probable or confirmed diagnosis. Dr Thavendiranathan and colleagues[32] addressed the relationship of palpitations to cardiac arrhythmias. Both male gender and age more than 60 years were associated with a higher likelihood of palpitations caused by a cardiac arrhythmia.[3,4] Moreover, regular rapid-pounding sensation in the neck[44] or visible neck pulsation[46] during palpitations made the diagnosis of AVNRT more likely. The clinical examination was not sufficiently accurate in excluding clinically significant arrhythmias in most patients. Therefore, for most patients, confirmation with electrocardiographic (EKG) monitoring to demonstrate symptoms with rhythm changes is necessary to establish a diagnosis of cardiac arrhythmia in patients who present with palpitations.[32]

The likelihood of cardiac arrhythmia associated with palpitations is higher in patients with cardiac disease,[3] those with palpitations during sleep,[4] and in those who experience palpitations at work.[4] Palpitations that last less than 5 minutes[3] and in patients with a known history of panic disorder are less likely to be associated with a cardiac arrhythmia.[39] **Table 2** summarizes the accuracy of clinical evaluation in identifying clinically significant arrhythmias based on multiple studies.[4,7,15,32]

STANDARD 12-LEAD EKG

The 12-lead EKG is an essential first step in the diagnostic evaluation of palpitations. An EKG obtained during palpitations allows the ED physician to analyze and correlate any abnormal findings with the symptoms. The diagnostic accuracy of a 12-lead EKG is in the range of 3% to 26%.[3,4,7]

AMBULATORY MONITORING

Ambulatory cardiac monitoring allows for more detailed and real-time data. Many patients do not present to the ED in time to get an EKG as they are experiencing the palpitations. Ambulatory monitoring allows the providers to document the cardiac rhythm in these patients, especially when symptoms do not last very long. Two types of ambulatory monitoring devices are available: external or implantable. Implantable

Table 1
Symptom presentation and associated cardiac arrhythmias in older people

Arrhythmia	Average Age of Onset (y)	Description	Possible Associated Symptoms	Findings on EKG	Underlying Condition
Paroxysmal SVT	All ages	Sudden onset regular, with periods of palpitations, sudden termination	Polyuria, diaphoresis	Pre-excitation common in AVNRT	None
Atrial fibrillation	≥60	Irregular, variable rate,	Polyuria	Signs of left ventricular hypertrophy, nonspecific repolarization, discrete P waves absent, irregularly irregular rhythm, inconsistent R-R interval	Hypertension, ischemic heart disease, valvular heart disease
Atrial flutter/atrial tachycardia	≥60	Mostly regular with elevated heart rate	None	A regular rhythm with P waves that can appear saw-toothed, atrial rates of between 240–400 beats per min	Same as for AF
Ventricular tachycardia	≥50	Rapid heart rate	Signs and symptoms of hemodynamic instability	Pathologic Q waves are common	Ischemic heart disease

Abbreviations: AVNRT, AV nodal reentrant tachycardia; EKG, electrocardiogram.

Table 2
Predictive value of clinical features in diagnosing clinically significant arrhythmias

Clinical Features	Positive Likelihood Ratio (95% CI)	Negative Likelihood Ratio (95% CI)
Cardiac disease	0.42	1.07
Age >60 y	1.89	0.77
Family history of palpitations	1.07	0.98
Psychiatric disorder	0.67	1.12
Duration >5 min	0.79	1.23
Heart rate >100/min	1.08	0.86
Affected by sleep	2.44	0.63
Palpitations at work	1.54	0.86
Pounding neck sensation	177	0.07
Dizzy spells	1.34	0.67
Chest pain	0.92	1.02
Presyncope	1.04	0.95
Dyspnea	0.27	1.12
Obesity	3.00	0.78
Hypertension on examination	1.01	1.00

Abbreviation: CI, confidence interval.
Data from Cooper JM. Cardiology patient page. Palpitations. Circulation 2005;112(18):e299–301.

monitors are used in patients with unexplained recurrent palpitations, severe in symptoms, and when all other diagnostic workup has been negative.[34,47]

EXTERNAL MONITORS

These external monitors include Holter monitors, event recorders, external loop recorders (ELRs), and mobile cardiac outpatient telemetry.[34] Holter monitors use external recorders connected to a patient by skin electrodes. For patients with complaints of palpitations who underwent 24-hour Holter monitoring, the yield for explained or diagnosed arrhythmias was 34%.[48] Event recorders are portable devices that are applied to patients' skin when the symptoms occur. The yield for event recorders ranges from 30% to 60% for any arrhythmia and from 17% to 19% for clinically significant arrhythmias, such as AF, atrial flutter, PSVT, and VT.[4,49] ELRs continuously record by skin electrodes. These monitors record 1 to 3-lead EKG recordings and are activated by patients. Newer models can also trigger automatically. The mobile cardiac outpatient telemetry is an ELR that transmits EKG tracings to a remote center or Web site. This transmission allows monitoring of the rhythm in real time.

The newer devices can continuously monitor and record EKG for up to 30 days and do not require patient activation or transmission of data. The data are immediately transmitted to a central site where it is analyzed by a technician. The technician can contact the patient and/or physician if any urgent intervention is needed. A randomized controlled trial with 266 patients compared real-time telemetry devices with ELRs in patients with a high clinical suspicion for a malignant arrhythmia, history of syncope, presyncope, or severe infrequent palpitations with a nondiagnostic 24-hour Holter. The study showed that 41.4% of patients in the real-time telemetry group had detection of a clinically significant arrhythmia compared with 14.6% in the ELR group.[50]

IMPLANTABLE MONITORS

The implantable loop recorder (ILR) is implanted under the skin through a small incision. The ILR is useful in patients with unexplained palpitations after a non-diagnostic conventional work up. Giada and colleagues[47] compared the use of ILRs with conventional management in patients with unexplained palpitations. The study found that in people without severe heart disease and with infrequent palpitations, ILRs are safer and more cost-effective than traditional strategy.[47] Traditional strategy in participants with recurrent unexplained palpitations included 24-hour Holter, loop recorder evaluation for 4 weeks, and an electrophysiology study. In these patients, ILRs provided a diagnostic yield of 73% compared with 21% in the group evaluated with standard conventional therapy.[47]

Pacemakers are permanent implantable devices that can also be used as intracardiac monitors. They are able to detect and record atrial and ventricular rhythms.[34] They are not indicated for a routine diagnostic workup in patients with palpitations.

Many of these patients will be discharged for follow-up for further cardiac monitoring. Follow-up of these patients is often unreliable. ED physicians may or may not be able to access the ambulatory monitoring recorders at times. When they can, they can use the information recorded for patients who present with recurrent palpitations. A novel recording patch has been developed and tested that can be used in patients with palpitations who are discharged from the ED.[51] These devices are similar to event recorders and can be worn for 14 days. However, their use in the ED has not been widely tested.

CHOICE OF DEVICE

The new devices offer a higher diagnostic yield but place the burden on the clinician to be available for constant review of the data. In addition, the standard devices are less expensive than the newer continuous monitors. The duration of monitoring needed depends on the frequency of presenting symptoms. Patients who present with palpitations and have daily symptoms can be discharged from the ED with a Holter monitor. Palpitations that occur less frequently are more challenging. In a study in which patients with palpitations were prescribed an event monitor, the highest diagnostic yield was within the first week when 80% of patients transmitted at least one rhythm strip corresponding to their symptoms. During the next 3 weeks of a standard 1-month monitoring period, only an additional 3.9% of patients received a diagnosis, and no patients received a diagnosis after week 2.[52] In studies directly comparing a Holter with 48-hour monitoring and a longer evaluation with a loop recorder, the diagnostic yield of a loop recorder in detecting a cardiac arrhythmia was up to 83% compared with 39% for Holter monitoring in patients presenting with palpitations.[52–55]

Evaluating and managing ambulatory cardiac monitors can be very difficult in the ED. In practice, the monitoring companies have standard rules for recommending that patients seek emergency treatment and allow ED physicians to tailor the criteria for which they wish to be notified for non–life-threatening arrhythmias.

In patients with a diagnosis of palpitations, the authors recommend discharge with a Holter, standard continuous loop or postevent recorder, because of the low cost and the ability to provide a direct symptom-rhythm correlation. Patients should follow up with their primary care physicians within 48 to 72 hours, although there are no data to support this recommendation. If patients are unable to manage the technical requirements of a standard loop recorder, a real-time continuous telemetry device may be best, ordered in conjunction with a cardiology evaluation before ED discharge.

Table 3 summarizes the diagnostic yield, limitations, and indications of different types of devices.[32,34,47]

EMERGENCY DEPARTMENT MANAGEMENT

The goals of patients presenting to the ED with palpitation are to (1) identify patients at a high risk of cardiac arrhythmia; (2) obtain an EKG during symptoms to confirm or refute arrhythmia; (3) treat life-threatening cardiac arrhythmias, such as VT or very rapid atrial tachycardia; and (4) select the most appropriate follow-up and consider ambulatory cardiac event recorder monitoring, if the diagnosis remains elusive.

In the ED, the first step for older patients who present with complaints of palpitations is to evaluate the hemodynamic status and obtain a 12-lead EKG. Those that are hemodynamically unstable likely have a cardiac arrhythmia and need emergent management based on the type of arrhythmia and rate identified. These cases are managed based on ACLS guidelines.[56] The next step is to obtain a detailed history and physical examination, including an in-depth detail of the medications that patients are taking.

The following section reviews the ED approach to elderly patients with some common dysrhythmias.

ATRIAL FIBRILLATION

AF is the most common dysrhythmia in the elderly. It is an independent risk factor for cardiac and overall mortality,[57] with the prevalence close to 10% in all patients older than 80 years.[58,59] The prevalence of AF increases with older age, ranging from 0.1% among patients younger than 55 years to 9.0% among patients aged 80 years or older; among patients aged 60 years or older, 3.8% have AF.[58] The estimated prevalence of AF in the overall ED population is 1.1% (95% confidence interval [CI], 1.03–1.17). Among patients undergoing EKG evaluation in the ED, the prevalence of AF was reported as high 5.68% (95% CI, 5.32–6.05). In this study population, the mean age was 74.5 ± 12.9 years (median, 77.4). This high rate is mostly likely the result of the increased frequency of cardiovascular disease in patients presenting to the ED.[60]

The underlying pathophysiology is complex and can involve multiple causes.[61,62] **Fig. 3** shows the mechanisms that can produce AF.[63] Aging is associated with anatomic and histologic changes in the atria that may arise from underlying disease, such as hypertension, coronary artery disease, heart failure, valvular disease, or cardiomyopathies.[64] As the atria dilate with fibrosis and inflammation, there is a difference in the refractory periods within the tissue that promotes electrical reentry. This process results in AF. The rapidly firing foci are usually in the pulmonary veins and can trigger AF.[65] In the clinical setting, the most common causes are acute myocardial infarction and cardiothoracic surgery.[66,67] Patients commonly present in the setting of hypertension and coronary artery disease. Those who have congestive heart failure are at a higher risk of developing this arrhythmia.[68] AF is associated with a higher risk of stroke and thromboembolism.[69] Pooled data from multiple trials showed that the risk of stroke increases by 1.4% per decade of age and by 3 clinical risk factors: hypertension, prior stroke or transient ischemic attack, and diabetes.[70] The CHADS$_2$ is a stroke risk index that has been validated in the Medicare population. It estimates the risk of stroke in patients with nonrheumatic AF in the absence of anticoagulation based on their clinical risk factors and age.[71] CHADS$_2$ is helpful in assessing treatment options for elderly patients who present with AF to the ED. **Table 4** defines this risk assessment score and its components in detail.[71–73]

AF decreases the quality of life and mental function in the elderly. The Rotterdam study showed that both Alzheimer disease and senility were more common in elderly

Table 3
Types of devices for ambulatory cardiac monitoring

Device	Diagnostic Yield for any Arrhythmia (%)	Diagnostic Yield for Clinically Significant Arrhythmia (%)	Advantages	Limitations	Indications
Holter monitor	34	3–24	Low cost	24 h, 7 d; size may prevent activities that may trigger arrhythmias; patients often fail to complete the clinical diary to correlate between symptoms and the arrhythmias recorded is based	Daily to weekly palpitations; unable to use other devices
External Loop monitors	34–84	8–36	Records retrospective and prospective EKG records	3–4 wk; maintenance required; uncomfortable to wear; poor EKG records	Weekly to monthly, short-lasting palpitations associated to hemodynamic impairment; very compliant patients
Event recorders	30–60	17–19	Low cost and easy to use	3–4 wk; very brief arrhythmias are not recorded; arrhythmic triggers unknown; poor EKG records	Weekly to monthly, long-lasting palpitations; no associated hemodynamic impairment; compliant patients
Implantable loop recorders	N/A	73	Retrospective and prospective EKG records; good EKG records; monitoring capability up to 36 mo	Invasive; risk of local complications at implantation site; higher cost; limited memory	Monthly to yearly palpitations; hemodynamic compromise, when all other examination proves inconclusive; noncompliant patients without hemodynamic compromise when a clinically significant arrhythmic cause is likely or must be ruled out

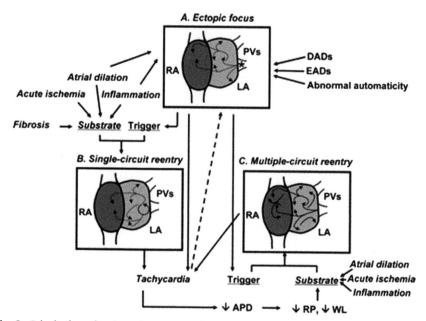

Fig. 3. *Principal mechanisms that can produce AF.* Reentry involves a vulnerable substrate, which requires a trigger for reentry initiation. Ischemia, inflammation, and dilation make atria more vulnerable to AF. AF that results from any mechanism causes tachycardia-induced remodeling. APD, action potential duration; DADs, delayed after depolarizations; EADs, early after depolarizations; LA, left atrium; PVs, pulmonary veins; RA, right atrium; RP, refractory period; WL, wavelength. (*From* Nattel S, Burstein B, Dobrev D. Atrial remodeling and atrial fibrillation: mechanisms and implications. Circ Arrhythm Electrophysiol 2008;1(1):62–73.)

patients with AF.[74,75] This common arrhythmia can be acute, chronic, or paroxysmal; in addition to palpitations, it may be associated with shortness of breath, stroke, or even death. It is extremely important to exclude this arrhythmia as a cause of palpitations in all elderly patients presenting to the ED.

Table 4				
CHADS$_2$: cardiac failure, hypertension, age, diabetes, stroke system				
Recent cardiac failure				1 point
Hypertension				1 point
Age >75 y				1 point
Diabetes				1 point
Prior stroke or TIA				2 points
CHADS$_2$ Score	Treatment Recommendation	Risk of Stroke with Aspirin (%)	Risk of Stroke with Warfarin (%)	Risk of Stroke with No Treatment (%)
0	ASA alone	1.0	1.0	1.9
1	ASA or warfarin	1.5	1.4	2.8
2	Warfarin	2.5	2.0	4.0
3	Warfarin	5.0	3.0	5.9
4+	Warfarin	$\geq$7.0	$\geq$4.3	$\geq$8.5

Initial Management of AF

Treatment ranges from immediate cardioversion to chronic rate control. Jacoby and colleagues[76] looked at ED synchronized cardioversion in patients with new-onset AF and compared it with a control group management with rate control and hospitalization. They found that there was a significantly shorter length of stay in the hospital for the cardioversion group. They found no complications after the 4-week follow-up. However, the mean age of the population studied was about 63 years. The Ottawa Aggressive Protocol includes chemical cardioversion or electrical cardioversion, if needed, and then discharge home.[77] This protocol was evaluated in a large study involving 660 patients of whom 95% had AF. In this study, 243 patients required cardioversion with a success rate of about 92%. Again, the overall mean age was 64.5 years. It is unclear if these protocols can be applied to older patient populations. Further studies in those older than 65 years can give us some insight into ED cardioversion as one of the initial steps in the management of new-onset AF.

For patients in whom the time of onset of newly diagnosed AF is unknown or for elderly patients with chronic AF who present with episodes of uncontrolled AF or for those in whom cardioversion is deemed too risky, the usual treatment is rate control. Medications, such as digoxin, have long been out of favor, except for use in patients with congestive heart failure. The drug of choice for rate control in the ED is a calcium channel blocker, typically diltiazem or verapamil. If a patient's blood pressure is low, consider giving calcium gluconate before calcium channel blocker to limit the adverse effect of hypotension. Although this has been shown to be effective with verapamil,[78] evidence is lacking to support this practice of calcium pretreatment when using diltiazem in the ED.[79] Diltiazem can be given as small boluses or an infusion titrated to a target heart rate of fewer than 110 beats per minute.[80] Beta-blockers may also be used. Because of the additive effects of the calcium channel blocker and beta-blockers, therapy is started with one class of drugs, and the second class is not added until the first has been maximized. In patients who are already taking beta-blockers, it is often prudent to start intravenous beta-blocker treatment for rate control.

Currently, in the elderly, the mainstay of treatment has been to use drug therapy.[81] However, AF with rapid ventricular rate requires prompt attention. Patients with hypotension will require emergency synchronized cardioversion. Despite the risk of embolic stroke inherent in cardioversion of patients in AF with unknown duration of dysrhythmia, hemodynamic instability mandates emergent cardioversion. Stroke risk is as high as 5% in patients who are not anticoagulated. For those who are already on warfarin for anticoagulation, the international normalized ratio should at least be 2.5 to confer a significant reduction of stroke risk.[82] Uretsky and colleagues[83] studied the reliability of a transthoracic echo (TTE) in reliably identifying echocardiograph features that could assist in decision making for patients with AF for anticoagulation. They found that the left atrial appendage velocity is a parameter that can be used with a TTE for risk stratification of AF. Whether these findings apply to the ED setting is unknown. ED physicians would need to be trained to accurately determine features of a TTE that can assist in the evaluation of a cardiac thrombus. For AF that lasts more than 48 hours, transesophageal echocardiography (TEE) is still recommended before cardioversion.[84] Successful cardioversion will often restore the heart to normal sinus rhythm. However, in patients with chronic AF or underlying valvular heart disease, electrical cardioversion may not successfully convert AF to normal sinus rhythm.

For elderly patients in rapid AF who have normal blood pressure, the initial treatment depends on whether the dysrhythmia is new onset or paroxysmal and if the time of onset of the AF is known or unknown. Patients who can provide a clear history of the time of onset of AF, which is less than 48 hours, may be candidates for electrical or chemical cardioversion. Because of the risk for embolic stroke in cardioversion, it is common practice to obtain a TEE to evaluate for blood clots in the atria before cardioversion, unless the time of onset is very clear. TEE requires moderate sedation; and the procedure itself has some inherent risks, so some elderly patients may not be safe candidates for TEE. In the absence of atrial clots, synchronized cardioversion is performed immediately while patients are still sedated, with the objective to restore the heart to normal sinus rhythm. Studies comparing the superior 100% sensitivity and 100% specificity of TEE to detect atrial thrombi as opposed to the lower 69% sensitivity and equivalent specificity of noninvasive TTE are often done on structurally abnormal hearts.[85] A study looking at TTE versus TEE specifically to detect thrombi in patients with AF with planned electrical cardioversion found that, although TTE did not detect all thrombi, it was able to determine if the heart was structurally normal or not. No structurally normal hearts had thrombi. All the structurally abnormal hearts had TEE done, and thrombi were only detected via TEE from the group that was first identified as structurally abnormal. These investigators suggested that TTE may first be used as a screening test before cardioversion and TEE may only be necessary for those patients with structural abnormalities.[86]

The benefit of cardioversion for AF is the prompt restoration of normal sinus rhythm, which obviates prolonged medications for rate control and anticoagulation, as well as the potential detrimental structural changes to the heart with long-term cardiac remodeling caused by chronic AF. Chemical conversion of new-onset AF is an alternative to electrical cardioversion or is used if prior electrical cardioversion has failed, often using drugs, such as ibutilide, procainamide, or amiodarone. These drugs have variable success rates in the ED.

Ibutilide has a conversion rate of 70%.[87] Procainamide is less effective, with a conversion rate of 53%.[88] An analysis of many trials of amiodarone for acute AF in the ED shows a conversion rate of 80%, but these studies used high-dose amiodarone and exclude patients with an ejection fraction less than 40% with acute decompensated heart failure.[89] Despite the potential for rapid restoration of cardiac rhythm with electrical or chemical cardioversion, both methods have risks. Electrical conversion often necessitates sedation. Given the comorbidities of elderly patients as well as physiologic changes of the elderly, geriatric patients are at risk for oversedation. Antidysrhythmia drugs themselves cause adverse drug events. Therefore, many clinicians have traditionally taken a more conservative approach of rate control as described later. However, recent studies have shown that cardioversion is successful and decreases hospital admissions, even for the geriatric population. In Canada, clinical researchers successfully performed ED cardioversion in patients as old as 92 years who presented with new-onset AF. Patients were first given a trial of chemical conversion with procainamide. If that failed, they received electrical cardioversion; 93% of patients were discharged home in sinus rhythm.[77]

Patients with new-onset or uncontrolled AF are generally admitted to the hospital for titration of rate-control medications. Other objectives of admission are to further evaluate the cause of the AF and contemplate rhythm control versus rate control. All patients with disabling or severe AF symptoms are admitted, including those with congestive heart failure or ischemic symptoms.

Anticoagulation in the Elderly

One of the preventive strategies for AF is the institution of anticoagulation. Data regarding anticoagulation in those older than 80 years are equivocal. Fang and colleagues[90] studied the risk of warfarin-associated hemorrhage with age. They found that those older than 80 years had a significantly higher rate of intracranial hemorrhage than those younger than 80 years. Conversely, patients older than 75 years are also a high-risk group for AF-related stoke; the highest benefit for anticoagulation is in the oldest age category (85 years and older). Additionally, one study found the net benefit for the 85 years and older to be significantly more than for those aged between 75 and 84 years.[91] Many providers are hesitant to prescribe anticoagulation in elderly people because of the risk of falls. However, a recent prospective study found no significant difference in major bleeds among patients with a high risk of falls. Instead, the investigators found that the number of medications is an independent risk factor for major bleeds, with each additional drug posing a 12% risk. The risk of bleeding was also significantly increased among women.[92] Current anticoagulation recommendations are based on the American Chest Physician's guidelines.[73] If there are no contraindications to anticoagulation, patients are often treated with anticoagulation medication in the acute hospital setting with consideration of long- or short-term anticoagulation. Anticoagulation decisions in the elderly for AF should incorporate both the risk of stroke from thromboembolism and the risk of bleeding.

Role of the CHADS$_2$ Score in the Emergency Department

The goals of AF management are rate and rhythm control and prevention of thromboembolism. The CHADS$_2$ score can help risk stratify patients in the ED with AF who are hemodynamically stable and with minimal symptoms. Assessing the risk of stroke in patients with AF is critical to its management in the ED. However, the CHADS$_2$ score may underestimate the score in some patients who have only had a prior transient ischemic attack (TIA) or have other risk factors not included in the scoring system.[93] Therefore, the risk stratification in the ED should not be limited to the CHADS$_2$ score and should be patient centered and take into account both the risk of stroke and the risk of intracranial hemorrhage.

Effectiveness of Anticoagulation Therapy

The morbidity and mortality associated with AF is mainly caused by the potential risk of thromboembolic events resulting in an ischemic stroke. Areas of stasis in the atria during AF provide the environment for thrombus formation, especially in the left atrial appendage. Antiplatelet therapy and anticoagulation prevent formation of this thrombus and, thus, reduce the risk of ischemic stroke. The risk of thromboembolic stroke is increased 3 to 5 times in patients with nonvalvular AF.[94] AF is responsible for about 15% of all ischemic strokes. In the elderly, AF is the leading cause of ischemic strokes in women older than 75 years. An analysis of pooled date from 5 randomized control trials showed that warfarin reduced the risk of stroke in patients with AF by 68%.[70] Another study showed a 51% reduction in stroke risk with anticoagulation.[95] The effectiveness of anticoagulation has been shown in multiple studies. It is up to the provider to individualize the treatment of elderly patients.

Long-term Management of AF

Despite the risks of anticoagulation, rate control with anticoagulation for thromboembolic stroke prevention may be a better choice than chronic rhythm control given the adverse proarrhythmic effects of antidysrhythmic drugs.[96] In the elderly, the rate-control strategy is a very acceptable approach, with beta-blockers, calcium channel blockers, and digitalis, or a combination of these. In patients for whom digitalis is considered, renal function must be taken into account because of the high risk of digitalis toxicity in the elderly. For patients in whom symptoms persist, correction of the rhythm may be desired, and referral to an electrophysiologist is recommended to determine if patients are candidates for an ablation procedure. AF ablation is a therapeutic technique that uses radiofrequency energy or freezing to destroy atrial tissue that is involved in the propagation of the dysrhythmia. Catheter ablation is indicated to prevent the recurrence of symptomatic AF in patients in whom medical therapy has been ineffective. Ablation is most effective in patients with paroxysmal AF and less effective in patients with persistent AF, heart failure, or valvular disease. Regardless of the apparent efficacy of ablation, the guidelines recommend that anticoagulation in the long term (after 2 months) should be based on the risk of stroke as predicted by the $CHADS_2$ score.[97]

In summary, the goals of treatment include (1) rate control to avoid tachycardia-associated cardiomyopathy; (2) anticoagulation if no contraindications are identified, to reduce the risk of stroke and thromboembolism; and (3) maintenance of sinus rhythm to prevent adverse atrial modeling. In patients in whom rate control is not achieved, referral to a specialist for nodal ablation and permanent pacemaker implantation can be considered. These interventions should be individualized based on the patient's functional status, comorbid conditions, and goals of care.

ATRIAL FLUTTER

Atrial flutter is a common arrhythmia in older people. It is caused by a reentrant macro-circuit usually in the right atrium and can be cured with catheter ablation, which is considered the first-line therapy.[98] Medical treatment of atrial flutter follows that of AF. All recommendations for AF are considered applicable to atrial flutter. The initial treatment may depend on patient presentation.

Paroxysmal Supraventricular Tachycardia

PSVT has an increased incidence in elderly patients compared with those younger than 65 years.[99] AVNRT is the most common form of non-AF, non–atrial flutter SVT in adults. The calcification of the AV conduction system with aging may increase the likelihood of the recognition of Wolff-Parkinson-White syndrome (WPW) in the elderly.[100] Nonpharmacologic techniques to abort SVT by increasing vagal tone with the Valsalva maneuver may be attempted before using medications. Carotid massage is cautioned in the elderly because of the high incidence of carotid atherosclerosis and fear of disrupting a cholesterol plaque and causing a stroke[101] However, the risk of persistent neurologic complications from carotid massage is less than 0.25%.[102]

Fortunately, SVT caused by AV nodal reentrant tachycardia is often amenable to immediate termination with intravenous adenosine. Because this drug blocks the AV node, during the conversion from SVT to normal sinus rhythm, patients often have extreme bradycardia, during which they often report feeling as if they are going to die. This sensation resolves within seconds, but practitioners should prepare patients for this sensation before giving the medication. If 6 mg of adenosine fails initially, the dose is doubled to 12 mg to achieve rhythm conversion. If adenosine fails, other intravenous medications include calcium channel blockers, such as verapamil or diltiazem, or beta-blockers. Adenosine and verapamil have similar success rates for terminating SVT. Adenosine has more adverse effects but they are ephemeral. Verapamil is more likely to cause hypotension.[103]

If medications fail to terminate the SVT or if patients are hemodynamically unstable (including pulmonary edema or ischemic chest pain) as a result of the SVT, then synchronized cardioversion should be performed. Typically, 50 J is sufficient to cardiovert patients in SVT to normal sinus rhythm. Patients with recurrent SVT are often placed on calcium channel blockers or beta-blockers to prevent future episodes of SVT.[104] Referral to an electrophysiologist is indicated in cases of recurrent SVT. Catheter ablation has been shown to be effective in the elderly for the treatment of SVT[105,106] and is becoming more widely used. There is a slight increase in the risk of complications associated with an invasive procedure, but the proarrhythmic nature of antiarrhythmic medications makes ablation a good solution for the elderly.[105,106]

For older patients, observation in the hospital is appropriate because post-SVT cardioversion recurrence rates of 19% have been reported within 24 hours.[107] Luber and colleagues[107] found that patients discharged after treatment of SVT had a recurrence within 24 hours. All patients were stable, but the mean age of discharged patients was 49 years compared with the mean age of 65 years for those admitted to the hospital that had a 19% SVT recurrence rate. In geriatric patients with poor home social support or those who live alone or with frail caregivers, hospitalization for patients with severely symptomatic SVT should be considered.

INAPPROPRIATE SINUS TACHYCARDIA

Inappropriate sinus tachycardia refers to episodes of tachycardia in situations that should not induce an elevated heart rate and in which other medical causes, such as dehydration, fever, orthostatic hypotension, anemia, and thyrotoxicosis, are excluded. This disorder has been documented in the elderly, sometimes associated with anxiety. Beta-blockers or calcium channel blockers have been the traditional initial therapy and recently ivabradine, an inhibitor of the I_f current in the sinus node, has been shown to relieve this condition[108] The I_f current influences diastolic depolarization of the sinoatrial node.[109] Referral to an electrophysiologist for consideration of AV node ablation is an option but is a risky procedure for an otherwise rather benign condition.[110,111]

PREMATURE VENTRICULAR AND ATRIAL CONTRACTIONS

Premature ventricular contractions (PVC) and premature atrial contractions (PAC) are frequently found on EKG or captured on the cardiac monitor of patients complaining of palpitations. In addition, these are commonly seen on outpatient Holter monitor and event recorder readings. These ectopic atrial and ventricular beats, even those resulting in brief runs of nonsustained VT (less than 30 seconds duration), are not life threatening in patients without structural cardiac anomalies.[112]

In patients with PVC and PAC, electrolytes should be corrected as needed to keep them in the normal range to limit ectopy. Patients with PACs and PVCs should be reassured that the cause of their palpations is benign and seldom requires treatment. However, if patients are very symptomatic, a trial of beta-blockers is a reasonable therapy. Antiarrhythmic drugs can be used in particularly symptomatic patients. These medications should be administered under the direction of a cardiologist or electrophysiologist because of the association of class IC antiarrhythmic medications, which were found to be proarrhythmic in the Cardiac Arrhythmia Suppression (CAST) trial of patients with coronary artery disease who were given these drugs to suppress ventricular ectopy. The CAST trial studied the effects of encainide and flecainide versus placebo in post–myocardial infarction patients who had multiple PVCs. The hypothesis was that these drugs would suppress the PVCs and short runs of VT, thus preventing deaths. The study was stopped before the completion of the 3-year enrollment period after preliminary results showed that there was an excess of mortality often caused by dysrhythmias in the treatment arm compared with the placebo group.[113]

NONSUSTAINED VENTRICULAR TACHYCARDIA

Nonsustained VT is defined as 3 or more ectopic ventricular beats in a row at a rate faster than 120 beats per minutes, which lasts less than 30 seconds.[114] Asymptomatic healthy patients do not require any treatment because this does not increase the risk of death.[112] However, many elderly patients do not have normal hearts. A reduced left ventricular ejection fraction is the most accurate predictor of mortality related to ventricular arrhythmia.[115] Patients with a low ejection fraction or ischemic heart disease without contraindications for beta-blockers should be treated with beta-blockers for ventricular ectopy.[116] If the cardiac status of a patient is unknown and the presenting palpitation complaint is secondary to witnessed nonsustained VT, then the patient should be observed in the hospital to evaluate for ischemia and low ejection fraction.

VENTRICULAR TACHYCARDIA

VT is considered life threatening because of the high risk of causing sudden cardiac death. This risk is especially true if VT occurs in the setting of coronary artery disease or heart failure. VT is often caused by scarring of the heart from prior infarct; structural heart disease; or electrolyte abnormalities, such as hypokalemia, hypomagnesemia, or hypocalcaemia. Elderly patients on diuretics are certainly at risk for these electrolyte disorders, which can trigger VT; and electrolytes should be checked and corrected in all patients with VT. Digoxin toxicity can also trigger VT or ventricular fibrillation.

Treatment for VT should follow current ACLS recommendations. Stable VT is treated with antiarrhythmic medications and then synchronized cardioversion, if medications fail or patients become unstable. All patients with VT should be admitted to the hospital after conversion for further treatment with antidysrhythmic drugs and evaluation. Implantable cardioverter defibrillators (ICD) should be considered in all patients with VT presenting with irreversible cause. ICDs reduce the incidence of death from recurrent VT. In patients with a history of ventricular arrhythmias or cardiac arrest, ICDs reduce overall mortality by 25% to 30% in comparison with antiarrhythmic drugs.[117] The evidence to show a benefit in the elderly population older than 65 years is less robust, so this is an area where geriatric clinical expertise must transcend gaps in evidence-based medicine. ICD survival benefit may be limited because of the presence of other comorbid conditions. In one study, the overall mortality from these in patients aged 75 years or older was triple than in younger patients.[118] However, another trial showed a greater reduction in overall mortality in those older than 75 years (>45%) when compared with younger patients (34%).[119] An additional study in octogenarians did not show a difference in efficacy and safety when compared with those aged 70 to 79 years.[120]

SUMMARY OF ED MANAGEMENT

In summary, most patients who present with the complaint of palpitations will be asymptomatic at the time of medical evaluation. The evidence does not warrant further evaluation if patients have a normal EKG and do not have any heart disease or risk factors for rhythm disorder. EKG findings suspicious for life-threatening dysrhythmias include short PR interval, delta waves (WPW), prolonged QT interval, bundle branch blocks, peaked P waves, and left ventricular hypertrophy.[20]

For those with risk factors and EKG changes or very anxious patients who insist on further workup, patients should be referred for ambulatory cardiac monitoring. Patients with significant abnormal findings on ambulatory monitoring should be referred to a cardiologist for further evaluation. In addition, patients can be referred to a specialist for electrophysiological studies and advice regarding the treatment of atrial and ventricular arrhythmias. Although there are no randomized controlled studies of optimal an follow-up time for patients with palpitations who are discharged from the ED, the authors recommend that patients see their primary care doctor or a cardiologist within 1 week of ED discharge. The authors recommend that those who are discharged with cardiac ambulatory monitoring should follow up within 48 to 72 hours. Patients whose ED workup suggests an underlying psychiatric disorder or other noncardiac causes, a follow-up within 1 week ensures the evaluation of future symptom recurrence and gives the provider an opportunity to discuss and plan long-term management.

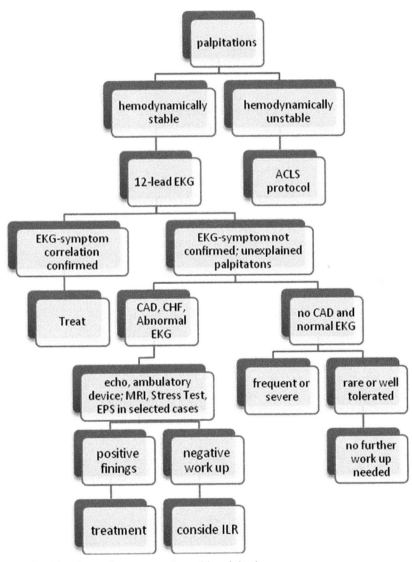

Fig. 4. Algorithm for patients presenting with palpitations.

The details of the history and physical, a copy of the EKG and any treatment given in the ED should be communicated to the primary care physician for an appropriate management plan to be made on an outpatient basis. In addition, it may be helpful to provide patients or families with a copy of their EKG to take to their physician and to inform patients that a cardiologist may decide to do further testing, such as ambulatory cardiac monitoring, to determine the type and frequency (or absence) of any potential dysrhythmia. The safe and effective ED discharge must address all of these issues in an efficient manner that can be tailored to the particular learning needs of individual patients. Patients need structured content presented verbally and with written and visual cues to enhance recall. Written instructions need to be provided in the patients' language and at an appropriate reading level.

Specific investigations are sometimes recommended based on individual patient assessment. Stress testing is recommended for patients who have palpitations associated with physical exertion or when underlying coronary artery disease is suspected. Echocardiogram is recommended in patients when underlying structural heart disease is suspected. Cardiac magnetic resonance imaging (MRI) or catheterizations are indicated only in patients with suspected or confirmed coronary artery disease.[34] Outpatient management is appropriate for most patients with palpitations, and ambulatory cardiac monitoring is frequently used for outpatient evaluation. The algorithm in **Fig. 4** summarizes the approach to patients presenting with palpitations.[34]

Criteria for Hospital Admission

Palpitations are a frequent dilemma in older patients presenting to the ED. Before sending elderly patients home from the ED with plans for further outpatient follow-up with ambulatory cardiac monitoring, the physician should consider whether the patients' history and risk factors are sufficiently concerning to warrant observation in the hospital. Historical clues exist to identify patients who might benefit from short-term observation in the hospital rather than with the risk of a lethal event in the case of a ventricular dysrhythmia. Examples include family history of sudden death, palpitations associated with syncope or near syncope, chest pain, shortness of breath, structural heart disease, and congestive heart failure.[34] Hospitalization is also needed for patients who either lack availability of ambulatory cardiac monitoring or have a disabling symptom in severity or frequency. Lastly, hospitalization is recommended if the initial ED evaluation reveals significant cardiac risk factors.

SUMMARY

The rapidly growing aging population will result in a higher prevalence of elderly patients presenting to the ED with complaints of palpitations. These patients should be sought for any underlying medical conditions that increase the likelihood of cardiac arrhythmias. In the ED, the most common reason for palpitations is a primary cardiac diagnosis. However, anxiety and panic disorders are also common. Attributing palpitations to an anxiety disorder should be done only after all possible causes are excluded. In the elderly, initial management is based on hemodynamic status. Long-term management should be individualized and patient centered.

REFERENCES

1. Cooper JM. Cardiology patient page. Palpitations. Circulation 2005;112(18): e299–301.
2. Barsky AJ, et al. Predictors of persistent palpitations and continued medical utilization. J Fam Pract 1996;42(5):465–72.

3. Weber BE, Kapoor WN. Evaluation and outcomes of patients with palpitations. Am J Med 1996;100(2):138–48.
4. Summerton N, et al. New-onset palpitations in general practice: assessing the discriminant value of items within the clinical history. Fam Pract 2001;18(4): 383–92.
5. Zeldis SM, et al. Cardiovascular complaints. Correlation with cardiac arrhythmias on 24-hour electrocardiographic monitoring. Chest 1980;78(3):456–61.
6. Barsky AJ. Palpitations, arrhythmias, and awareness of cardiac activity. Ann Intern Med 2001;134(9 Pt 2):832–7.
7. Hoefman E, et al. Predictive value of history taking and physical examination in diagnosing arrhythmias in general practice. Fam Pract 2007;24(6):636–41.
8. Barsky AJ, et al. The accuracy of symptom reporting by patients complaining of palpitations. Am J Med 1994;97(3):214–21.
9. O'Mahony D, Foote C. Prospective evaluation of unexplained syncope, dizziness, and falls among community-dwelling elderly adults. J Gerontol A Biol Sci Med Sci 1998;53(6):M435–40.
10. Fragakis N, Katsaris G. Arrhythmias in the elderly: modern management. Hellenic J Cardiol 2006;47(2):84–92.
11. Lakatta EG. Arterial and cardiac aging: major shareholders in cardiovascular disease enterprises: part III: cellular and molecular clues to heart and arterial aging. Circulation 2003;107(3):490–7.
12. Manolio TA, et al. Cardiac arrhythmias on 24-h ambulatory electrocardiography in older women and men: the cardiovascular health study. J Am Coll Cardiol 1994;23(4):916–25.
13. Abbott AV. Diagnostic approach to palpitations. Am Fam Physician 2005;71(4): 743–50.
14. Lessmeier TJ, et al. Unrecognized paroxysmal supraventricular tachycardia. Potential for misdiagnosis as panic disorder. Arch Intern Med 1997;157(5): 537–43.
15. Barsky AJ, et al. Psychiatric disorders in medical outpatients complaining of palpitations. J Gen Intern Med 1994;9(6):306–13.
16. Barsky AJ, et al. The clinical course of palpitations in medical outpatients. Arch Intern Med 1995;155(16):1782–8.
17. Barsky AJ, et al. Differential diagnosis of palpitations. Preliminary development of a screening instrument. Arch Fam Med 1997;6(3):241–5.
18. Thompson J. Psychological and physical etiologies of heart palpitations. Holist Nurs Pract 2006;20(3):107–15 [quiz: 116–7].
19. Brugada P, et al. Investigation of palpitations. Lancet 1993;341(8855):1254–8.
20. Zimetbaum P, Josephson ME. Evaluation of patients with palpitations. N Engl J Med 1998;338(19):1369–73.
21. Giada F, Raviele A. Diagnostic management of patients with palpitations of unknown origin. Ital Heart J 2004;5(8):581–6.
22. Pickett CC, Zimetbaum PJ. Palpitations: a proper evaluation and approach to effective medical therapy. Curr Cardiol Rep 2005;7(5):362–7.
23. Lev M. Aging changes in the human sinoatrial node. J Gerontol 1954;9(1):1–9.
24. Najjar SS, Scuteri A, Lakatta EG. Arterial aging: is it an immutable cardiovascular risk factor? Hypertension 2005;46(3):454–62.
25. Tallis R, Fillit HM. Brocklehurst's textbook of geriatric medicine and gerontology. 6th edition. Churchill Livingstone; 2003.
26. Mayou R. Chest pain, palpitations and panic. J Psychosom Res 1998;44(1): 53–70.

27. Sprague JE. Teaching cardiac arrhythmias: a focus on pathophysiology and pharmacology. Am J Pharm Educ 2001;65(2).

28. Demling RH, Wilson RF. Decision making in surgical critical care. Clinical decision making series. Toronto; Philadelphia; St Louis (MO): B.C. Decker; Mosby [distributor, U.S. and possessions]; 1988. p. 247.

29. Kroenke K, Arrington ME, Mangelsdorff AD. The prevalence of symptoms in medical outpatients and the adequacy of therapy. Arch Intern Med 1990; 150(8):1685–9.

30. Knudson MP. The natural history of palpitations in a family practice. J Fam Pract 1987;24(4):357–60.

31. Schellings DA, et al. Clinical cardiology consultation at non-cardiology departments: stepchild of patient care? Neth Heart J 2012;20(6):260–3.

32. Thavendiranathan P, et al. Does this patient with palpitations have a cardiac arrhythmia? JAMA 2009;302(19):2135–43.

33. Mayou R, et al. Characteristics of patients presenting to a cardiac clinic with palpitation. QJM 2003;96(2):115–23.

34. Raviele A, et al. Management of patients with palpitations: a position paper from the European Heart Rhythm Association. Europace 2011;13(7):920–34.

35. Naranjo CA, et al. A method for estimating the probability of adverse drug reactions. Clin Pharmacol Ther 1981;30(2):239–45.

36. Furlanello F, et al. Illicit drugs and cardiac arrhythmias in athletes. Eur J Cardiovasc Prev Rehabil 2007;14(4):487–94.

37. Lange RA, Hillis LD. Cardiovascular complications of cocaine use. N Engl J Med 2001;345(5):351–8.

38. Gordon M. Occult cardiac arrhythmias associated with falls and dizziness in the elderly: detection by Holter monitoring. J Am Geriatr Soc 1978;26(9): 418–23.

39. Barsky AJ, et al. Panic disorder, palpitations, and the awareness of cardiac activity. J Nerv Ment Dis 1994;182(2):63–71.

40. Hermida JS, et al. Familial incidence of late ventricular potentials and electrocardiographic abnormalities in arrhythmogenic right ventricular dysplasia. Am J Cardiol 1997;79(10):1375–80.

41. Marcus GM, et al. A first-degree family history in lone atrial fibrillation patients. Heart Rhythm 2008;5(6):826–30.

42. Abe H, et al. Neurohumoral and hemodynamic mechanisms of diuresis during atrioventricular nodal reentrant tachycardia. Pacing Clin Electrophysiol 1997; 20(11):2783–8.

43. Laurent G, et al. Influence of ventriculoatrial timing on hemodynamics and symptoms during supraventricular tachycardia. J Cardiovasc Electrophysiol 2009;20(2):176–81.

44. Gursoy S, et al. Brief report: the hemodynamic mechanism of pounding in the neck in atrioventricular nodal reentrant tachycardia. N Engl J Med 1992; 327(11):772–4.

45. Delacretaz E. Clinical practice. Supraventricular tachycardia. N Engl J Med 2006;354(10):1039–51.

46. Sakhuja R, et al. Test characteristics of neck fullness and witnessed neck pulsations in the diagnosis of typical AV nodal reentrant tachycardia. Clin Cardiol 2009;32(8):E13–8.

47. Giada F, et al. Recurrent unexplained palpitations (RUP) study comparison of implantable loop recorder versus conventional diagnostic strategy. J Am Coll Cardiol 2007;49(19):1951–6.

48. Scalvini S, et al. Cardiac event recording yields more diagnoses than 24-hour Holter monitoring in patients with palpitations. J Telemed Telecare 2005; 11(Suppl 1):14–6.
49. Arjona Barrionuevo Jde D, et al. Utility of cardiac event recorders in diagnosing arrhythmic etiology of palpitations in patients without structural heart disease. Rev Esp Cardiol 2002;55(2):107–12 [in Spanish].
50. Rothman SA, et al. The diagnosis of cardiac arrhythmias: a prospective multi-center randomized study comparing mobile cardiac outpatient telemetry versus standard loop event monitoring. J Cardiovasc Electrophysiol 2007;18(3):241–7.
51. Steven Higgins M, Drigalla D, Sattar A, et al. Use of a novel ambulatory cardiac monitor to detect arrhythmias in discharged ED patients. AB38–04. La Jolla (CA); Temple (TX); Stanford (CA): Scripps Memorial Hospital; Scott & White Healthcare, Texas A&M University Health Science Center College of Medicine; Stanford University School of Medicine; 2012.
52. Zimetbaum PJ, et al. Diagnostic yield and optimal duration of continuous-loop event monitoring for the diagnosis of palpitations. A cost-effectiveness analysis. Ann Intern Med 1998;128(11):890–5.
53. Zimetbaum PJ, Josephson ME. The evolving role of ambulatory arrhythmia monitoring in general clinical practice. Ann Intern Med 1999;130(10):848–56.
54. Kinlay S, et al. Cardiac event recorders yield more diagnoses and are more cost-effective than 48-hour Holter monitoring in patients with palpitations. A controlled clinical trial. Ann Intern Med 1996;124(1 Pt 1):16–20.
55. Fogel RI, Evans JJ, Prystowsky EN. Utility and cost of event recorders in the diagnosis of palpitations, presyncope, and syncope. Am J Cardiol 1997;79(2): 207–8.
56. Field JM, et al. Part 1: executive summary: 2010 American Heart Association Guidelines for cardiopulmonary resuscitation and emergency cardiovascular care. Circulation 2010;122(18 Suppl 3):S640–56.
57. Benjamin EJ, et al. Impact of atrial fibrillation on the risk of death: the Framingham Heart Study. Circulation 1998;98(10):946–52.
58. Go AS, et al. Prevalence of diagnosed atrial fibrillation in adults: national implications for rhythm management and stroke prevention: the AnTicoagulation and Risk Factors in Atrial Fibrillation (ATRIA) Study. JAMA 2001;285(18):2370–5.
59. Kannel WB, et al. Epidemiologic features of chronic atrial fibrillation: the Framingham study. N Engl J Med 1982;306(17):1018–22.
60. Scott PA, et al. Prevalence of atrial fibrillation and antithrombotic prophylaxis in emergency department patients. Stroke 2002;33(11):2664–9.
61. Fuster V, et al. ACC/AHA/ESC guidelines for the management of patients with atrial fibrillation: executive summary. A report of the American College of Cardiology/American Heart Association Task Force on Practice Guidelines and the European Society of Cardiology Committee for Practice Guidelines and Policy Conferences (committee to develop guidelines for the management of patients with atrial fibrillation): developed in collaboration with the North American Society of Pacing and Electrophysiology. J Am Coll Cardiol 2001;38(4):1231–66.
62. Falk RH. Atrial fibrillation. N Engl J Med 2001;344(14):1067–78.
63. Nattel S, Burstein B, Dobrev D. Atrial remodeling and atrial fibrillation: mechanisms and implications. Circ Arrhythm Electrophysiol 2008;1(1):62–73.
64. Lafuente-Lafuente C, Mahe I, Extramiana F. Management of atrial fibrillation. BMJ 2009;339:b5216.
65. Haissaguerre M, et al. Spontaneous initiation of atrial fibrillation by ectopic beats originating in the pulmonary veins. N Engl J Med 1998;339(10):659–66.

66. Sugiura T, et al. Atrial fibrillation in acute myocardial infarction. Am J Cardiol 1985;56(1):27–9.
67. Goldberg RJ, et al. Impact of atrial fibrillation on the in-hospital and long-term survival of patients with acute myocardial infarction: a community-wide perspective. Am Heart J 1990;119(5):996–1001.
68. Allessie MA, et al. Pathophysiology and prevention of atrial fibrillation. Circulation 2001;103(5):769–77.
69. Camm AJ, et al. Guidelines for the management of atrial fibrillation: the Task Force for the Management of Atrial Fibrillation of the European Society of Cardiology (ESC). Eur Heart J 2010;31(19):2369–429.
70. Risk factors for stroke and efficacy of antithrombotic therapy in atrial fibrillation. Analysis of pooled data from five randomized controlled trials. Arch Intern Med 1994;154(13):1449–57.
71. Gage BF, et al. Validation of clinical classification schemes for predicting stroke: results from the National Registry of Atrial Fibrillation. JAMA 2001;285(22): 2864–70.
72. Health, B.C.M.o. Stroke and transient ischemic attack - management and prevention; Guidelines. 2009. Available at: www.bcguidelines.ca/guideline_stroke.html. Accessed September 20, 2012.
73. Albers GW, et al. Antithrombotic therapy in atrial fibrillation. Chest 2001; 119(Suppl 1):194S–206S.
74. Sabatini T, et al. Atrial fibrillation and cognitive disorders in older people. J Am Geriatr Soc 2000;48(4):387–90.
75. Ott A, et al. Atrial fibrillation and dementia in a population-based study. The Rotterdam Study. Stroke 1997;28(2):316–21.
76. Jacoby JL, et al. Synchronized emergency department cardioversion of atrial dysrhythmias saves time, money and resources. J Emerg Med 2005;28(1):27–30.
77. Stiell IG, et al. Association of the Ottawa Aggressive Protocol with rapid discharge of emergency department patients with recent-onset atrial fibrillation or flutter. CJEM 2010;12(3):181–91.
78. Haft JI, Habbab MA. Treatment of atrial arrhythmias. Effectiveness of verapamil when preceded by calcium infusion. Arch Intern Med 1986;146(6):1085–9.
79. Kolkebeck T, et al. Calcium chloride before i.v. diltiazem in the management of atrial fibrillation. J Emerg Med 2004;26(4):395–400.
80. Van Gelder IC, et al. Lenient versus strict rate control in patients with atrial fibrillation. N Engl J Med 2010;362(15):1363–73.
81. Yadav A, Scheinman M. Atrial fibrillation in the elderly. Am J Geriatr Cardiol 2003;12(1):49–56.
82. Gallagher MM, et al. Embolic complications of direct current cardioversion of atrial arrhythmias: association with low intensity of anticoagulation at the time of cardioversion. J Am Coll Cardiol 2002;40(5):926–33.
83. Uretsky S, et al. Assessment of left atrial appendage function with transthoracic tissue Doppler echocardiography. Eur J Echocardiogr 2009;10(3):363–71.
84. Silverman DI, Manning WJ. Role of echocardiography in patients undergoing elective cardioversion of atrial fibrillation. Circulation 1998;98(5):479–86.
85. Lin SL, et al. Usefulness of transesophageal echocardiography for the detection of left atrial thrombi in patients with rheumatic heart disease. Echocardiography 1992;9(2):161–8.
86. Sharifi M, et al. Is transesophageal echocardiography necessary before D.C. cardioversion in patients with a normal transthoracic echocardiogram? Echocardiography 2007;24(4):397–400.

87. Mountantonakis SE, et al. Ibutilide to expedite ED therapy for recent-onset atrial fibrillation flutter. Am J Emerg Med 2006;24(4):407–12.

88. Stiell IG, et al. Emergency department use of intravenous procainamide for patients with acute atrial fibrillation or flutter. Acad Emerg Med 2007;14(12): 1158–64.

89. Slavik RS. Intravenous amiodarone for acute pharmacological conversion of atrial fibrillation in the emergency department. CJEM 2002;4(6):414–20.

90. Fang MC, et al. Age and the risk of warfarin-associated hemorrhage: the antico- agulation and risk factors in atrial fibrillation study. J Am Geriatr Soc 2006;54(8): 1231–6.

91. Singer DE, et al. The net clinical benefit of warfarin anticoagulation in atrial fibril- lation. Ann Intern Med 2009;151(5):297–305.

92. Donze J, et al. Risk of falls and major bleeds in patients on oral anticoagulation therapy. Am J Med 2012;125(8):773–8.

93. Adlan AM, Lip GY. Role of the CHADS2 score in acute coronary syndromes: with or without atrial fibrillation. Chest 2012;141(6):1375–6.

94. Kannel WB, et al. Prevalence, incidence, prognosis, and predisposing condi- tions for atrial fibrillation: population-based estimates. Am J Cardiol 1998; 82(8A):2N–9N.

95. Go AS, et al. Anticoagulation therapy for stroke prevention in atrial fibrillation: how well do randomized trials translate into clinical practice? JAMA 2003; 290(20):2685–92.

96. Wyse DG, et al. A comparison of rate control and rhythm control in patients with atrial fibrillation. N Engl J Med 2002;347(23):1825–33.

97. Wazni O, Wilkoff B, Saliba W. Catheter ablation for atrial fibrillation. N Engl J Med 2011;365(24):2296–304.

98. Poty H, et al. Radiofrequency catheter ablation of type 1 atrial flutter. Prediction of late success by electrophysiological criteria. Circulation 1995;92(6):1389–92.

99. Orejarena LA, et al. Paroxysmal supraventricular tachycardia in the general population. J Am Coll Cardiol 1998;31(1):150–7.

100. Fan W, et al. Age-related changes in the clinical and electrophysiologic charac- teristics of patients with Wolff-Parkinson-White syndrome: comparative study between young and elderly patients. Am Heart J 1991;122(3 Pt 1):741–7.

101. Bastulli JA, Orlowski JP. Stroke as a complication of carotid sinus massage. Crit Care Med 1985;13(10):869.

102. Walsh T, et al. Carotid sinus massage–how safe is it? Age Ageing 2006;35(5): 518–20.

103. Delaney B, Loy J, Kelly AM. The relative efficacy of adenosine versus verapamil for the treatment of stable paroxysmal supraventricular tachycardia in adults: a meta-analysis. Eur J Emerg Med 2011;18(3):148–52.

104. Blomstrom-Lundqvist C, et al. ACC/AHA/ESC guidelines for the management of patients with supraventricular arrhythmias–executive summary. A report of the American College of Cardiology/American Heart Association task force on practice guidelines and the European Society of Cardiology committee for practice guidelines (writing committee to develop guidelines for the management of patients with supraventricular arrhythmias) developed in collaboration with NASPE-Heart Rhythm Society. J Am Coll Cardiol 2003; 42(8):1493–531.

105. Smith PN, et al. Catheter ablation in the elderly in the United States: use in the Medicare population from 1991 to 1998. Pacing Clin Electrophysiol 2001;24(1): 66–9.

106. Zado ES, et al. Efficacy and safety of catheter ablation in octogenarians. J Am Coll Cardiol 2000;35(2):458–62.
107. Luber S, et al. Paroxysmal supraventricular tachycardia: outcome after ED care. Am J Emerg Med 2001;19(1):40–2.
108. Sette A, et al. Efficacy of ivabradine in a case of inappropriate sinus tachycardia and ventricular dysfunction. J Cardiovasc Electrophysiol 2010;21(7):815–7.
109. Sulfi S, Timmis AD. Ivabradine – the first selective sinus node I(f) channel inhibitor in the treatment of stable angina. Int J Clin Pract 2006;60(2):222–8.
110. Shen WK. Modification and ablation for inappropriate sinus tachycardia: current status. Card Electrophysiol Rev 2002;6(4):349–55.
111. Lopera G, et al. Chronic inappropriate sinus tachycardia in elderly females. Ann Noninvasive Electrocardiol 2003;8(2):139–43.
112. Kennedy HL, et al. Long-term follow-up of asymptomatic healthy subjects with frequent and complex ventricular ectopy. N Engl J Med 1985;312(4):193–7.
113. Echt DS, et al. Mortality and morbidity in patients receiving encainide, flecainide, or placebo. The Cardiac Arrhythmia Suppression Trial. N Engl J Med 1991;324(12):781–8.
114. Buxton AE, et al. Nonsustained ventricular tachycardia. Cardiol Clin 2000;18(2):327–36, viii.
115. Caruso AC, et al. Predictors of arrhythmic death and cardiac arrest in the ESVEM trial. Electrophysiologic study versus electromagnetic monitoring. Circulation 1997;96(6):1888–92.
116. Aronow WS. Management of the older person with ventricular arrhythmias. J Am Geriatr Soc 1999;47(7):886–95.
117. A comparison of antiarrhythmic-drug therapy with implantable defibrillators in patients resuscitated from near-fatal ventricular arrhythmias. The Antiarrhythmics versus Implantable Defibrillators (AVID) Investigators. N Engl J Med 1997;337(22):1576–83.
118. Panotopoulos PT, et al. Efficacy of the implantable cardioverter-defibrillator in the elderly. J Am Coll Cardiol 1997;29(3):556–60.
119. Huang DT, Sesselberg H, Salam T, et al. Survival benefits associated with defibrillator implant in elderly patients enrolled in MADIT II [abstract: 1790]. Circulation 2003;108(Suppl IV):IV-386.
120. Noseworthy PA, et al. Feasibility of implantable cardioverter defibrillator use in elderly patients: a case series of octogenarians. Pacing Clin Electrophysiol 2004;27(3):373–8.

Treating the Elderly Stroke Patient
Complications, Controversies, and Best Care Metrics

Laura E. Heitsch, MD[a],*, Peter D. Panagos, MD[b]

KEYWORDS

- Acute ischemic stroke • Elderly stroke • Thrombolysis • Emergency care/treatment
- tPA • Intra-arterial

KEY POINTS

- Acute stroke is a devastating disease that affects almost 800,000 Americans annually. It is the number one cause of adult disability and inflicts suffering for patients and families that is unlike most other diseases. Worldwide, the incidence of stroke is rapidly increasing and outpacing the growth rates of North America. Although stroke can affect all age groups, patients over age 80 are at much higher risk for ischemic stroke due to accumulated vascular risk factors.
- Intravenous (IV) thrombolysis with tissue plasminogen activator (tPA), is the only US Food and Drug Administration (FDA)–approved therapy for acute ischemic stroke (AIS). Unfortunately, it is severely underused due to myriad factors: lack of symptom recognition leading to delays in presentation to the hospital, lack of physician awareness of treatment options, and disorganization with local and regional stroke systems of care.
- Almost all the research studies involving IV or intra-arterial (IA) thrombolysis have excluded patients over age 80. Therefore, definitive statements on the true efficacy and safety of thrombolysis within this age group are lacking.

OVERALL BURDEN OF ISCHEMIC STROKE

Acute ischemic stroke (AIS) is the fourth leading cause of mortality and the leading cause of serious long-term disability in the United States.[1,2] Approximately 795,000 people experience a stroke every year in the United States, with projections that by 2030, there will be a 24.9% increase in the incidence of stroke.[3] Stroke imparts a tremendous medical, emotional, and fiscal burden to society. Annual costs for stroke care in the United States alone exceed $73 billion.[3]

Conflict of Interest: Heitsch—None; Panagos—Speakers Bureau, Genentech and Consultant—American Heart Association/American Stroke Association.
[a] Division of Emergency Medicine, Washington University School of Medicine, 660 S Euclid, CB 8072, St Louis, MO 63110, USA; [b] Division of Emergency Medicine and Department of Neurology, Washington University School of Medicine, 660 S Euclid, CB 8072, St Louis, MO 63110, USA
* Corresponding author.
E-mail address: heitschl@wusm.wustl.edu

According to World Health Organization statistics, the incidence and prevalence of stroke are 9.0 million and 30.7 million, respectively, with a higher incidence found in the Western Pacific, Europe, and Southeast Asia. Compared with other causes of death worldwide, stroke accounts for 10% (5.5 million) compared with 12% (7.1 million) for cancer. Due to advances in Western health care, the prevalence of stroke since 1970 has decreased 42% whereas it is has more than doubled in low-income to middle-income countries.[4]

The predominant subtype of stroke is ischemic stroke, accounting for 87% of all strokes in the United States. Currently, the only FDA-approved medication for treatment of AIS is IV tPA within a 3-hour therapeutic window. Additional therapies, such as IA fibrinolysis, are also promising treatments for acute stroke patients. The safety and efficacy in the elderly population, however, have not been adequately studied because most randomized clinical trials have excluded very elderly patients ($\geq$80 years).

STROKE WITHIN THE ELDERLY COMMUNITY

Stroke is common within the elderly population. The highest prevalence and annual rate of first-ever strokes are reported in those 80 years or older.[3] An analysis of 502,036 ischemic stroke admissions from 1256 hospitals in the Get With the Guidelines–Stroke program from 2003 to 2009 found that more than 30% of patients were 80 years or older.[5] A similar percentage (33.6%) of patients 80 years or older was found in a recent analysis of the Registry of the Canadian Stroke Network.[6]

Because of the aging population, it has been projected that significant increases in the number of worldwide elderly will occur in the future. Increases up to 300% in the overall number of elderly are anticipated among the inhabitants of many developing countries.[7] There are projections of a 75% increase in the proportion of those aged 80 years or older in Canada by 2026.[6] Thus, the global occurrence of stroke is expected to concomitantly increase in the future.

It is well known that elderly patients have poor outcomes associated with ischemic stroke. They have significantly higher in-hospital and 3-month mortality rates and are less likely to be discharged to home than their younger counterparts.[5,8–10] Inequities in active medical care and inpatient management have been proposed as contributors to the age-related differences in outcome. Analysis of a large Canadian registry, however, found that, despite reaching similar rates of stroke care quality metrics, patients older than 80 years of age still had higher in-hospital mortality, were more likely to have significant disability at discharge and were less likely to be discharged home.[6] Elderly patients are also more likely to present with severe neurologic deficits, have preadmission dementia and dependency, and have higher prevalence of comorbidities (especially atrial fibrillation).[6,10,11]

Given the higher rates of morbidity and mortality due to ischemic stroke among the elderly and the projected growth in the number of adults within this population, how best to acutely manage their treatment in the emergency department (ED) has become a pressing concern for practicing physicians. The purpose of this article is to highlight the age-specific challenges facing the elderly entering the medical system with an acute stroke.

DISPARITIES IN TREATMENT RATES BETWEEN THE ELDERLY AND THEIR YOUNGER COUNTERPARTS

Despite this higher burden of disease, there is a disparity in thrombolytic treatment rates between the elderly and their younger counterparts. This is the case even when there are similar eligibility profiles between the 2 groups.[12] As discussed previously, more than 30% of ischemic strokes occur in patients 80 years or older.[5,8,9,13] Yet, the percentage of elderly patients within the treatment population varies from 6.5% to 32.4%, depending on the time interval and country of origin of the reported rates (**Table 1**). In addition, it has been demonstrated that older patients are less likely to receive timely administration of tPA on arrival to the ED.[5,40–42]

Even more telling is that analysis of the US National Inpatient Sample database (2000–2006) revealed that tPA treatment rates, although increasing over the study period, were still only 1.05% in the elderly population versus 1.72% in the younger population.[13] Similar discrepancies in treatment rates have been reported by Singer et al.[43] Meanwhile, percentages of patients eligible for IV tPA have been reported comparable between the 2 groups in other countries (14.2% in age <80 and 12.4% in age ≥80, $P = .35$).[31]

Age alone has been reported as reason for exclusion of potentially eligible patients from treatment within the 3-hour window.[23,44,45] This hesitation to treat elderly patients may be rooted in several factors. Elderly subjects were under-represented or excluded from randomized controlled trials. Some studies that did include them have suggested worse outcomes when compared with younger subjects and potentially increased rates of hemorrhagic transformation. In addition, tPA was not approved for treatment of elderly patient in Europe, so physicians practicing in those countries must decide whether to treat elderly patients off label.

SMALL NUMBERS OF ELDERLY SUBJECTS IN RANDOMIZED CONTROLLED TRIALS

Despite the higher burden of stroke and growing population of elderly patients, there have been surprisingly few elderly patients included in randomized controlled trials. The pivotal NINDS study enrolled only 42 patients who were 80 years old or older, representing only 7% of the study population, and subgroup analysis indicated that older age with higher baseline National Institutes of Health Stroke Scale (NIHSS) predicted less favorable outcomes overall.[46] This same analysis, however, reported that there was no influence on the likelihood of a differential response to tPA in this group and a treatment benefit was even suggested. Unfortunately, other randomized trials have excluded elderly patients from enrollment.[38,47–50] Thus, there was little information regarding safety and efficacy in this subgroup to guide treating physicians during the early stages of incorporating tPA into general acute stroke management.

In addition, in part because of these issues, the license for tPA treatment in Europe was restricted to patients less than or equal to 80 years of age by the European Medicine Evaluation Agency. Many centers in Europe have been treating the elderly in an off-label capacity as a result. One center reported that more than 50% of its off-label treatment group was composed of patients older than 80 years of age.[34] Although the treatment window for IV tPA was recently approved for expansion to 4.5 hours in the European Union, the exclusion of elderly patients remains.

Given the controversy surrounding acute treatment of elderly ischemic stroke patients, a number of observational studies and registry analyses have been published. A majority of these studies have evaluated the response to treatment within the elderly cohort by comparing them with their younger counterparts. Fewer studies have made the comparison between treatment with IV tPA and no acute intervention within the elderly population. Although observational studies can potentially be skewed by observer and selection bias in comparison to randomized controlled trials, these types of studies were the only source of data on the elderly cohort until recently.

Table 1
Comparison of outcomes between patients 80 and older and those less than 80 years old treated with IV tPA

	N		sICH		mRS 0–1 @ 90 d		Mortality @ 90 d	
	Age <80	Age ≥80	Age <80	Age ≥80	Age <80	Age ≥80	Age <80	Age ≥80
Tanne et al,[14] 2000 (discharge endpoints)	159	30 (15.8)	10 (6%)[a]	1 (3%)[a]	30%	37%	12 (8%)[d]	6 (20%)[d]
Simon et al,[15] 2004 (only pts ≥80 analyzed)	265	62 (23%)	NR	6 (9.7%)[b]	NR	(19.7%)	NR	20 (32.8%)
Vatankhah et al,[16] 2005 (only pts >75)	NR	29 (21.2%)	NR	1 (3.4%)	NR	NR	NR	6 (20.7%)
Berrouschot et al,[17] 2005, German centers	190	38 (16.7)	5 (2.6%)[b]	1 (2.6%)[b]	89 (46.8%)	10 (26.3%)	10 (5.3%)	8 (21.1%)
Mouradian et al,[18] 2005, Canada (mRS 0–2)	65	31 (32.3%)	4 (6.2%)[c]	3 (9.7%)[c]	38 (58.5%)	5 (16.1%)	7 (10.8%)	10 (32.3%)
Chen et al,[19] 2005[d]	127	56 (30.6%)	8 (6.3%)[b]	4 (7.1%)[b]	NR	NR	14 (11%)[d]	11 (20%)[d]
Engelter et al,[20] 2005, Swiss survey	287	38 (12%)	24 (8%)[a]	5 (13%)[a]	107 (37%)	11 (29%)	35 (12%)	12 (32%)
Sylaja et al,[21] 2006, CASES database	865	270 (23.8%)	40 (4.6%)[a]	12 (4.4%)[a]	(40%)	(25.9%)	157 (18.2%)	95 (35.3%)
van Oostenbrugge et al,[22] 2006, the Netherlands	139	45 (24.5%)	4 (2.9%)[a]	5 (11.1%)[a]	62 (45%)	12 (27%)	22 (16%)	18 (40%)
Zeevi et al,[23] 2007, Connecticut[d]	690	341 (33%)	6 (5.0%)[b]	1 (2.2%)[b]	NR	NR	21 (18%)[d]	15 (33%)[d]
Meseguer et al,[24] 2008 Paris	107	22 (17%)	8 (7.5%)[b]	3 (13.6%)[b]	40 (37.4%)	6 (27.3%)	12 (11.2%)	6 (27.3%)
Uyttenboogaart et al,[25] 2007, the Netherlands	111	31 (22%)	4 (3.6%)	3 (9.7%)	40 (36.0%)	5 (16.1%)	14 (12.6%)	14 (45.2%)
Toni et al,[26] 2008, Italy (≤80 yo, mRS 0–2)	207	41 (16.5%)	10 (4.8%)[b]	2 (4.8%)[b]	121 (58.5%)	18 (44%)	22 (10.6%)	14 (34.1%)
Gomez-Choco et al,[27] 2008, Barcelona	108	49 (31.2%)	6 (6%)[b]	3 (6%)[b]	39 (37%)	12 (25%)	11 (10%)	3 (6%)
Pundik et al,[28] 2008, Cleveland	404	78 (16.2%)	(4.92%)	(9.09%)	NR	NR	12.2%	NR
Ford et al,[29] 2010, SITS-ISTR	19411	1831 (8.6%)	7.6%[a] 1.6%[c]	9.5%[a] 1.8%[c]	40.6%	24.7%	12.2%	30.2%

Alshekhlee et al,[13] 2010, NIS database (US)	6291	1659 (20.8%)	NR	NR	NR	NR	721 (11.5%)[d]	280 (16.9%)[d]
Forster et al,[30] 2011, single center, Germany (mRS ≤2)	178	59 (24.9%)	2 (1.1%)[c]	6 (10.5%)[c]	50.0%	20.0%	6.2%[d]	20.3%[d]
Martins et al,[31] 2011, Porto Alegre Stroke Network, Brazil	183	55 (23.1%)	12 (6.6%)[b]	6 (11%)[b]	58%	42%	13%	24%
Dharmasaroja et al,[32] 2011, Thailand	244	17 (6.5%)	7.8%[a] 3.8%[b]	0[a] 0[b]	49.8%	42.9%	9.7%	21.4%
Boulouis et al,[33] 2012, Lille, France (mRS ≤2; return to premorbid)	302	98 (25%)	29 (10%)[a] 18 (6%)[b] 12 (4%)[c]	12 (12%)[a] 6 (6%)[b] 4 (4%)[c]	189 (70%)	33 (52%)	33 (11%)	34 (35%)
Guillan et al,[34] 2012, Madrid (mRS 0–2; 4.5 window)	241	129 (25%)	6 (2.2%)[c]	3 (2.3%)[c]	173 (64.3%)	47 (40%)	30 (11.1%)	31 (24%)
Costello et al,[35] 2012, single center, Australia	141	65 (31.5%)	4 (2.8%)[b]	0[b]	NR	NR	NR	NR
Cronin et al,[36] 2012, single center, Maryland	160	31 (16%)	7 (4.4%)	2 (6.5%)	NR	NR	6 (3.8%)[d]	NR
Willey et al,[37] 2012, US SPOTRIAS centers	2283	1095 (32.4%)	NR	NR	NR	NR	NR	NR

Abbreviations: NR, information or data not reported in the published manuscript; NIS, National Inpatient Sample; pts, patients; yo, years old.

[a] NINDS-type sICH: any new hemorrhage on CT scan associated with any decline in neurologic status.[2]

[b] ECASS-type sICH: any hemorrhage on imaging that is associated with an increase in the NIHSS by at least 4 points from baseline.[38]

[c] SITS-MOST-type: local or remote type 2 parenchymal hematoma combined with a neurologic worsening of 4 or more points from baseline NIHSS, or from the lowest NIHSS score between baseline and 24 h, or any hemorrhage associated with death.[39]

[d] In-hospital mortality only.

OUTCOMES BASED ON COMPARISON OF TREATED PATIENTS GREATER THAN 80 VERSUS LESS THAN 80 YEARS OF AGE

In total, there are 6200 elderly patients included in studies comparing the outcome of IV tPA treatment in elderly patients to younger patients (see **Table 1**). These studies differ in the endpoints (ie, in-hospital mortality vs 90-day mortality) as well as the definition of symptomatic intracranial hemorrhage (sICH) used. The studies also range in sample size from small single-center observational studies to large national registries.

A higher in-hospital mortality rate (16%–33% in older vs 4%–18% in younger) has been consistently reported for octogenarians compared with younger patients.[13,14,18,19,23,30,36,37] This seems due to several factors, including worse premorbid functioning,[23,30] more severe strokes/larger infarct size,[14,18,30,37] higher prevalence of comorbidities (especially atrial fibrillation),[23,30] and higher rates of secondary complications.[14,30] A German center recently reported that significantly more in-hospital complications unrelated to thrombolytic administration were seen in the elderly population (44.1% vs 27.0%, odds ratio [OR] 2.72, $P = .01$).[30] Pneumonia, in particular, is a more frequent complication during hospitalization for elderly compared with younger patients.[6,29,33]

In addition to higher in-hospital mortality rates, octogenarians were more often discharged to a location other than home when compared with younger patients.[13,14,19,37] Despite similarities between distributions of favorable outcome (modified Rankin Scale [mRS] 0–1) **(Table 2)**, degree of neurologic improvement, and severe residual neurologic deficit (NIHSS $\geq$11) **(Table 3)** at hospital discharge, significantly more elderly patients were less frequently discharged home compared with those aged less than 80 years.[14] Similar findings have been reported elsewhere.[19] It is likely that factors beyond the persistent neurologic deficit are responsible for this disparity. Social factors, such as lack of support or socioeconomic resources, affect frailty and may play a role in discharge location for the elderly.[52,53] A complex interplay of comorbidity, dementia, and functional and cognitive impairment as well these social factors affect recovery after stroke in the elderly.[8,32,54]

Worse outcomes at 3 months in elderly patients have also been reported in the literature as well as increased mortality rates during that time period.[17,18,21,22,24,25,29,30,33,34] Although not all studies have found this to be true. Despite a higher 3-month mortality rate among elderly patients in several studies, there was no significant difference in the rate of a favorable outcome among the survivors.[20,26,32] Another study failed to

Table 2
Explanation of scoring in modified Rankin Scale (mRS)

Level	Description
0	No symptoms
1	No significant disability, despite symptoms; able to perform all usual duties and activities
2	Slight disability; unable to perform all previous activities but able to look after own affairs without assistance
3	Moderate disability; requires some help but able to walk without assistance
4	Moderately severe disability; unable to walk without assistance and unable to attend to own bodily needs without assistance
5	Severe disability; bedridden and requiring constant nursing care and attention
6	Death

Table 3
Components and scoring of the NIHSS

Item #	Component	Responses and Scores
1A	Level of consciousness	0—Alert 1—Drowsy 2—Obtunded 3—Coma/unresponsive
1B	Orientation questions (2)	0—Answers both correctly 1—Answers one correctly 2—Answers neither correctly
1C	Response to commands (2)	0—Performs both tasks correctly 1—Performs one task correctly 2—Performs neither
2	Gaze	0—Normal horizontal movements 1—Partial gaze palsy 2—Complete gaze palsy
3	Visual fields	0—No visual field defect 1—Partial hemianopia 2—Complete hemianopia 3—Bilateral hemianopia
4	Facial movement	0—Normal 1—Minor facial weakness 2—Partial facial weakness 3—Complete unilateral palsy

5	Motor function (arm)
	   a. Left
	   b. Right
		0—No drift
		1—Drift before 5 s
		2—Falls before 10 s
		3—No effort against gravity
		4—No movement

6	Motor function (leg)
	   a. Left
	   b. Right
		0—No drift
		1—Drift before 5 s
		2—Falls before 5 s
		3—No effort against gravity
		4—No movement

7	Limb ataxia	0—No ataxia 1—Ataxia in 1 limb 2—Ataxia in 2 limbs
8	Sensory	0—No sensory loss 1—Mild sensory loss 2—Severe sensory loss
9	Language	0—Normal 1—Mild aphasia 2—Severe aphasia 3—Mute or global aphasia
10	Articulation	0—Normal 1—Mild dysarthria 2—Severe dysarthria
11	Extinction or inattention	0—Absent 1—Mild (loss 1 sensory modality) 2—Severe (loss 2 modalities)

Note: The NIHSS is a 42-point scale that quantifies neurologic deficits in 11 categories. It is used as a serial measurement of deficits and is reproducible among clinicians and investigators.[51]

find a difference in mortality or rates of favorable outcome despite longer times to treatment in the elderly patients (147 minutes vs 133 minutes, $P = .034$).[27] In addition, many studies reported that more patients in the older cohort had more severe neurologic deficits at presentation, higher rates of comorbid conditions and more pre-existing disability.[18,21,24,29,30,32–34]

OUTCOMES BASED ON TREATED VERSUS NOT TREATED IN GREATER THAN 80 YEARS OLD COHORT

In contrast to the body of literature focused on comparing outcomes between older and younger patients, there are few publications comparing outcomes between treated and nontreated elderly patients (**Table 4**). In addition, different endpoints for outcome analyses were used between studies, making it difficult to draw comparisons between findings.

Two analyses with small sample sizes did not find any difference in outcome measures between treatment and control groups and reported conflicting results in regard to risk of hemorrhage.[55,57] A subsequent pooled analysis of elderly in randomized controlled trials (including one of the previous analyses) found a significant imbalance in baseline neurologic deficits and that adjusting for this imbalance lead to a suggestion of benefit from treatment.[58] Analysis of a Dutch registry also indicated that there was a suggestion of benefit for treatment with tPA in patients 80 years and older.[56] Other studies have reported a significantly increased chance of a favorable outcome and neurologic improvement with treatment in the elderly when compared with nonthrombolytic medical therapy.[58–60] The association between thrombolysis and favorable outcome was similar in magnitude to that found in the younger patients (**Table 5**).[58,59] According to one of these analyses, 8.5 patients aged 80 years or younger need to be treated for 1 more patient to achieve an mRS of 0 to 2 whereas 8.2 patients aged older than 80 need to be treated to achieve the same endpoint.[59] Where reported, this benefit was not offset by an excess of mortality or symptomatic hemorrhage among elderly with tPA use.[23,59,60]

Recently reported results from a large international randomized study and an updated meta-analysis have been able to provide additional compelling evidence of treatment benefit in the elderly (discussed later).[61,62]

EARLY NEUROLOGIC IMPROVEMENT IN THE ELDERLY

As discussed previously, a subanalysis of the NINDS trials found no difference in the likelihood of a response to tPA in the elderly and a treatment benefit was suggested.[46] Other, more recent studies, have reported similar proportions of elderly and younger patients achieving early neurologic improvement (**Table 6**) as well as regaining similar number of points on the NIHSS at 24 hours.[26,29,33] The change in baseline to 24 hours NIHSS has been used in stroke trials to measure treatment efficacy and has been established as a clinical biomarker of successful recanalization and effective reperfusion from thrombolytic therapy.[2,49,63,64] This suggests that elderly have similar rates of recanalization as those of their younger counterparts and is consistent with findings reported elsewhere (discussed next).[28]

ENDOVASCULAR TREATMENT IN THE ELDERLY

Although IA recanalization techniques are promising for the treatment of select patients with ischemic stroke, there are few data on the outcome and efficacy of IA recanalization techniques in patients older than 80. Due to a growing number of elderly patients and the increasing availability of endovascular interventions for AIS, under-standing the existing data concerning both safety and efficacy is important. Yet, most clinical trials in acute stroke have excluded octogenarians.[49,65] Several recent studies have attempted to shed light on this topic.

In a large Specialized Program of Translational Research in Acute Stroke (SPOTRIAS) consortium registry, acute endovascular therapy (IA tPA, endovascular intervention alone, or bridging therapy with both IV tPA and endovascular intervention) was not associated with an increase in in-house mortality in patients 80 years old or older when compared with IV tPA treatment in the same age group.[37] A total of 3768 patients, the largest study of endovascular therapy in patients 80 years or older, were included in the study that concluded that IA therapy (IAT) does not seem to increase the risk of in-hospital mortality among those 80 years or older compared with IV thrombolysis alone.

In a much smaller study, Kim and colleagues[66] retrospectively compared patients age 80 years or older (n = 33) with patients aged less than 80 years (n = 81) from a registry of consecutive patients treated with IA thrombolysis over a 9-year period at a single institution. They concluded that IAT can achieve recanalization rates and hemorrhage rates equal to a younger patient population. Additionally, although the octogenarian group had higher mortality rates and less robust functional outcomes, nondisabling outcomes were achieved 25% of the time. Therefore, from the few data available, it is evident that endovascular therapy in older patients may have higher mortality rates and lower likelihood of clinical benefit. A properly selected subgroup in the older age group may benefit from endovascular therapy.

Questions still left to answer are how to use advanced brain imaging, such as CT angiography or magnetic resonance angiography, to select patients most likely to benefit from IAT and how to reasonably triage prehospital stroke patients to high-volume comprehensive stroke centers with neurointerventional expertise. It is esti-mated that less than 10% of all US hospitals perform more than 100 cervicocerebral angiograms and other interventional procedures.[67] Unlike the extensive cardiac catheterization models for acute myocardial infarction and much larger number of interventional cardiologists in the United States, acute stroke interventionalist services are scarcer and geographically imbalanced, favoring larger urban, tertiary centers. Therefore, many patients do not have readily available neurointerventional service within their community. Yet, it is encouraging that the numbers of some neurointerven-tional procedures and centers has been increasing over the past several years.

EVEN SMALLER COHORT OF PATIENTS GREATER THAN 90 YEARS OLD

Because 1 in every 9 baby boomers lives to at least the age of 90 years,[68] it is esti-mated that by 2050 there will be more than 55 million nonagenarians wordwide.[69] Although age is a known risk factor for stroke, clinical trials have excluded any patient older than 90 years old. Little information is known about the outcomes after treatment with IV thrombolysis in this age group. As part of the Canadian Activase for Stroke Effectiveness Study (CASES) national registry,[70] 28 nonagenarians were identified who had received IV tPA. Compared with 242 octogenarians also treated with IV tPA, the older cohort did not have a significant difference in 90-day mortality or 30-day functional outcome or an increased rate of sICH. In a smaller cohort of Mayo Clinic or University of Alberta patients treated with IV tPA, 22 patients were identified.[71] These patients had higher 30-day and 90-day mortality rates (55% and 59%, respec-tively) than any other similar patients available in the literature. Most of the patients aged 90 days or older who received IV tPA in this group had poor 30-day outcomes or died. Given the limited amount of clinical experience in this age group, it is

Table 4
Comparison between tPA treated and nontreated within elderly patient cohort

Authors/Journal	Patient Population	N >/≥80 y		Data Collection Period (OTT)	Endpoints
		tPA	Non-tPA		
Longstreth et al,[55] 2010	Post hoc analysis NINDS trial (RCT– North America)	25	19	1991–1994 (3-h tPA)	90-d mRS 90-d NIHSS 90-d Barthel 90-d GOS ICH

Major findings:
No significant difference in all 4 measured outcomes (shift analysis)
6 Hemorrhages in 25 tPA treated
1 Hemorrhage in 19 placebo
>80 Cohort 2.87 times more likely to have sICH than <80

| Dirks et al,[56] 2011 | Observational cohort study (12 hospitals Netherlands) | 163 | 283 | 2005–2007 (not explicit, upper limit SD 209 min) | 90-d mRS
sICH[a]
Death |

Major findings:
Good outcome (mRS ≤2; no shift): 96 tPA vs 46 placebo; adjusted OR 1.19 (0.71–1.98)
sICH: 7.4% in tPA (none in placebo)

| Sung et al,[57] 2011 | Observational cohort study (single center, Taiwan) | 30 | 41 | 2006–2009 (3-h tPA) | Discharge home
mRS ≤2 @ d/c
sICH[c] |

Major findings:
Discharge home: 59.2% tPA vs 61.0% non-tPA
mRS ≤2 @ d/c: 20.0% tPA vs 17.1% non-tPA Shift analysis
sICH: 6.7% tPA vs 2.4% non-tPA

Study	Design	N	N	Period	Outcomes
Mishra et al,[58] 2010	VISTA (pooled data from neuroprotection RCTs)	301	893	1998–2007 (not given)	90-d mRS 90-d NIHSS Survival

Major findings: (for tPA treatment)
Good outcome:
1. Shift analysis: more favorable distribution of mRS (P = .002, adjusted OR 1.52 [1.05–1.70])
2. mRS ≤1 @ 90d: OR 1.46 (0.97–2.20), P = .07
3. mRS ≤2 @ 90d: OR 1.52 (1.06–2.17), P = .022
4. Survival: OR 1.20 (0.90–1.65), P = .20

Study	Design	N	N	Period	Outcomes
Mishra et al,[59] 2010	SITS-ISTR registry for tPA (Europe), VISTA for controls	2235	1237	SITS-ISTR: 2002–2009 (not given) VISTA: 1998–2007 (not given)	90d mRS

Major findings: (for tPA treatment)
Good outcome:
1. Shift analysis: more favorable distribution of mRS (adjusted OR 1.4 (1.3–1.6), P<.001)
2. mRS ≤1 @ 90 d: OR 1.9 (1.5–2.3)
3. mRS ≤2 @ 90 d: OR 2.1 (1.7–2.5)
4. Mortality: OR 0.89 (0.76–1.04)
Notes that 8.2 patients aged >80 need to be treated to achieve mRS score 0–2.

Study	Design	N	N	Period	Outcomes
Zacharatos et al,[60] 2012	Observational cohort study (3 hospitals, MN)	66	44 (IV) [also 46 IR]	2007–2009 (3-h tPA)	NIHSS improved by 4+ or 0 @ 7 d/d/c mRS ≤2 @ d/c sICH[c]

Major findings:
mRS ≤2 @ d/c: 17 (39%) tPA vs 24 (36%) non-tPA; adjusted OR 5.6 (1.8–17.5)
NIHSS improvement ≥4 or 0 @ 7d or d/c: 27 (61%) tPA vs 20 (30%) non-tPA; adjusted OR 7.2 (2.7–19.5)
sICH: 2% in IV tPA, none in non-tPA

Abbreviations: OTT, onset of symptoms to time of treatment (onset to treatment); RCT, randomized controlled trial; h, hours; d, day; d/c, discharge; GOS, Glasgow Outcome Scale; IR, interventional radiology; MN, Minnesota; SD, standard deviation; VISTA, Virtual International Stroke Trials Archive (www.vista.gla.ac.uk).

a NINDS-type sICH: any new hemorrhage on CT scan associated with any decline in neurologic status.[2]

b ECASS-type sICH: any hemorrhage on imaging that is associated with an increase in the NIHSS by at least 4 points from baseline.[38]

c SITS-MOST–type: local or remote type 2 parenchymal hematoma combined with a neurologic worsening of 4 or more points from baseline NIHSS, or from the lowest NIHSS score between baseline and 24 h, or any hemorrhage associated with death.[39]

Table 5
Comparison of magnitude of outcome between elderly and younger patients when compared with their nontreated age cohorts

Study/Outcomes	Age >80 Odds Ratio (95% CI)	Age ≤80 Odds Ratio (95% CI)
Mishra et al,[58] *Stroke* 2010		
mRS 0–1 at 90 d	1.46 (0.97–2.20)	1.31 (1.12–1.53)
mRS 0–2 at 90 d	1.52 (1.06–2.17)	1.54 (1.33–1.79)
Mishra et al,[59] *BMJ* 2010		
mRS 0–1 at 90 d	1.9 (1.5–2.3)	1.6 (1.4–1.7)
mRS 0–2 at 90 d	2.1 (1.7–2.5)	1.9 (1.7–2.0)

concluded that although some patients do benefit from receiving IV tPA, the overall functional outcome is poor (**Fig. 1**).

AGE AND RISK OF HEMORRHAGIC TRANSFORMATION AFTER THROMBOLYSIS

It is controversial whether elderly age is a risk factor for sICH in the setting of thrombolytic treatment. There is concern that aging itself incurs an inherently increased risk due to underlying changes in physiology, such as impaired clearance of medications, increased vascular frailty, and the development of age-related white matter disease and cerebral amyloid angiopathy.[7,26,72]

There is some evidence that age may play a role in sICH. Post hoc analysis of both European Cooperative Acute Stroke Study (ECASS) I and ECASS II as well as a pooled analysis of randomized controlled trials reported advanced age was associated with an increased risk of parenchymal hemorrhage.[73–75] A few observational studies have reported increased risk of any hemorrhage with increasing age.[76] Significantly higher rates of sICH have also been reported in some observational studies, although often with significant imbalances in at least several of the baseline variables.[22,30] Also, 2 recent publications include age in a risk score for sICH but neither has been prospectively validated (**Table 7**).[77,78]

Alternatively, there have been many observational and registry studies published that do not show a significant difference in sICH rates between patients 80 years old or older and patients younger than 80 years old (see **Table 1**).[14,17–21,23–28,32–34,37] Two large systematic reviews of observational studies did not find an increased likelihood of sICH in the cohort of elderly patients.[79,80] An analysis of a large registry (*Safe Implementation of Thrombolysis in Stroke–International Stroke Thrombolysis Register* [SITS-ISTR]) reported that after adjustment for baseline factors (including independence before stroke, comorbidities, and degree of neurologic deficit at presentation), there was no significant difference in sICH between the elderly and younger patients.[29]

A majority of studies have shown that the increased mortality among the elderly does not seem related to bleeding complications associated with thrombotic therapy.

Table 6
Early neurologic improvement in elderly patients

Early Neurologic Improvement[a]	Elderly[b]	Younger	P
Toni et al,[26] *Cerebrovasc Dis* 2008	85/207 (41%)	13/41 (31.7%)	0.26
Boulouis et al,[33] *J Neurol* 2012	129/302 (43%)	37/98 (38%)	0.39

[a] Early neurologic improvement at hour 24 = NIHSS 0 or 1, or improvement by >4 points on NIHSS.
[b] Elderly = age >80 years in Toni et al, age ≥80 years in Boulouis et al.[33]

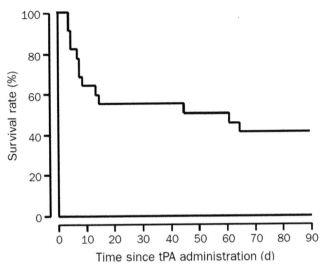

Fig. 1. Survival of patients aged 90 years or older, after administration of IV tPA for AIS (n = 22). (*From* Mateen FJ, Nasser M, Spencer BR, et al. Outcomes of intravenous tissue plasminogen activator for acute ischemic stroke in patients aged 90 years or older. Mayo Clin Proc 2009;84:334–8; with permission.)

Despite the increased mortality rate, 16.5% to 52% of the elderly patients maintained a good outcome or functional independence at 3 months (see **Tables 1** and **4**). This is often in spite of severe neurologic deficits at presentation, poor premorbid functioning, and high rates of comorbidities. Elderly patients consistently have higher rates of atrial fibrillation, a condition that has been associated with more severe stroke, increased risk of hemorrhage, and the development of cognitive and functional decline (independent of stroke).[54,65,81,82]

RECENT ADVANCES IN KNOWLEDGE

The results of the third International Stroke Trial, an international, multicenter, randomized, open-treatment trial, were recently published.[61] This trial was designed to provide outcomes and safety information for a wide range of patients previously excluded from treatment with tPA. As such, 1617 patients (53%) enrolled in the trial were older than 80 years of age. It was determined that 223 out of the 817 treated with tPA (27.3%) and 188 out of the 799 not treated with tPA (23.5%) were alive and independent at 3 months.[61] This difference was found to favor treatment with tPA (adjusted OR 1.35; 99% CI, 0.97–1.88).[61] This gives a number needed to treat (NNT) of 17 for one more elderly patient to be alive and independent at 3 months (calculated using http://ktclearinghouse.ca/cebm/practise/ca/calculators/ortonnt). (NNT and number needed to harm [NNH] for all age groups subdivided by time segments can be found in **Table 8**.)

A subsequent updated meta-analysis reported a significant difference in the percentages of elderly patients achieving an mRS less than or equal to 2 (ie, good functional outcome) at the end of follow-up (28.9% tPA vs 19.3% controls; OR 1.56; 95% CI, 1.28–1.90; $P<.0001$).[62] Both publications reported that the benefit seen in the elderly population was similar to that seen in patients younger than 80 years of age, especially when treated within 3 hours of symptom onset.[61,62] An ongoing open-label randomized trial, Thrombolysis in Elderly Stroke Patients in Italy, is investigating IV tPA treatment within 3 hours for patients older than 80 years of age and should

Table 7
Proposed risk scores for symptomatic hemorrhage after thrombolysis

Risk Score	SITS Symptomatic Intracerebral Hemorrhage Risk Score[77]		The SEDAN Score[78]		
Score components	Risk factor	Points	Risk Factor	Category	Points
	Aspirin + clopidogrel	3	Sugar	≤144 mg/dL	0
	Aspirin monotherapy	2		145–216 mg/dL	1
	NIHSS ≥13	2		>216 mg/dL	2
	NIHSS 7–12	1	Early infarct signs of HCT	No	0
	Glucose ≥180 mg/dL	2		Yes	1
	Age ≥72 y	1	Hyperdense on MCA HCT	No	0
	Systolic BP ≥146 mm Hg	1		Yes	1
	Weight ≥95 kg	1	Age	≤75 y	0
	OTT ≥180 min	1		>75 y	1
	History of hypertension	1	NIHSS on admission	0–9 points	0
				≥10 points	1
Interpretation	Total Score	sICH rate (95% CI)	Total Score	LR for sICH (95% CI)	
	0–2	0.4% (0.2–0.6%)	0	0.14 (0.03–0.75)	
	3–5	1.5% (1.3–1.7%)	1	0.52 (0.27–0.95)	
	6–8	3.6% (3.1–4.1%)	2	0.77 (0.45–1.23)	
	≥9	9.2% (5.9–12.5%)	3	1.46 (0.93–2.17)	
			4	2.92 (1.65–4.91)	
			5	5.51 (2.08–14.03)	
Derivation population	31,627 Patients treated with IV tPA in the SITS-ISTR		974 Patients treated with IV tPA at the Helsinki University Central Hospital		
Discriminating capability	C statistic 0.69 in internal validation cohort		AUC-ROC 0.77 (95% CI, 0.71–0.83) in external validation cohort		

Abbreviations: AUC-ROC, area under a receiving operating characteristic curve; BP, blood pressure; HCT, head computed tomography scan; MCA, middle cerebral artery; OTT, onset to treatment timel; y, years old; CI, confidence intervals; sICH, symptomatic intracranial hemorrhage.

Table 8 NNT and NNH per 90-minute segments for all patients			
Treatment Time (min)	Adjusted Odds Ratio for Benefit[75] (95% CI)	NNT[83]	NNH[83]
0–90	2.81 (1.75–4.50)	3.6	65
91–180	1.55 (1.12–2.15)	4.3	38
181–270	1.40 (1.05–1.85)	5.9	30
271–360	1.15 (0.90–1.47)	19.3	14

Benefit = favorable outcome (mRS 0–1, Barthel Index 95–100, or NIHSS 0–1) at 90 days.

further augment the information on treatment outcomes and safety in elderly stroke patients.[84]

ED MANAGEMENT OF STROKE: A BRIEF OVERVIEW

The successful treatment of AIS is dependent on a narrow therapeutic window. There-fore, it is imperative that hospitals and EDs create and maintain efficient pathways and processes designed to properly identify, evaluate, and treat acute stroke patients. In 1995, a consensus panel was convened by the National Institute of Neurological Disorders and Stroke (NINDS) to establish goals for the early management of stroke patients in EDs.[85] Additional guidance has been provided by the American Stroke Association and is outlined in the advanced cardiac life support curriculum (**Fig. 2**). Key points of this early ED evaluation are

- Initial evaluation and stabilization of the ABCs followed by a secondary assessment of neurologic deficits and comorbidities
- A history of the presenting complaint focused on determining when the patient was last known normal
- A focused physical examination
- A brief but thorough neurologic examination using a formal stroke score or scale, such as the NIHSS (see **Table 3** for parts of the score)
- Routine diagnostic testing to help identify comorbidity or systemic conditions that may mimic stroke
- Brain imaging, such as noncontrast CT scanning, to help differentiate ischemic from hemorrhagic stroke. Use of other advanced imaging modalities are often not necessary but may be useful in a selected patient population.
- Neurologic consultation. Although not absolutely necessary, the complexity of stroke presentation is sometimes better understood by a consultant trained in the subtleties of brain injury.

During the early phase of the ED evaluation of a stroke patient, it is useful to consider and review the widely accepted IV thrombolysis inclusion and exclusion characteristics (**Box 1**), both within the FDA-approved 3-hour window and the more stringent 3-hour to 4.5-hour window (**Box 2**). Although this extended IV window is not currently FDA approved in the United States, it has European approval and is widely used at many high-volume US stroke centers.

FUTURE DIRECTIONS

The future of stroke clinical care is exciting because of the exponential increase in un-derstanding of the stroke pathophysiology, diagnosis, management, and prevention. Yet, the only FDA-approved treatment of AIS is IV tPA, which was approved in 1996.

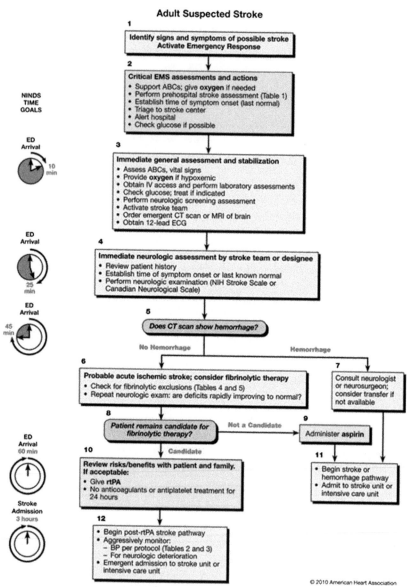

Fig. 2. Algorithm on how to approach a suspected stroke patient. (*From* Jauch EC, Cucchiara B, Adeoye O, et al. Part 11: adult stroke: 2010 American Heart Association Guidelines for Cardio-pulmonary Resuscitation and Emergency Cardiovascular Care. Circulation 2010;122:S818–28; with permission.)

Every few years, a group of academic physicians, industry representatives, and regu-lators meet to discuss ways to enhance the development of acute and restorative stroke therapies. In 2010, the seventh meeting of the Stroke Treatment Academic Industry Roundtable set forth the conceptual research agenda for the next several years.[86] This panel recognized that despite the tremendous advances in the under-standing of the pathophysiology of brain ischemia and investment in acute therapeutic trials, only a fraction of all eligible patients with ischemic stroke receive this care. The

---

Box 1
Inclusion and exclusion characteristics of patients with ischemic stroke potentially eligible for tPA within 3 hours from symptom onset

Inclusion Criteria

- Diagnosis of ischemic stroke causing measurable neurologic deficit
- Onset of symptoms <3 hours before beginning treatment
- Age ≥18 years

Exclusion Criteria

- Head trauma or prior stroke in previous 3 months
- The symptoms are suggestive of subarachnoid hemorrhage
- Gastrointestinal or urinary tract hemorrhage in previous 21 days
- Major surgery in the previous 14 days
- Arterial puncture at a noncompressible site in the previous 7 days
- History of previous intracranial hemorrhage
- Elevated blood pressure (systolic ≥185 mm Hg or diastolic ≥110 mm Hg)
- Evidence of active bleeding on examination
- Acute bleeding diathesis, including but not limited to
  - Platelet count <100,000/mm^3
  - Heparin received within 48 hours, resulting inn aPTT greater than upper limit of normal
  - Current use of anticoagulant with an INR >1.7 or PT >15 seconds
- Blood glucose concentration <50 mg/dL (2.7 mmol/L)
- CT demonstrates multilobar infarction (hypodensity greater than one-third the cerebral hemisphere)

Relative Exclusion Criteria

Recent experience suggests that under some circumstances—with careful consideration and weighing of risk to benefit—patients may receive fibrinolytic therapy despite one or more relative contraindications. Consider the risk to benefit of tPA administration carefully if any of these relative contraindications is present:

- Only minor or rapidly improving stroke symptoms (clearing spontaneously)
- Seizure at onset with postictal residual neurologic impairments
- Within 14 days of major surgery or serious trauma
- Recent gastrointestinal or urinary tract hemorrhage (within previous 21 days)
- Recent acute myocardial infarction (within previous 3 months)

Abbreviations: aPTT, activated partial thromboplastin time; INR, international normalized ratio; PT, partial thromboplastin time.

---

main recommendations of this group and the current direction of stroke care are as follows:

1. Maximize strategies in the use of IV thrombolytics through direct targeted public education. Failure of patients to recognize stroke symptoms and present to the ED within the 3-hour window is the number one reason for exclusion from treatment.

Box 2
Additional inclusion and exclusion characteristics of patients with ischemic stroke who could be treated with tPA from 3 to 4.5 hours from symptom onset (ECASS-3 Criteria)

Inclusion Criteria

- Diagnosis of ischemic stroke causing measurable neurologic deficit
- Onset of symptoms 3–4.5 hours before beginning treatment

Exclusion Criteria

- Age >80 years
- Severe stroke (NIHSS >25)
- Taking an oral anticoagulant regardless of INR
- History of both diabetes and prior ischemic stroke

Notes

- The checklist includes some FDA-approved indications and contraindications for tPA administration for AIS. Recent guideline revisions have modified the original FDA criteria. A physician with expertise in acute stroke care may modify this list.
- Onset time is either witnessed onset or last known normal.
- In patients without recent use of oral anticoagulants or heparin, treatment with tPA can be initiated before availability of coagulation study results but should be discontinued if the INR is >1.7 or PT is elevated by local laboratory standards.
- In patients without history of thrombocytopenia, treatment with tPA can be initiated before availability of platelet count but should be discontinued if the platelet count is less than 100,000/mm³.

Abbreviations: aPTT, activated partial thromboplastin time; INR, international normalized ratio; PT, partial thromboplastin time.
Data from Hacke W, Kaste M, Bluhmki E, et al. Thrombolysis with alteplase 3–4.5 hours after acute ischemic stroke. N Engl J Med 2008;359:1317–29.

---

2. Refinement of the current treatment exclusion criteria: many of the current thrombolysis exclusion criteria from the original NINDS trial published in 1995 were created from consensus opinion or adapted from the cardiac literature.
3. Increase the use of mechanical devices and IA recanalization: this will be accomplished by obtaining more definitive data on safety and efficacy in well-designed clinical trials.
4. Improved ability to identify particular characteristics associated with treatment efficacy: this can mean clinical scales, advanced imaging, or serum markers.
5. Further clarification of the true patient-specific effective time window for thrombolytic efficacy.
6. Optimization of the technical approaches to IA procedures.
7. Development of procedures to limit procedure and treatment complications.
8. Continue the elusive search for the ideal neuroprotective strategies to be provided concurrently or in lieu of thrombolysis. The ideal agent would need to be rapidly administered, directed toward the prevention of complications associated with early reperfusion, have multiple mechanisms of action, and avoid possible interactions between neuroprotective and thrombolytic therapies.
9. Further refine and define the roles of primary stroke centers, comprehensive stroke centers, and organized stroke systems of care so that patients, emergency medical services, and hospitals can provide seamless and efficient stroke care.

Although this is an extensive research agenda, many of these areas of research focus are well developed and currently being studied in clinical trials. The future of stroke care is exciting.

CONTROVERSIES IN TREATMENT

The use of thrombolytic therapy, specifically tPA, in patients with ischemic stroke is not without controversy within the field of emergency medicine. It has been 17 years since publication of the NINDS study,[2] the trial on which FDA approval for tPA in ischemic stroke was based. The findings of the trial were validated on reanalysis by independent observers[87] and a considerable amount of postmarketing evidence has accumulated in support of the NINDS conclusions.[38,39,48–50] Nevertheless, tPA for ischemic stroke 17 years post-NINDS remains hotly debated in some circles of medicine.

Today, several professional and community organizations have endorsed tPA use in stroke, including the American Academy of Neurology, American College of Chest Physicians, American Heart Association/American Stroke Association, Canadian Stroke Consortium, National Stroke Association, and many others. Additionally, the National Institutes of Health (NIH) sponsored national symposia on promoting treatment of acute stroke in 1997 and in 2002. There are more than 800 primary stroke centers certified by The Joint Commission and now a mechanism for comprehensive stroke centers certification is available to larger tertiary centers providing advanced cerebrovascular care. The cornerstone of these centers is the ability to provide timely and efficient IV thrombolysis to all eligible patients under 1 hour from ED arrival.

Yet, given the preponderance of evidence, why do some physicians still debate the safety and efficacy of the treatment? To answer this question, one must first understand the early history of tPA after FDA approval in 1996. Absent from the original list of endorsing professional organizations was emergency medicine representation. In 1996, the American College of Emergency Physicians (ACEP) agreed "with reservations" to the new stroke guidelines. In 2002, the ACEP issued a policy statement indicating, "intravenous tPA may be an efficacious therapy" but that "there is insufficient evidence to endorse the use of tPA when systems are not in place to ensure that NINDS guidelines are followed." The decision to use tPA "should begin at the institutional level." The American Academy of Emergency Medicine issued a position statement in 2002 to address issues of medical-legal liability. Their position paper stated, "Debate on the safety, efficacy and applicability of tPA has limited its widespread use. Nonetheless, an increasing number of liability suits are emerging against physicians for not administering tPA" and stated that there was insufficient evidence to classify tPA use in stroke as a standard of care.

The ACEP statement has since been removed from the ACEP Web site and is under revision to reflect the realities of stroke care in the twenty-first century. Yet, these ambivalent statements set the tone of doubt and resistance for some physicians for more than a decade.

Additionally, several emergency medicine leaders have repeatedly questioned the validity of the NINDS trial based on perceived conflicts between the American Heart Association, the major publisher of US stroke guidelines, and Genentech, the manufacturer of tPA. The implications are that the relationship between the pharmaceutical company, stroke physician thought leaders, and the American Heart Association places any results in serious question. The influence and persuasiveness of these physicians have caused many practicing emergency physicians to adopt a cautionary stance around IV thrombolysis for stroke.

Given the recent positive results of ECASS-3[50] and SITS–Monitoring Study (MOST),[39] which have provided additional reassurance about the safety and efficacy of tPA in ischemic stroke, and the wave of organized stroke systems of care throughout the United States, Canada, and Europe, it is only a matter of time before these voices of dissent are tempered by the overwhelming clinical data supportive of IV tPA, and, more particularly, organized stroke care designed on the foundations of education, stroke recognition, diagnosis, treatment, prevention, and rehabilitation.

SUMMARY

As discussed previously, elderly ischemic stroke patients have higher in-hospital and 3-month mortality compared with their younger counterparts. Treatment with tPA does not mitigate this outcome. Those patients 80 years old or older who have received acute treatment, either IV or IA thrombolysis, continue to have higher in-hospital and 3-month mortality rates than treated patients who are younger than 80 years old.[14,17–20,24–26] There is no excess mortality associated with tPA use in elderly patients, however. In-hospital mortality rates are similar for treated and nontreated elderly patients.[23] Patients 80 years or older seem to benefit from tPA therapy in a fashion similar to younger groups. Although older patients may have overall higher risk for complications and mortality, there is no reason to withhold treatment in any patient otherwise eligible for thrombolytic treatment.

REFERENCES

1. Centers for Disease Control and Prevention (CDC). Prevalence of stroke—United States, 2006-2010. MMWR Morb Mortal Wkly Rep 2012;61:379–82.
2. Tissue plasminogen activator for acute ischemic stroke. The national institute of neurological disorders and stroke rt-PA stroke study group. N Engl J Med 1995;333:1581–7.
3. Roger VL, Go AS, Lloyd-Jones DM, et al. Heart disease and stroke statistics—2012 update: a report from the American Heart Association. Circulation 2012;125:e2–220.
4. Kim AS, Johnston SC. Global variation in the relative burden of stroke and ischemic heart disease. Circulation 2011;124:314–23.
5. Fonarow GC, Reeves MJ, Zhao X, et al. Age-related differences in characteristics, performance measures, treatment trends, and outcomes in patients with ischemic stroke. Circulation 2010;121:879–91.
6. Saposnik G, Black SE, Hakim A, et al. Age disparities in stroke quality of care and delivery of health services. Stroke 2009;40:3328–35.
7. Asdaghi N, Butcher KS, Hill MD. Risks and benefits of thrombolysis in the elderly. Int J Stroke 2012;7:142–9.
8. Di Carlo A, Lamassa M, Pracucci G, et al. Stroke in the very old: clinical presentation and determinants of 3-month functional outcome: a European perspective. European BIOMED study of stroke care group. Stroke 1999;30:2313–9.
9. Marini C, Baldassarre M, Russo T, et al. Burden of first-ever ischemic stroke in the oldest old: evidence from a population-based study. Neurology 2004;62:77–81.
10. Kammersgaard LP, Jorgensen HS, Reith J, et al. Short- and long-term prognosis for very old stroke patients. The copenhagen stroke study. Age Ageing 2004;33:149–54.
11. Denti L, Scoditti U, Tonelli C, et al. The poor outcome of ischemic stroke in very old people: a cohort study of its determinants. J Am Geriatr Soc 2010;58:12–7.

12. Hills NK, Johnston SC. Why are eligible thrombolysis candidates left untreated? Am J Prev Med 2006;31:S210–6.
13. Alshekhlee A, Mohammadi A, Mehta S, et al. Is thrombolysis safe in the elderly? Analysis of a national database. Stroke 2010;41:2259–64.
14. Tanne D, Gorman MJ, Bates VE, et al. Intravenous tissue plasminogen activator for acute ischemic stroke in patients aged 80 years and older: the tPA stroke survey experience. Stroke 2000;31:370–5.
15. Simon JE, Sandler DL, Pexman JH, et al. Is intravenous recombinant tissue plasminogen activator (rt-PA) safe for use in patients over 80 years old with acute ischaemic stroke? The calgary experience. Age Ageing 2004;33:143–9.
16. Vatankhah B, Dittmar MS, Fehm NP, et al. Thrombolysis for stroke in the elderly. J Thromb Thrombolysis 2005;20:5–10.
17. Berrouschot J, Rother J, Glahn J, et al. Outcome and severe hemorrhagic complications of intravenous thrombolysis with tissue plasminogen activator in very old (> or = 80 years) stroke patients. Stroke 2005;36:2421–5.
18. Mouradian MS, Senthilselvan A, Jickling G, et al. Intravenous rt-PA for acute stroke: comparing its effectiveness in younger and older patients. J Neurol Neurosurg Psychiatr 2005;76:1234–7.
19. Chen CI, Iguchi Y, Grotta JC, et al. Intravenous TPA for very old stroke patients. Eur Neurol 2005;54:140–4.
20. Engelter ST, Reichhart M, Sekoranja L, et al. Thrombolysis in stroke patients aged 80 years and older: swiss survey of IV thrombolysis. Neurology 2005;65:1795–8.
21. Sylaja PN, Cote R, Buchan AM, et al. Thrombolysis in patients older than 80 years with acute ischaemic stroke: canadian alteplase for stroke effectiveness study. J Neurol Neurosurg Psychiatr 2006;77:826–9.
22. van Oostenbrugge RJ, Hupperts RM, Lodder J. Thrombolysis for acute stroke with special emphasis on the very old: experience from a single Dutch centre. J Neurol Neurosurg Psychiatr 2006;77:375–7.
23. Zeevi N, Chhabra J, Silverman IE, et al. Acute stroke management in the elderly. Cerebrovasc Dis 2007;23:304–8.
24. Meseguer E, Labreuche J, Olivot JM, et al. Determinants of outcome and safety of intravenous rt-PA therapy in the very old: a clinical registry study and systematic review. Age Ageing 2008;37:107–11.
25. Uyttenboogaart M, Schrijvers EM, Vroomen PC, et al. Routine thrombolysis with intravenous tissue plasminogen activator in acute ischaemic stroke patients aged 80 years or older: a single centre experience. Age Ageing 2007;36:577–9.
26. Toni D, Lorenzano S, Agnelli G, et al. Intravenous thrombolysis with rt-PA in acute ischemic stroke patients aged older than 80 years in Italy. Cerebrovasc Dis 2008;25:129–35.
27. Gomez-Choco M, Obach V, Urra X, et al. The response to IV rt-PA in very old stroke patients. Eur J Neurol 2008;15:253–6.
28. Pundik S, McWilliams-Dunnigan L, Blackham KL, et al. Older age does not increase risk of hemorrhagic complications after intravenous and/or intra-arterial thrombolysis for acute stroke. J Stroke Cerebrovasc Dis 2008;17:266–72.
29. Ford GA, Ahmed N, Azevedo E, et al. Intravenous alteplase for stroke in those older than 80 years old. Stroke 2010;41:2568–74.
30. Forster A, Szabo K, Kreisel S, et al. Thrombolysis in very old people with stroke: stroke subtypes, patterns, complications, and clinical outcome. J Am Geriatr Soc 2011;59:178–80.

31. Martins SC, Friedrich MA, Brondani R, et al. Thrombolytic therapy for acute stroke in the elderly: an emergent condition in developing countries. J Stroke Cerebrovasc Dis 2011;20:459–64.
32. Dharmasaroja PA, Muengtaweepongsa S, Dharmasaroja P. Intravenous thrombolysis in thai patients with acute ischemic stroke: role of aging. J Stroke Cerebrovasc Dis 2011;300:74–7.
33. Boulouis G, Dumont F, Cordonnier C, et al. Intravenous thrombolysis for acute cerebral ischaemia in old stroke patients >/=80 years of age. J Neurol 2012; 259:1461–7.
34. Guillan M, Alonso-Canovas A, Garcia-Caldentey J, et al. Off-label intravenous thrombolysis in acute stroke. Eur J Neurol 2012;19:390–4.
35. Costello CA, Campbell BC, Perez de la Ossa N, et al. Age over 80 years is not associated with increased hemorrhagic transformation after stroke thrombolysis. J Clin Neurosci 2012;19:360–3.
36. Cronin CA, Shah N, Morovati T, et al. No increased risk of symptomatic intracerebral hemorrhage after thrombolysis in patients with European cooperative acute stroke study (ECASS) exclusion criteria. Stroke 2012;43:1684–6.
37. Willey JZ, Ortega-Gutierrez S, Petersen N, et al. Impact of acute ischemic stroke treatment in patients >80 years of age: the specialized program of translational research in acute stroke (SPOTRIAS) consortium experience. Stroke 2012;43: 2369–75.
38. Hacke W, Kaste M, Fieschi C, et al. Randomised double-blind placebo-controlled trial of thrombolytic therapy with intravenous alteplase in acute ischaemic stroke (ECASS II). Second European-Australasian acute stroke study investigators. Lancet 1998;352:1245–51.
39. Wahlgren N, Ahmed N, Davalos A, et al. Thrombolysis with alteplase for acute ischaemic stroke in the Safe Implementation of Thrombolysis in Stroke-Monitoring Study (SITS-MOST): an observational study. Lancet 2007;369:275–82.
40. Mikulik R, Kadlecova P, Czlonkowska A, et al. Factors influencing in-hospital delay in treatment with intravenous thrombolysis. Stroke 2012;43:1578–83.
41. Saver JL, Smith EE, Fonarow GC, et al. The "golden hour" and acute brain ischemia: presenting features and lytic therapy in >30,000 patients arriving within 60 minutes of stroke onset. Stroke 2010;41:1431–9.
42. Kleindorfer D, Lindsell CJ, Brass L, et al. National US estimates of recombinant tissue plasminogen activator use: ICD-9 codes substantially underestimate. Stroke 2008;39:924–8.
43. Singer OC, Hamann GF, Misselwitz B, et al. Time trends in systemic thrombolysis in a large hospital-based stroke registry. Cerebrovasc Dis 2012;33: 316–21.
44. Barber PA, Zhang J, Demchuk AM, et al. Why are stroke patients excluded from TPA therapy? an analysis of patient eligibility. Neurology 2001;56:1015–20.
45. Huang P, Chen CH, Yang YH, et al. Eligibility for recombinant tissue plasminogen activator in acute ischemic stroke: way to endeavor. Cerebrovasc Dis 2006;22: 423–8.
46. Generalized efficacy of t-PA for acute stroke. Subgroup analysis of the NINDS t-PA stroke trial. Stroke 1997;28:2119–25.
47. Hacke W, Kaste M, Fieschi C, et al. Intravenous thrombolysis with recombinant tissue plasminogen activator for acute hemispheric stroke. The European cooperative acute stroke study (ECASS). JAMA 1995;274:1017–25.
48. Clark WM, Wissman S, Albers GW, et al. Recombinant tissue-type plasminogen activator (Alteplase) for ischemic stroke 3 to 5 hours after symptom onset. The

ATLANTIS Study: a randomized controlled trial. Alteplase thrombolysis for acute noninterventional therapy in ischemic stroke. JAMA 1999;282:2019–26.

49. Clark WM, Albers GW, Madden KP, et al. The rtPA (alteplase) 0- to 6-hour acute stroke trial, part A (A0276g): results of a double-blind, placebo-controlled, multi-center study. Thromblytic therapy in acute ischemic stroke study investigators. Stroke 2000;31:811–6.

50. Hacke W, Kaste M, Bluhmki E, et al. Thrombolysis with alteplase 3 to 4.5 hours after acute ischemic stroke. N Engl J Med 2008;359:1317–29.

51. Lyden P, Brott T, Tilley B, et al. Improved reliability of the NIH stroke scale using video training. NINDS TPA stroke study group. Stroke 1994;25:2220–6.

52. Rockwood K, Stolee P, McDowell I. Factors associated with institutionalization of older people in Canada: testing a multifactorial definition of frailty. J Am Geriatr Soc 1996;44:578–82.

53. Lang IA, Hubbard RE, Andrew MK, et al. Neighborhood deprivation, individual socioeconomic status, and frailty in older adults. J Am Geriatr Soc 2009;57:1776–80.

54. Marzona I, O'Donnell M, Teo K, et al. Increased risk of cognitive and functional decline in patients with atrial fibrillation: results of the ONTARGET and TRANSCEND studies. CMAJ 2012;184:E329–36.

55. Longstreth WT Jr, Katz R, Tirschwell DL, et al. Intravenous tissue plasminogen activator and stroke in the elderly. Am J Emerg Med 2010;28:359–63.

56. Dirks M, Koudstaal PJ, Dippel DW, et al. Effectiveness of thrombolysis with intra-venous alteplase for acute ischemic stroke in older adults. J Am Geriatr Soc 2011;59:2169–71.

57. Sung PS, Chen CH, Hsieh HC, et al. Outcome of acute ischemic stroke in very elderly patients: is intravenous thrombolysis beneficial? Eur Neurol 2011;66:110–6.

58. Mishra NK, Diener HC, Lyden PD, et al. Influence of age on outcome from throm-bolysis in acute stroke: a controlled comparison in patients from the virtual inter-national stroke trials archive (VISTA). Stroke 2010;41:2840–8.

59. Mishra NK, Ahmed N, Andersen G, et al. Thrombolysis in very elderly people: controlled comparison of SITS international stroke thrombolysis registry and virtual international stroke trials archive. BMJ 2010;341:c6046.

60. Zacharatos H, Hassan AE, Vazquez G, et al. Comparison of acute nonthrombo-lytic and thrombolytic treatments in ischemic stroke patients 80 years or older. Am J Emerg Med 2012;30:158–64.

61. Sandercock P, Wardlaw JM, Lindley RI, et al. The benefits and harms of intrave-nous thrombolysis with recombinant tissue plasminogen activator within 6 h of acute ischaemic stroke (the third international stroke trial [IST-3]): a randomised controlled trial. Lancet 2012;379:2352–63.

62. Wardlaw JM, Murray V, Berge E, et al. Recombinant tissue plasminogen activator for acute ischaemic stroke: an updated systematic review and meta-analysis. Lancet 2012;379:2364–72.

63. Parsons M, Spratt N, Bivard A, et al. A randomized trial of tenecteplase versus alteplase for acute ischemic stroke. N Engl J Med 2012;366:1099–107.

64. Kharitonova T, Mikulik R, Roine RO, et al. Association of early national institutes of health stroke scale improvement with vessel recanalization and functional outcome after intravenous thrombolysis in ischemic stroke. Stroke 2011;42:1638–43.

65. Seet RC, Zhang Y, Wijdicks EF, et al. Relationship between chronic atrial fibrilla-tion and worse outcomes in stroke patients after intravenous thrombolysis. Arch Neurol 2011;68:1454–8.

66. Kim D, Ford GA, Kidwell CS, et al. Intra-arterial thrombolysis for acute stroke in patients 80 and older: a comparison of results in patients younger than 80 years. AJNR Am J Neuroradiol 2007;28:159–63.

67. Grigoryan M, Chaudhry SA, Hassan AE, et al. Neurointerventional procedural volume per hospital in United States: implications for comprehensive stroke center designation. Stroke 2012;43:1309–14.

68. JC T. Testimony on the graying of nations. In: Senate special committee on aging. Available at: http://www.hhs.gov/asl/testify/t980608b.html. 1998. Accessed September 21, 2012.

69. International Day of Older Persons. Available at: http://www.un.org/en/events/olderpersonsday/background.shtml. Accessed September 21, 2012.

70. Mateen FJ, Buchan AM, Hill MD. Outcomes of thrombolysis for acute ischemic stroke in octogenarians versus nonagenarians. Stroke 2010;41:1833–5.

71. Mateen FJ, Nasser M, Spencer BR, et al. Outcomes of intravenous tissue plasminogen activator for acute ischemic stroke in patients aged 90 years or older. Mayo Clin Proc 2009;84:334–8.

72. Palumbo V, Boulanger JM, Hill MD, et al. Leukoaraiosis and intracerebral hemorrhage after thrombolysis in acute stroke. Neurology 2007;68:1020–4.

73. Larrue V, von Kummer R, del Zoppo G, et al. Hemorrhagic transformation in acute ischemic stroke. Potential contributing factors in the European cooperative acute stroke study. Stroke 1997;28:957–60.

74. Larrue V, von Kummer RR, Muller A, et al. Risk factors for severe hemorrhagic transformation in ischemic stroke patients treated with recombinant tissue plasminogen activator: a secondary analysis of the European-Australasian acute stroke study (ECASS II). Stroke 2001;32:438–41.

75. Hacke W, Donnan G, Fieschi C, et al. Association of outcome with early stroke treatment: pooled analysis of ATLANTIS, ECASS, and NINDS rt-PA stroke trials. Lancet 2004;363:768–74.

76. Tanne D, Kasner SE, Demchuk AM, et al. Markers of increased risk of intracerebral hemorrhage after intravenous recombinant tissue plasminogen activator therapy for acute ischemic stroke in clinical practice: the multicenter rt-PA stroke survey. Circulation 2002;105:1679–85.

77. Mazya M, Egido JA, Ford GA, et al. Predicting the risk of symptomatic intracerebral hemorrhage in ischemic stroke treated with intravenous alteplase: safe implementation of treatments in stroke (SITS) symptomatic intracerebral hemorrhage risk score. Stroke 2012;43:1524–31.

78. Strbian D, Engelter S, Michel P, et al. Symptomatic intracranial hemorrhage after stroke thrombolysis: the SEDAN score. Ann Neurol 2012;71:634–41.

79. Engelter ST, Bonati LH, Lyrer PA. Intravenous thrombolysis in stroke patients of > or = 80 versus <80 years of age–a systematic review across cohort studies. Age Ageing 2006;35:572–80.

80. Bhatnagar P, Sinha D, Parker RA, et al. Intravenous thrombolysis in acute ischaemic stroke: a systematic review and meta-analysis to aid decision making in patients over 80 years of age. J Neurol Neurosurg Psychiatr 2011;82:712–7.

81. Sanak D, Herzig R, Kral M, et al. Is atrial fibrillation associated with poor outcome after thrombolysis? J Neurol 2010;257:999–1003.

82. Tu HT, Campbell BC, Churilov L, et al. Frequent early cardiac complications contribute to worse stroke outcome in atrial fibrillation. Cerebrovasc Dis 2011;32:454–60.

83. Lansberg MG, Schrooten M, Bluhmki E, et al. Treatment time-specific number needed to treat estimates for tissue plasminogen activator therapy in acute stroke

based on shifts over the entire range of the modified rankin scale. Stroke 2009;40: 2079–84.

84. Lorenzano S, Toni D. TESPI (Thrombolysis in Elderly Stroke Patients in Italy): a randomized controlled trial of alteplase (rt-PA) versus standard treatment in acute ischaemic stroke in patients aged more than 80 years where thrombolysis is initiated within three hours after stroke onset. Int J Stroke 2012;7:250–7.

85. Proceedings of a national symposium on rapid identification and treatment of acute stroke. 1996. Available at: http://www.ninds.nih.gov/news_and_events/ proceedings/stroke_proceedings/contents.html. Accessed September 21, 2012.

86. Albers GW, Goldstein LB, Hess DC, et al. Stroke treatment academic industry roundtable (STAIR) recommendations for maximizing the use of intravenous thrombolytics and expanding treatment options with intra-arterial and neuroprotective therapies. Stroke 2011;42:2645–50.

87. Ingall TJ, O'Fallon WM, Asplund K, et al. Findings from the reanalysis of the NINDS tissue plasminogen activator for acute ischemic stroke treatment trial. Stroke 2004;35:2418–24.

Elder Abuse and Neglect
Definitions, Epidemiology, and Approaches to Emergency Department Screening

Michael C. Bond, MD*, Kenneth H. Butler, DO

KEYWORDS

- Elder abuse • Neglect • Geriatrics • Abuse

KEY POINTS

- Elder abuse and neglect is estimated to affect approximately 700,000 to 1.2 million elderly people a year with an estimated annual cost of tens of billions of dollars.[1,2]
- Elder abuse can take many forms (physical, neglect, financial, and so forth), the perpetrator is most commonly a family member, and elders that are maltreated are 3.1 times more likely to die in the next 3 years.[3–5]
- Despite the large population at risk, its significant morbidity and mortality, and substantial cost to society, elder abuse continues to be underrecognized and underreported. In one study, physicians reported only 1.4% of the abuse cases referred to adult protective services.[6]

> Every person…deserves to be treated with respect and with caring.
> Everyone, no matter how young or old, deserves to be safe from harm by those who live with them, care for them, or come in day-to-day contact with them
> —American Psychological Association[3]

INTRODUCTION

According to the US Census Bureau's national population projections, the structure of the United States population is aging steadily.[1–6] The first among the baby boomer generation reached retirement age in 2011, and the last will hit retirement age in 2029. Members of this generation currently account for 25% of the total population in the United States.[7] The elderly population has become more visible, more active, and more independent than ever before. Because of advances in health care, they

Conflict of interest: The authors have no conflict of interest to report.
Department of Emergency Medicine, University of Maryland School of Medicine, Baltimore, MD, USA
* Corresponding author. Department of Emergency Medicine, University of Maryland School of Medicine, 110 South Paca Street, Sixth Floor, Suite 200, Baltimore, MD 21201.
E-mail address: mbond007@gmail.com

Clin Geriatr Med 29 (2013) 257–273
http://dx.doi.org/10.1016/j.cger.2012.09.004   geriatric.theclinics.com

are living longer. But as this population grows, so do the hidden problems of elder abuse, exploitation, and neglect.

Research suggests that 700,000 to 1.2 million elderly people (ie, 4% of all adults older than 65) are subjected to mistreatment in the United States and that there are 450,000 new cases annually.[2] Sadly, this statistic is an inaccurate underestimation, because for every case of elder abuse and neglect that is reported to authorities, as many as 5 cases are not reported.[2] Abused elderly have a higher mortality rate, and tend to die earlier, than elderly people who are not abused, even those without chronic illnesses or life-threatening diseases.[8]

It is estimated that elder abuse costs Americans tens of billions of dollars annually, including health care, social service, investigative and legal costs, and lost income and assets.[1] In fact, the financial abuse of seniors is estimated to cost more than $2.6 billion per year and is more often perpetrated by family members and caregivers.[9]

The global economic recession has weighed heavily on this issue. In the United States, more family members are living under one roof, increasing demands on the caregiver. More elderly have had to make difficult financial decisions, and many cannot afford health care on their limited resources. Nationwide, 2 million adults leave Medicaid and become uninsured every year.[10]

Elder abuse, like other forms of abuse, is a complex problem, and many physicians understandably have misconceptions about it. In the emergency department, elder abuse and neglect are less evident than child abuse and domestic violence. Emergency providers tend to think of elder abuse and neglect as affecting people living in nursing homes with poor health care service. Unfortunately, elder abuse and neglect are much more common and could be happening right next door. The American Psychological Association has presented a more accurate picture of elder abuse[3]:

- *Most incidents of elder abuse do not occur in nursing homes.* Occasionally, shocking reports of nursing home residents who are mistreated by the staff are brought to the public's attention. No doubt such abuse does occur, but it is not the most common type of elder abuse. Only about 4% of older adults live in nursing homes,[11] and the vast majority of nursing home residents are being cared for without being subjected to abuse or neglect.
- *Most elder abuse and neglect occur in the home.* Ninety-five percent of individuals over age 65 live on their own or with their spouses, children, siblings, or other relatives, not in institutional settings.[12] When elder abuse happens, the abuser is usually a household member (89.7%) or a paid caregiver (4.2%).[13] Although there are extreme cases of elder abuse, the abuse is often subtle, and it is not always easy to distinguish normal interpersonal stress from abuse.
- *There is no single pattern of elder abuse in the home.* Sometimes the abuse is a continuation of long-standing patterns of physical or emotional abuse within the family. Alternatively, abuse can develop in response to changes in the family's living situation and relationships, brought about by the older person's increasing frailty and dependence on others for companionship and fulfillment of basic needs.
- *Infirm and mentally impaired people are not the only elderly who are vulnerable to abuse.* Elders who are ill, frail, disabled, mentally impaired, or depressed are at greater risk of abuse, but those who do not have these obvious risk factors can also find themselves in abusive situations and relationships.[6]

Like other forms of violence, elder abuse is never an acceptable response to any problem or situation, however stressful it may be. Effective interventions are available to prevent or stop elder abuse. By increasing awareness among and effective communication between physicians, mental health professionals, home health care workers, and others who provide services to the elderly and family members, patterns of abuse or neglect can be broken.

HISTORY

Since the first reports of elder abuse appeared in the medical literature more than 30 years ago,[14] studies from various disciplines—medicine, nursing,[15,16] social work,[17] and law enforcement[18,19]—have attempted to define the problem. While complex related issues are being debated and interventions evaluated, the importance of the problem and the need to identify elders at risk are clear. The uniqueness of the patient's home as the site of care has important implications for detecting and managing elder abuse and neglect. Family members and paid caregivers are more likely to be present during a home visit than during an office visit or a hospital encounter, so the interaction between the elderly person and his/her caregiver can be observed. Suspicions can be corroborated or diminished during visits, discussions can be undertaken with people entering the home (aides, therapists), and observations can be made over time. The need for support services, caregiver respite, or even emergency protection from harm can be overt, or the signs can be subtle, requiring a long-term relationship before they are identified.[3]

Elder abuse is now recognized internationally as a pervasive and growing problem, deserving the attention of clinicians who provide acute and chronic medical care for the elderly as well as that of the general public.[20] A report from the World Health Organization on violence and health prominently featured elder abuse and highlighted the range of harmful activities covered by this term throughout the world. Examples ranged from outright physical assault of old people in modernized cultures, which, sadly, has been acculturated into so-called traditional forms of family violence, to the systematic ostracization of tribal elders by the community in some less developed countries as a form of scapegoating (eg, levying charges of witchcraft against elderly Tanzanian women and then abandoning them as retribution for natural events such as drought or famine).

The establishment of the International Network for the Prevention of Elder Abuse in 1997,[21] with representation from more and less developed countries throughout the world, indicates the increasing concern about elder abuse. Along with this rising public interest, a slowly improving body of scientific work on the subject has been published. Although most research has been criticized as biased and methodologically flawed, recent investigations have used more rigorous approaches with concomitant gains in knowledge of elder abuse.[4] Much of the published research comes from the United States, Canada, the United Kingdom, and other European countries,[22] but additional countries are beginning to address this problem as well. For example, the World Health Association and the International Network for the Prevention of Elder Abuse held focus groups in Kenya, Lebanon, Argentina, India, and Brazil as a prelude to international collaborative research on the topic in 2001.[23] Several incidence and prevalence studies have been done throughout the world, using standard case definitions and, in some studies, scientifically acceptable research methods.[24] More rigorously designed risk-factor and natural-history studies have been done,[22] and there are calls for intervention studies that involve rigorous randomized designs, observer masking, and attempts to standardize interventions.[24] In the United States, a National Academy of Sciences panel was convened to assess the state of research on the abuse of elderly people.[22] Fortunately, elder abuse is being recognized as a threat to well-being and healthy aging, worthy of interest by clinicians, epidemiologists, and health-service researchers; however, these research advances create a quandary for the busy clinician.

Research into the detection and prevention of elder abuse is complex and sometimes contradictory, and a gap exists between basic research and clinical application.[25] Much of the epidemiologic and risk-factor research has been done by social scientists who have no first-hand familiarity with the ergonomically efficient practice of medicine, whereas clinical guidelines come mainly from the specialties of medicine and nursing. Several emergency medicine textbooks also advocate for elder abuse screening, but these lack a solid evidentiary basis or efficient protocol.[26,27] Elder abuse is one of a mounting list of family and social problems that encompass the scope of contemporary medical practice, yet the time and resources needed to address them are increasingly constrained in health systems in virtually all countries.

DEFINITION OF KEY TERMS

Various definitions of elder abuse have been developed, separating physical, psychological, and financial acts from omissions. A general definition is the following: intentional actions that cause harm or a serious risk of harm to a vulnerable elder by a caregiver or person who stands in a trust relationship with the elder, or failure by a caregiver to satisfy the elder's basic needs or to protect the elder from harm.[22] This definition encompasses 2 key ideas: that the old person has suffered injury, deprivation, or unnecessary danger, and that a specific individual (or individuals) is responsible for causing or failing to prevent it. It is important to consider the many forms that these acts or omissions can take and to be aware of subtle signs of abuse and neglect.

The National Center on Elder Abuse developed the following definitions for the 8 types of elder abuse and neglect (**Table 1**)[28]:

- *Abandonment* is the desertion of an older person by an individual who has assumed responsibility for providing care for the older adult or by a person with physical custody.

| Table 1 | |
| Types of elder abuse | |
Term	Definition
Abandonment	The desertion of an older person by an individual who has assumed responsibility for providing care for the older adult or by a person with physical custody
Emotional or psychological abuse	The infliction of anguish, pain, or distress through verbal or nonverbal acts
Financial or material exploitation	The illegal or improper use of an older adult's funds, property, or assets
Neglect	The refusal or failure to fulfill any part of a person's obligations or duties to an older adult
Physical abuse	The use of physical force that can result in bodily injury, physical pain, or impairment
Sexual abuse	Nonconsensual sexual contact of any kind with an older adult
Self-neglect	A person's refusal or failure to provide himself/herself with adequate food, water, clothing, shelter, personal hygiene, medication, and safety precautions
Resident-to-resident aggression	Negative and aggressive physical, sexual, or verbal interactions between long-term care residents

Adapted from National Center on Elder Abuse. Major types of elder abuse. Available at: www.ncea.aoa.gov. Accessed August 7, 2012.

- *Emotional or psychological* abuse is the infliction of anguish, pain, or distress through verbal or nonverbal acts. It is the second most common form of elder abuse. It can take the form of verbal harassment, belittling, threatening, and scolding, and may be overt or subtle. The victim's reactions can include withdrawal, apathy, rapid worsening of cognitive function, or new repetitive movements, such as rocking in place. Because many of these signs have a long differential diagnosis in geriatrics, a comprehensive approach is necessary, and full assessment may require several home visits.
- *Financial or material exploitation* is the illegal or improper use of an older adult's funds, property, or assets. It involves the breaking of trust through a manipulative or exploitive (possibly illegal) act. This type of abuse is suggested by sudden changes in bank accounts or banking practices, abrupt changes in the elder's will or other financial documents, and shortcomings in the care being provided (eg, lack of appropriate clothing) or failure to pay bills despite the availability of adequate finances. This type of abuse affects individuals from all socioeconomic statuses. Even small amounts of money or a monthly income can be a target.
- *Neglect* is the refusal or failure to fulfill any part of a person's obligations or duties to an older adult. It can be an intentional failure to provide goods and services that are necessary for optimal health and safety, or it can be unintentional, related to a lack of resources and knowledge. This type of neglect often involves the inadequate provision of life necessities such as food, water, and appropriate living conditions. Neglect is the most common type of harm (**Fig. 1**).[29] Unfortunately, it is also the hardest to prove.[13]

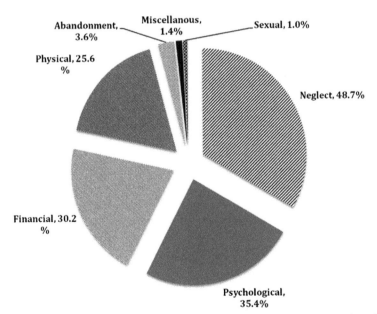

Fig. 1. Types of elder abuse and their incidence. (*Data from* US Department of Health and Human Services Administration on Aging and the Administration for Children and Families. The national elder abuse incidence study. Washington, DC: National Center for Elder Abuse; 1998; and Geroff AJ, Olshaker JS. Elder abuse. Emerg Med Clin North Am 2006;24:491–505.)

- ○ Psychological neglect includes the failure to provide social stimulation, imposed isolation, and restrictions on social interactions.
- ○ Financial neglect includes the failure to use available funds (often done with the intent to preserve a presumed inheritance) for goods and services needed for an elder's health and safety.

Neglect is usually not a willful act; it often occurs because of a lack of resources (eg, food, money, shelter) and lack of knowledge about how to request and receive assistance. Many care providers are doing the best they can, but they are physically, financially, or mentally unable to care for their loved one. The caregiver's guilt, pride, or shame might prevent him or her from seeking help, and others do not seek help for fear of losing their loved one to a nursing home or hospital. The same psychology can be seen with victims of neglect. Fear that they will lose the companionship of their family or fear of being sent to a nursing home may prevent them from reporting that they are living in substandard or unsafe conditions. Other factors that contribute to the underreporting of elder abuse and neglect are highlighted in **Box 1**.

- • *Physical abuse* is the use of physical force that can result in bodily injury, physical pain, or impairment. Physical abuse is probably the easiest to recognize,

---

Box 1
Factors affecting the reporting and recognition of elder abuse and neglect

- • Elderly people might not report or admit abuse for the following:
  - ○ Fear of retaliation
  - ○ Fear of being placed in a nursing home
  - ○ Fear that the care provider, usually a family member, will get in trouble
  - ○ Denial
  - ○ Blaming themselves for being a burden on their care provider
  - ○ Embarrassment and shame over being abused
  - ○ Poor self-esteem and feeling that the abuse is deserved
  - ○ Inability to communicate effectively, as in patients with aphasia or dementia
  - ○ Not having knowledge of available resources
- • Medical care providers might not report abuse for the following reasons
  - ○ Might not recognize the abuse/neglect and therefore attribute the patient's medical condition to another cause
  - ○ Might feel constrained by time
  - ○ Might be concerned about offending the patient and family or in denial that a family member is abusing, especially if the potential abuser is also a patient of the physician
  - ○ Is unfamiliar with mandatory reporting laws
  - ○ Is unfamiliar with available resources
  - ○ Is concerned about personal safety and have a fear of involvement
  - ○ Is unfamiliar with screening tools
  - ○ Misinterprets the patient's signs as indicative of another disease process

Data from Abbey L. Elder abuse and neglect: when home is not safe. Clin Geriatr Med 2009;25:47–60; and Kleinschmidt KC. Elder abuse: a review. Ann Emerg Med 1997;30:463–72.

although a victim's reluctance or inability to report it make even this form a challenge to prove. It can be extremely difficult or impossible to differentiate injuries sustained in a fall from those caused by being thrown to the ground. Physical abuse involves force or contact that is intended to cause intimidation, injury, impairment, physical suffering, or bodily harm.[30] It can take many forms, including kicking, biting, slapping, punching, cutting, burning, shoving, shaking, force feeding, pulling hair, pinching, striking with objects, and choking.[31] It can also include subtle forms of abuse such as forced isolation, the use of physical and chemical restraints, or not being allowed to bathe or use the restroom. Depending on the nature of the abuse, a health care provider might not see any physical indicators of it, or the caregiver and even the victim might provide a fictitious account of how the injuries occurred. Because of the potential lag between the time of injury and presentation to a medical care provider, it is imperative that the patient be interviewed separately from the care providers and asked about the infliction of abuse.

- *Sexual abuse* is nonconsensual sexual contact of any kind with an older adult. This type of intrusion should be considered if genital or breast injuries are discovered. Elders are often reluctant to admit that these acts have occurred. In some jurisdictions, suspicion of sexual abuse requires reporting to both law enforcement and social service officials. Sexual abuse is probably the least common and most understudied form of elder abuse. Tatara[32] estimated that 1% of elderly people in the United States are sexually assaulted. Sexual abuse can also take many forms. It can be physical, as rape and sodomy or subtle, as forced nudity, indecent exposure, and indecent speech. Unfortunately, the likelihood of proving sexual abuse is low. In 2001, Burgess and Hanrahan[33] reported the following:
  - The older the victim, the less likely that the offender will be convicted.
  - Offenders are more likely to be charged with a crime if the victim has signs of physical trauma.
  - Victims in assisted-living situations have a lower likelihood than those living independently that charges would be brought and the offender found guilty.
  - These results are particularly bothersome because the population that is least able to defend itself is the most likely to be sexually abused and the least likely to see justice served.

The elderly are certainly entitled to consensual sexual relations. Medical providers should not assume that this does not occur, and this topic should be broached in private as a routine inquiry. Furthermore, all cases of sexually transmitted disease in patients who, in the opinion of the medical care provider, lack the capacity to consent to sexual relations should be reported to the appropriate authorities as a potential sexual abuse case. The health care provider does not need to accuse or confront the potential abuser, but is obligated to alert authorities about a concern, which can then be investigated by trained professionals.

- *Self-neglect* is a person's refusal or failure to provide himself/herself with adequate food, water, clothing, shelter, personal hygiene, medication, and safety precautions. This could mean residing in deplorable conditions without heat or water, living in a home infested with insects, or not getting prescriptions filled. Elder self-neglect is an important public health concern and is the most common form of elder abuse and neglect reported to social services.[34] In fact, the number of reports of self-neglect to social services agencies is rising.[8] Self-neglect is associated with increased rates of hospitalization (rate ratio 1.47, 95% confidence interval 1.39–1.55), mortality and the severity of self-neglect is associated with the risk of death.[35] Self-neglect has great relevance to health care and social services agencies and to public health professionals, legal professionals, and community organizations. Many people with this type of neglect have underlying mental disorders (dementia, depression, psychosis, or substance abuse disorders) that prevent them from understanding that they need to seek assistance, although they tend to use outpatient, emergency, and hospital services more.[6,35,36]

- *Resident-to-resident aggression* is "negative and aggressive physical, sexual, or verbal interactions between long-term care residents that in a community setting would likely be construed as unwelcome and have high potential to cause physical or psychological distress to the recipient."[37]

Although this list of definitions is clear, each case may only have subtleties that make it difficult for the emergency physician to have an increased sense of suspicion (eg, lack of immediate family present, inconsistent visiting home health care providers, inability to know home environment, frequent provider changes or infrequent health maintenance visits, canceled visits, and vague or inconsistent details of injuries.) "It is very common for victims to move back and forth between acknowledging and denying mistreatment or accepting and refusing assistance."[38] These inconsistencies in their history should be a red flag to the physician and provide a sense of heightened awareness to suspect abuse or neglect.

Epidemiology

The true overall incidence and prevalence of elder abuse and neglect may never be known, as many cases go unreported or unrecognized, and research on this topic has been limited. The National Elder Mistreatment Study revealed that approximately 11% of United States elders surveyed had experienced some type of abuse or neglect over the previous year.[39] In 2004, Lachs and Pillemer[20] estimated the prevalence of elder abuse to be 2%–10%. The range was based on the sampling methods, survey methods, and case definitions used in the studies they reviewed. Even more worrisome is the estimation by several investigators that as few as 1 in 5 to 1 in 14 cases of elder abuse are reported to authorities and that the estimated prevalence has doubled over the past decade, from 3% to 5%.[13,40,41]

The best estimate of the incidence of elder abuse comes from a survey conducted by the National Center on Elder Abuse in 2000. The project coordinators reviewed the number of reports of elder abuse and neglect from 54 state regions (from a total of 56 "state regions" that have Adult Protective Services) for the most recent year available and found a total of 472,813.[34] A similar study published in 1998 estimated the incidence of elder abuse and neglect to be 551,000 cases involving more than 450,000 victims.[13,31] Finally, a survey of Adult Protective Services programs revealed approximately 381,430 reports of elder abuse and neglect in the United States in 2003.[42] Unfortunately, more recent data are not available. Most experts believe the incidence and prevalence are increasing, but it is not known if the increase is related to improved reporting and recognition or a true increase in the number.

To really comprehend the prevalence and incidence of elder abuse, the data must be analyzed in the context of our aging society. According to the 2010 United States census data, individuals age 65 years and over constitute the fastest growing segment of our population. Over the past decade (2000–2010), the population aged 65 and older grew 15.1% compared with a 9.7% increase in the total United States population. The number of individuals between the ages of 85 and 94 years increased 29.9% over the same decade. Individuals older than 65 years (numbering 40,267,984) now account for 13% of the United States population.[43] If abuse and neglect truly affect 11% of United States seniors, the number of victims is approximately 4.4 million every year. In reports published between 1993 and 2003, an estimated 1.5 to 2 million and 1 to 2 million elderly adults, respectively, were injured, exploited, or otherwise mistreated in the United States by someone they depend on for care or protection.[44,45]

Unfortunately, the most common perpetrators of elder abuse and neglect are family members, usually an adult child or a spouse (**Table 2**).[13,40,46] The risk is increased if the family member abuses alcohol or drugs. Many people worry about a family member being abused or taken advantage of by a paid care provider, but reports demonstrate that the elderly are actually safer when cared for by someone who is not a family member.

Elder abuse and neglect have a significant impact on morbidity and mortality rates among the elderly. One large study that adjusted for comorbidities and other factors associated with death showed that individuals who were maltreated were 3.1 times more likely to die during a 3-year period than those who were not abused. In the same study, after 13 years of follow-up, 9% of those who were maltreated were still alive compared with 41% of those who were not.[5] Elder abuse increases the risk of dementia, delusions, depression, and placement into a nursing home.[47–50] It is

Table 2 Characteristics of perpetrators of elder abuse	
Men[a]	52.5%
Abandonment	83.4%
Physical abuse	62.6%
Emotional abuse	60.1%
Financial exploitation	59.0%
Neglect	48.6%
Age	
41–59 y	38.4%
<40 y	27.4%
>60 y	34.3%
Race	
White	77.4%
Black	17.9%
Relationship	
Family member	89.7%
Adult child	47.3%
Spouse	19.3%
Other relatives	8.8%
Friend	6.2%
Home service provider	2.8%
Out-of-home service provider	1.4%

[a] Cases attributed to male perpetrators are listed by subcategory. Women had a lower incidence of abuse in all categories, except neglect, which was 52.4%.

Data from US Department of Health and Human Services Administration on Aging and the Administration for Children and Families. The national elder abuse incidence study. Washington, DC: National Center for Elder Abuse; 1998.

therefore clear that elder abuse has a significant effect on the life expectancy and quality of life of our senior citizens.

Legal Implications

Most states have mandatory reporting requirements for elder abuse and neglect. Physicians tend to be unfamiliar with these laws and less effective than other professional groups in identifying elder abuse.[51–53] A 2004 survey of state adult protective services programs showed that physicians made only 1.4% of the reports for elder abuse. The most common reporters of elder abuse were family members (17.0%), social services representatives (10.6%), friends (8.0%), law enforcement officers (5.3%), and nurses/aides (38%). This low level of reporting by physicians may be secondary to delegation of reporting to hospital or clinic staff, but it could also be related to the factors highlighted in **Box 1**.[6]

A medical care provider does not need to have definitive proof that abuse or neglect has occurred to file a report. A suspicion is all that is needed, and then the appropriate authorities, generally adult protective services, can investigate the claim. Most states that have mandatory-reporting status grant immunity to providers who report their suspicions in good faith. State-specific information on reporting requirements is available on the National Center for Elder Abuse Web site,[54] http://www.ncea.aoa.gov/ncearoot/Main_Site/Find_Help/State_Resources.aspx. Even if an investigation does not reveal intentional abuse or neglect, it can be extremely helpful to the patient and family by identifying resources that they did not know existed through other channels (Web search, social services, physician referral, and so forth). For instance, a family that is struggling to care for a loved one while they work during the day might learn about visiting nurses and adult daycare options.

However, medical care providers who believe that a patient is at risk of continued harm, whether it is from neglect, self-neglect, or abuse, are obligated to protect the patient. This might necessitate hospital admission to sort out the social situation, and it could require assessment of the patient's decision-making capacity if he or she wants to leave against medical advice.[55]

Risk Factors and Recognition

There is no stereotypical victim of elder abuse and neglect. Individuals from all races, cultures, and socioeconomic groups have been victims, and the abuse can occur anywhere (eg, in a personal home, a nursing home, or a hospital). Elderly women and the "old old" (>85 years old) are more likely to be victimized, though it is not clear if this higher risk stems from a decreased ability to defend oneself or the inability to escape from the situation. Most abusers (89%) are family members (see **Table 2**).[6]

Risk factors for elder abuse and neglect are presented in **Box 2**. Poor health and cognitive impairment probably increase the risk of maltreatment by reducing the elderly person's ability to report the abuse or defend himself or herself from it. Individuals who live alone are less likely to be abused, but elderly people who are socially isolated are at increased risk because they tend to have smaller support systems and the abuse is less likely to be noticed. A history of violence, mental illness, or alcohol/drug abuse increases the risk of abuse.[20,56–61] A good patient history, including an in-depth social history, can identify most of these risk factors. Unfortunately, these areas usually are not addressed in the Emergency Department.

Health care providers must be able to recognize the signs of elder abuse and neglect. Some red flags are highlighted in **Box 3**. Several screening tools have been designed to facilitate the detection of elder abuse. One that is easy to complete in the Emergency Department is the Elder Abuse Suspicion Index (EASI), which consists

Box 2
Risk factors for elder abuse and neglect

- Decreased physical health, (eg, requiring more assistance with activities of daily living)
- Dementia or cognitive impairment
- Female
- History of violence
- Increased age
- Shared living arrangements
- Social isolation
- Victim or caregiver with mental health or substance abuse issues

Data from Lachs MS, Pillemer K. Abuse and neglect of elderly persons. N Engl J Med 1995;332:437–43.

Box 3
Red flags of elder abuse and neglect

- Signs of neglect
  - Lack of medical aids (eg, medication, walker, cane, glasses)
  - Lack of adequate food, basic hygiene, heat, water, or appropriate clothing
  - Untreated medical issues (eg, pressure sores, Foley catheters, colostomy)
  - Confinement to a bed without assistance for long periods of time
- Signs of financial abuse
  - Excessive financial gifts or reimbursements for care provided or companionship
  - Lack of amenities the patient should be able to afford (eg, heat, water, food)
- Signs of psychological or emotional abuse
  - Unexplained changes in behavior (eg, depression, withdrawn, altered mental status)
  - Isolation from family members and friends
  - A caregiver who appears to be controlling, demeaning, overly concerned about spending money or is verbally or physically aggressive toward the patient
- Signs of physical or sexual abuse
  - Inadequately explained injuries (eg, fractures, sores, lacerations, welts, burns)
  - Delay in seeking medical attention after an injury
  - Unexplained sexually transmitted diseases
- General signs of abuse and neglect
  - Incongruity between accounts given by the patient and caregiver
  - Vague or improbable explanations for injuries
  - Presentation of a mentally impaired patient without a care provider
  - Laboratory or radiology findings that are not consistent with the history provided

Data from Lachs MS, Pillemer K. Abuse and neglect of elderly persons. N Engl J Med 1995;332:437–43; and Red flags of abuse. 2012. Available at: http://www.centeronelderabuse.org/docs/Red_Flags_2012.pdf.

of the 6 questions presented in **Box 4**.[62] Validation of the EASI occurred in family practice offices and ambulatory care settings, demonstrating a sensitivity and specificity of 0.47 and 0.75, respectively. The EASI requires less than 2 minutes to obtain. It was validated against a recognized, detailed elder abuse Social Work Evaluation (SWE).[62] An answer of "yes" to one or more of Questions 2 through 6 should prompt concern about abuse or neglect. A screening tool created by the American Medical Association (AMA) consists of the 9 questions presented in **Box 5**.[31] An answer of "yes" to any one of these questions should raise concern and prompt a more thorough evaluation.

The education of medical care providers and mandatory reporters is often promoted as a way of improving the recognition of elder abuse.[63] Educational interventions have been shown to increase knowledge, increase the use of assessment tools, and decrease reports of abusive actions by staff.[38,64,65] However, only Iowa requires that all mandatory reporters complete 2 hours of training within 6 months after initial employment and every 5 years thereafter.[38] Sadly though, there has been no change in the investigation and substantiation rates since the law was enacted.[66]

Education alone cannot increase the recognition of elder abuse, unless medical care providers actually have the time and resources to screen patients for this often occult problem. All medical providers should be educated on the screening for elder abuse. In the United States, the Joint Commission that accredits most hospitals already requires that Emergency Departments screen all patients to ensure that they are not a victim of abuse or neglect.[67] Typically, this is thought to be a domestic violence screen but it is also meant to identify elder abuse. Electronic medical records can also be designed to prompt for elder abuse.[68,69]

It is imperative that medical practitioners conduct a thorough history and physical examination, which could be instrumental in determining a patient's risk factors and identifying signs of abuse. At least a portion of the history should be conducted in

---

Box 4
Elder abuse suspicion index (EASI)

Questions 1 through 5 are answered by the patient. Question 6 is answered by the physician

1. Have you relied on people for any of the following: bathing, dressing, shopping, banking, or meals?

2. Has anyone prevented you from getting food, clothes, medication, glasses, hearing aids, or medical care or from being with people you wanted to be with?

3. Have you been upset because someone talked to you in a way that made you feel shamed or threatened?

4. Has anyone tried to force you to sign papers or to use your money against your will?

5. Has anyone made you afraid, touched you in ways that you did not want, or hurt you physically?

6. Doctor: Elder abuse may be associated with findings such as poor eye contact, withdrawn nature, malnourishment, hygiene issues, cuts, bruises, inappropriate clothing, or medication compliance issues. Did you notice any of these today or in the last 12 months?

The patient can answer "yes," "no," or "unsure." A response of "yes" on one or more of questions 2 through 6 should prompt concern for abuse or neglect.

Data from Yaffe MJ, Wolfson C, Lithwick M, et al. Development and validation of a tool to improve physician identification of elder abuse: the elder abuse suspicion index (EASI). J Elder Abuse Negl 2008;20:276–300.

> **Box 5**
> **American Medical Association screening questions for abuse**
>
> 1. Has anyone ever touched you without your consent?
> 2. Has anyone ever made you do things you didn't want to do?
> 3. Has anyone taken anything that was yours without asking?
> 4. Has anyone ever hurt you?
> 5. Has anyone ever scolded or threatened you?
> 6. Have you ever signed any documents you didn't understand?
> 7. Are you afraid of anyone at home?
> 8. Are you alone a lot?
> 9. Has anyone ever failed to help you take care of yourself when you needed help?
>
> *Data from* Geroff AJ, Olshaker JS. Elder abuse. Emerg Med Clin North Am 2006;24:491–505.

private, without family members or care providers present, so that the EASI or AMA screening questions can be asked. A thorough physical examination should then be conducted. This examination includes completely disrobing the patient to visualize any signs of abuse. Bruises or lacerations in various stages of healing, burns, or injuries that are not consistent with the mechanism reported should alert the provider to potential abuse. Decubitus ulcers, sores, dehydration, and poor hygiene should prompt concern for neglect or self-neglect. Again, one does not have to confirm that abuse occurred to make a report; you only need to have a legitimate concern, which will prompt a more thorough evaluation of the patient and his or her living situation. The provider should ensure that their note is factual, and does not make any accusations. The document should accurately reflect the concerns of the provider, and any physical examination or emotional findings that would make them suspect that abuse could be occurring. It is especially important to consider the diagnosis for patients who have frequent Emergency Department visits for dehydration or who show unexplained weight loss or a decline in physical and cognitive function.

SUMMARY

Elder abuse and neglect continue to be unrecognized and underreported. Increased educational efforts for health care providers, leading to increased awareness, of this societal problem, are needed to protect our elderly patients and decrease the incidence of abuse. Physicians can make a difference in the life of an elderly person by becoming familiar with the reporting requirements and the available assistance resources.

REFERENCES

1. 2005 White House Conference on Aging: post event summary report. 2005. Available at: http://www.preventelderabuse.org/whcoaging2005.html. Accessed September 1, 2012.
2. Report elder abuse, nursing home neglect and financial exploitation. Elder abuse reporting. Available at: http://www.elder-abuseca.com. Accessed August 10, 2012.

3. Elder abuse and neglect: in search of solutions. 2012. Available at: http://www.apa. org/pi/aging/resources/guides/elder-abuse.aspx. Accessed August 10, 2012.
4. WHO/INPEA. Missing voices: views of older persons on elder abuse. Geneva (Switzerland): World Health Organization; 2002.
5. Lachs MS, Williams CS, O'Brien S, et al. The mortality of elder mistreatment. JAMA 1998;280:428–32.
6. Abbey L. Elder abuse and neglect: when home is not safe. Clin Geriatr Med 2009; 25:47–60.
7. Rogers H. An aging population: demographic changes in America. 2012. Available at: http://ivn.us/2012/02/16/an-aging-population-demographic-changes-in-america. Accessed August 13, 2012.
8. Dong X, Simon M, Mendes de Leon C, et al. Elder self-neglect and abuse and mortality risk in a community-dwelling population. JAMA 2009;302: 517–26.
9. A study on elder financial abuse prevention. 2009. Available at: http://www. metlife.com/assets/cao/mmi/publications/studies/mmi-study-broken-trust-elders-family-finances.pdf. Accessed September 1, 2012.
10. Sommers BD. Loss of health insurance among non-elderly adults in Medicaid. J Gen Intern Med 2009;24:1–7.
11. A profile of older Americans. 2010. Available at: http://www.aoa.gov/aoaroot/ aging_statistics/Profile/2010/docs/2010profile.pdf. Accessed August 10, 2012.
12. Nasser HE. Fewer seniors live in nursing homes. U S A Today 2007. Available at: http://usatoday30.usatoday.com/news/nation/census/2007-09-27-nursing-homes_ N.htm. Accessed July 10, 2012.
13. US Department of Health and Human Services Administration on Aging and the Administration for Children and Families. The national elder abuse incidence study. Washington, DC: National Center for Elder Abuse; 1998.
14. Burston GR. Letter: granny-battering. Br Med J 1975;3:592.
15. Fulmer T, Guadagno L, Bitondo Dyer C, et al. Progress in elder abuse screening and assessment instruments. J Am Geriatr Soc 2004;52:297–304.
16. Fulmer T, Wetle T. Elder abuse screening and intervention. Nurse Pract 1986;11: 33–8.
17. Giordano NH, Giordana JA. Elder abuse: a review of the literature. Soc Work 1984;29:232–6.
18. Cooper GM, King MR. Interviewing the incarcerated offender convicted of sexually assaulting the elderly. J Forensic Nurs 2006;2:130–3, 146.
19. Morgan E, Johnson I, Sigler R. Public definitions and endorsement of the criminalization of elder abuse. J Crim Justice 2006;34:275–83.
20. Lachs MS, Pillemer K. Elder abuse. Lancet 2004;364:1263–72.
21. International Network for the Prevention of Elder Abuse. Available at: http://www. inpea.net. Accessed August 10, 2012.
22. Bonnie RJ, Wallace RB. Elder mistreatment: abuse, neglect, and exploitation in an aging America. Washington, DC: Panel to Review Risk and Prevalence of Elder Abuse and Neglect, The National Academies Press; 2003.
23. Krug EG, Dahlberg LL, Mercy JA, et al. World report on violence and health. Geneva (Switzerland): World Health Organization; 2002.
24. Thomas C. First national study of elder abuse and neglect: contrast with results from other studies. J Elder Abuse Negl 2000;12:15–7.
25. Carpenter CR, Gerson LW. Geriatric emergency medicine. In: Solomon DH, LoCicero J, Rosenthal RA, editors. New frontiers in geriatrics research. New York: American Geriatrics Society; 2008. p. 45–71.

26. Edwardsen ED. Elder abuse and neglect. In: Meldon S, Ma OJ, Woolard R, editors. Geriatric emergency medicine. 1st edition. New York: McGraw-Hill, Health Professions Division; 2004. p. 585, xix.

27. Jones JS. Abuse and neglect. In: Sanders AB, editor. Emergency care of the elder person Society for Academic Emergency Medicine Geriatric Emergency Medicine Task Force. St. Louis (MO): Beverly Cracom Publications; 1996. p. 171–96.

28. National Center on Elder Abuse. Major types of elder abuse. Available at: http://www.ncea.aoa.gov. Accessed August 7, 2012.

29. Lachs MS, Williams C, O'Brien S, et al. Risk factors for reported elder abuse and neglect: a nine-year observational cohort study. Gerontologist 1997;37: 469–74.

30. Physical abuse. Dorland's medical dictionary for health consumers. 2007. Available at: http://medical-dictionary.thefreedictionary.com/physical+abuse. Accessed July 5, 2012.

31. Geroff AJ, Olshaker JS. Elder abuse. Emerg Med Clin North Am 2006;24: 491–505.

32. Tatara T. Elder abuse in the United States: an issue paper. Washington, DC: National Aging Resource Center on Elder Abuse; 1990.

33. Burgess AW, Hanrahan NP. Identifying forensic markers in elder sexual abuse. Washington, DC: National Institute of Justice; 2001.

34. Teaster PB, Dugar T, Mendiondo M. The 2004 survey of State adult protective services: abuse of adults 60 years of age and older. 2006. Available at: http://www.apsnetwork.org/Resources/docs/AbuseAdults60.pdf. Accessed August 10, 2012.

35. Dong X, Simon MA, Evans D. Elder self-neglect and hospitalization: findings from the Chicago health and aging project. J Am Geriatr Soc 2012;60:202–9.

36. Dyer CB, Goodwin JS, Pickens-Pace S, et al. Self-neglect among the elderly: a model based on more than 500 patients seen by a geriatric medicine team. Am J Public Health 2007;97:1671–6.

37. Rosen T, Pillemer K, Lachs M. Resident-to-resident aggression in long-term care facilities: an understudied problem. Aggress Violent Behav 2008;13:77–87.

38. Daly JM. Evidence-based practice guideline: elder abuse prevention. J Gerontol Nurs 2011;37:11–7.

39. Acierno R, Hernandez MA, Amstadter AB, et al. Prevalence and correlates of emotional, physical, sexual, and financial abuse and potential neglect in the US: the national elder mistreatment study. Am J Public Health 2010;100: 292–7.

40. Pillemer K, Finkelhor D. The prevalence of elder abuse: a random sample survey. Gerontologist 1988;28:51–7.

41. Davidson JL. Elder abuse. In: Block MR, Sinnot JD, editors. The battered elder syndrome: an exploratory study. College Park (MD): University of Maryland; 1979. p. 49–66.

42. The 2004 Survey of State Adult Protective Services. Abuse of adults 60 years of age and older. Washington, D.C: National Center of Elder Abuse; 2006.

43. The older population: 2010. Washington, D.C: US Census Bureau; 2011.

44. Aravanis SC, Adelman RD, Breckman R, et al. Diagnostic and treatment guidelines on elder abuse and neglect. Arch Fam Med 1993;2:371–88.

45. Elder mistreatment: abuse, neglect and exploitation in an aging America. Washington, DC: National Research Council Panel to Review Risk and Prevalence of Elder Abuse and Neglect; 2003.

46. Paveza GJ, Cohen D, Eisdorfer C, et al. Severe family violence and Alzheimer's disease: prevalence and risk factors. Gerontologist 1992;32: 493–7.

47. Lachs MS, Williams CS, O'Brien S, et al. Adult protective service use and nursing home placement. Gerontologist 2002;42:734–9.

48. Coyne AC, Reichman WE, Berbig LJ. The relationship between dementia and elder abuse. Am J Psychiatry 1993;150:643–6.

49. Pillemer K, Suitor JJ. Violence and violent feelings: what causes them among family caregivers? J Gerontol 1992;47:S165–72.

50. Dyer CB, Pavlik VN, Murphy KP, et al. The high prevalence of depression and dementia in elder abuse or neglect. J Am Geriatr Soc 2000;48:205–8.

51. Blakely BE, Dolon R. The relative contributions of occupational groups in the discovery and treatment of elder abuse and neglect. J Gerontol Soc Work 1991;17:183–99.

52. Clark-Daniels CL, Baumhover LA, Daniels RS. To report or not to report: physicians' response to elder abuse. J Health Hum Resour Adm 1990;13:52–70.

53. Lachs MS, Pillemer K. Abuse and neglect of elderly persons. N Engl J Med 1995; 332:437–43.

54. State directory of helplines, hotlines, and elder abuse prevention resources. Available at: http://www.ncea.aoa.gov/ncearoot/Main_Site/Find_Help/State_Resources.aspx. Accessed August 10, 2012.

55. Sessums LL, Zembrzuska H, Jackson JL. Does this patient have medical decision-making capacity? JAMA 2011;306:420–7.

56. Williamson GM, Shaffer DR. Relationship quality and potentially harmful behaviors by spousal caregivers: how we were then, how we are now. The family relationships in late life project. Psychol Aging 2001;16:217–26.

57. Anetzberger G, Robbins JM. Podiatric medical considerations in dealing with elder abuse. J Am Podiatr Med Assoc 1994;84:329–33.

58. Compton SA, Flanagan P, Gregg W. Elder abuse in people with dementia in Northern Ireland: prevalence and predictors in cases referred to a psychiatry of old age service. Int J Geriatr Psychiatry 1997;12:632–5.

59. Grafstrom M, Nordberg A, Winblad B. Abuse is in the eye of the beholder. Report by family members about abuse of demented persons in home care. A total population-based study. Scand J Soc Med 1993;21:247–55.

60. Homer AC, Gilleard C. Abuse of elderly people by their carers. BMJ 1990;301: 1359–62.

61. Reay AM, Browne KD. Risk factor characteristics in carers who physically abuse or neglect their elderly dependants. Aging Ment Health 2001;5: 56–62.

62. Yaffe MJ, Wolfson C, Lithwick M, et al. Development and validation of a tool to improve physician identification of elder abuse: the Elder Abuse Suspicion Index (EASI). J Elder Abuse Negl 2008;20:276–300.

63. Hogan TM, Losman ED, Carpenter CR, et al. Development of geriatric competencies for emergency medicine residents using an expert consensus process. Acad Emerg Med 2010;17:316–24.

64. Pillemer K, Hudson B. A model abuse prevention program for nursing assistants. Gerontologist 1993;33:128–31.

65. Desy PM, Prohaska TR. The geriatric emergency nursing education (GENE) course: an evaluation. J Emerg Nurs 2008;34:396–402.

66. Jogerst GJ, Daly JM, Brinig MF, et al. Domestic elder abuse and the law. Am J Public Health 2003;93:2131–6.

67. Comply with the Joint Commission Standard PC.01.02.09 on Victims of Abuse. Available at: http://www.futureswithoutviolence.org/section/our_work/health/_health_material/_jcaho. Accessed July 7, 2012.
68. Bright TJ, Wong A, Dhurjati R, et al. Effect of clinical decision-support systems: a systematic review. Ann Intern Med 2012;157:29–43.
69. Kawamoto K, Houlihan CA, Balas EA, et al. Improving clinical practice using clinical decision support systems: a systematic review of trials to identify features critical to success. BMJ 2005;330:765.

APPENDIX

Sources of additional information on elder abuse and neglect:
National Center on Elder Abuse (NCEA) Program in Geriatric Medicine
University of California—Irvine
101 The City Drive South, 200 Building
Orange, CA 92868
1-855-500-3357 (ELDR)
www.ncea.aoa.gov
—*a national resource center dedicated to the prevention of the mistreatment of elders*

Clearinghouse on Abuse and Neglect of the Elderly (CANE)
Department of Consumer Studies and Research
University of Delaware, 297 Graham Hall
Newark, DE 19716
(302) 831-3525
www.cane.udel.edu
—*the nation's largest archive of published research, training resources, government documents, and other sources on elder abuse*

Eldercare Locator—
1-800-677-1116
www.eldercare.gov
—*a public service of the Administration on Aging, US Department of Health and Human Services; a nationwide service that connects older Americans and their caregivers with information on senior services*

Acute Kidney Injury, Sodium Disorders, and Hypercalcemia in the Aging Kidney
Diagnostic and Therapeutic Management Strategies in Emergency Medicine

Abdullah AlZahrani, MD[a], Richard Sinnert, DO[a,*],
Joel Gernsheimer, MD[b]

KEYWORDS

- Graying of America • Renal aging • Hyponatremia • Hypernatremia • Hypercalcemia
- Acute kidney injury • Hypovolemia • Hyperkalemia

KEY POINTS

- Structural and functional changes make the older patient more susceptible to acute kidney injury (AKI) and fluid and electrolyte disorders.
- When evaluating patients with hyponatremia, it is very important to classify the type of hyponatremia present. This classification is based on the patient's volume status, serum osmolarity, specific gravity of urine, and sodium concentration.
- Management is based on the type of hyponatremia the patient has and the patient's clinical status. For patients who have extremely low serum sodium levels and significant neurologic symptoms, such as seizures or altered mental status, treatment with hypertonic saline is the therapy of choice. Also, specific treatment of any underlying disorder should be given.
- Hypernatremia often presents in geriatric patients as dehydration and altered mental status.
- Management of severe hypercalcemia in geriatric patients should consist of hydration with normal saline, intravenous bisphosphonates, and calcitonin and treating the underlying cause.
- Underlying causes of acute renal failure, such as sepsis, hypovolemia, drug toxicity, and urinary obstruction, must be looked for and treated expeditiously.

[a] Department of Emergency Medicine, SUNY Downstate College of Medicine, 450 Clarkson Avenue, Brooklyn, NY 11203, USA; [b] Division of Geriatric Emergency Medicine, Department of Emergency Medicine, SUNY Downstate College of Medicine, 450 Clarkson Avenue, Brooklyn, NY 11203, USA
* Corresponding author.
E-mail address: nephron1@gmail.com

Clin Geriatr Med 29 (2013) 275–319
http://dx.doi.org/10.1016/j.cger.2012.10.007
0749-0690/13/$ – see front matter Published by Elsevier Inc.
geriatric.theclinics.com

INTRODUCTION

Improvements in sanitation and health care have led to a worldwide increase in human life expectancies. Simultaneously, lower growth rates in the developed world have contributed to the relative increase in the geriatric population. Thus, by 2030, there will be 71 million Americans aged 65 years or older accounting for approximately 20% of the US population.[1] The "Graying of America" is real and has a real effect on the medical care that is delivered.

An important geriatric medical issue with socioeconomic ramifications is that of renal diseases and electrolyte disorders associated with aging. According to the US Renal Data System, during 1995 to 2005, the adjusted point prevalence rates per million population of reported end-stage renal disease (ESRD) increased from 3627.5 to 5500.6 (51% increase) in the age group of 65 to 74 years and from 2762.4 to 4795.8 (73% increase) in those older than 75 years.[2] This increase seems to be because the management advances for cardiovascular and other diseases have prolonged the lives of older patients and given them the unfortunate opportunity to develop ESRD.

It may also be that new advances in screening for and diagnosing renal disease have increased the numbers of patients who are diagnosed with renal failure at earlier ages.

RENAL AGING

Aging in most species is associated with impaired adaptive and homeostatic mechanisms, leading to susceptibility to environmental or internal stresses that manifest clinically as increasing rates of disease, and the same is true of the kidney. Aging is associated with renal structural changes, functional decline and more difficulty in maintaining electrolyte balance.

STRUCTURAL CHANGES IN THE AGING KIDNEY

Grossly, the renal mass progressively decreases with age because the number and size of the glomeruli decrease with age. The average kidney weight progressively declines after the fifth decade of life,[3] with the renal cortex being affected more than the medulla.[4]

Vascular Changes

Arterial sclerosis is the main feature of the aging renal vasculature. The artery walls appear thick, and the vascular lumen is narrowed. This change is due to collagen increase in the media and intimal thickening, which is focal in its distribution, leading to heterogeneous cortical ischemia. None of these vascular changes are pathognomonic for aging and are often associated with several other conditions, including hypertension and diabetes.[5]

The aging kidney also contains a high percentage of afferent and efferent arterioles that communicate directly with each other ("aglomerular arterioles") because of loss of their glomeruli, particularly in the juxtamedullary location.[6] The aglomerular arterioles cause shunting of blood to the medulla, an increase in filtration fraction in the medulla, and medullary glomerular hypertrophy.[7]

Glomerular Changes

Nyengaard and Bendtsen[8] reported changes in glomerular number and size in relation to age. They showed that the number and the size of glomeruli were inversely proportional to age. Moreover, glomerular size was inversely proportional to kidney weight.[8] In addition, the percentage of glomeruli showing global glomerulosclerosis increases with age, and there are direct correlations between the number/percentage of globally sclerotic glomeruli and increasing age as well as between the number and percentage of globally sclerotic glomeruli and intrarenal arterial disease, particularly outer cortical arterial disease.[9] Up to 10% of the glomeruli may be globally sclerotic in "normal" subjects younger than 40 years.[10] Smith and colleagues[11] have suggested that beyond 40 years of age the percentage of "aging-related" sclerosed glomeruli is well represented by the formula (patient's age/2) − 10. Glomerular shape changes as well, with the spherical glomerulus in the fetal kidney developing lobular indentations as it matures. With aging, lobulation tends to diminish and the length of the glomerular tuft perimeter decreases relative to the total area.[12] Both diminished glomerular lobulation and sclerosis of glomeruli tend to reduce the surface area available for filtration and therefore contribute to the observed age-related decline in glomerular filtration rate (GFR).[13]

Tubulointerstitial Changes

Renal tubules undergo fatty degeneration and irregular thickening of their basal membrane with increasing zones of tubular atrophy and fibrosis.[5,14] The distal renal tubules develop diverticula that increase in number with advancing age. The diverticula in distal and collecting tubules may be precursors of the simple renal cysts that are seen in half of the subjects older than 40 years.[15,16] The number of renal cysts is greater in older patients than in younger patients. These cysts may cause complications such as rupture, infection, and obstruction. In addition, the aging human kidney is associated with mesangial matrix expansion and thickening of the glomerular basement membrane.[4]

FUNCTIONAL CHANGES IN THE AGING KIDNEY
Renal Hemodynamics

In 1940, Goldring and colleagues[17] reported a progressive decline of renal plasma flow (RPF) with aging in humans. Shock and colleagues[18] demonstrated a decreased clearance of p-aminohippurate in the older population, with the clearance decreasing from 600 mL/min per 1.73 m^2 in young adults to almost 300 mL/min per 1.73 m^2 by the age of 80 years.[19] The RPF is maintained through the fourth decade and then declines at the rate of 10% per decade.[20] The reduction in RPF is not entirely due to loss of renal mass, as xenon washout studies demonstrate a progressive reduction in blood flow per unit kidney mass with advancing age. The decrease in RPF is most profound in the renal cortex; redistribution of flow from cortex to medulla may explain the slight increase in filtration fraction seen in older patinets.[21]

Under normal conditions, the renal function reserve is the significant increase in the renal blood flow and GFR in response to renal vasodilation. The increase in RPF and GFR in response to maximum renal vasodilation induced by concurrent infusion of amino acids and dopamine is markedly reduced in healthy older individuals; this age-related impairment in renal hemodynamics is mainly because of morphologic changes, more specifically age-related renal vascular changes, rather than functional changes.[22,23] The reduction in renal hemodynamic and functional reserves can compromise renal adaptation to acute ischemia and as such can heighten susceptibility to acute renal injury in the geriatric population.

Glomerular Function

GFR is low at birth, approaches adult levels by the end of the second year of life, and is maintained at approximately 140 mL/min/1.73 m^2 until the fourth decade. As indicated by the classical inulin test, GFR declines by about 8 mL/min/1.73 m² per decade there-after.[18–24] Several studies have reported a decrease in GFR with age, with a delayed and slower decrease in women compared with men.[21–25]

In clinical practice, creatinine clearance is estimated in older patients using either the Cockcroft–Gault (CG) equation or the MDRD (modification of diet in renal disease) formula.[26] Creatinine clearance is influenced by the nutritional status, protein intake, and muscle mass and is therefore not an accurate measure of the GFR in geriatric patients.[27] A study showed more than 60% discordance in GFR estimation by the 2 equations in individuals older than 65 years. The MDRD equation generally yielded higher estimates of GFR than the CG equation.[28] This observation has important impli-cations, especially when calculating drug dosages in older patients. Overestimation of GFR can inadvertently result in unexpected drug toxicity. It was thus recommended that the CG equation should be used in preference to the MDRD equation to estimate GFR for drug dosage calculations in geriatric patients.[29]

Sodium Balance

The time required for the decrease in urinary sodium excretion in response to dietary sodium chloride deprivation is significantly prolonged in healthy older individuals when compared with young individuals.[30] The aging kidney also demonstrates an impaired capacity to respond to a sodium load. As shown by Luft and colleagues,[31] after a load of a 2-L saline infusion, older subjects excreted only 310 ± 9 mEq/24 h as opposed to 344 ± 5 mEq/24 h in subjects younger than 40 years. Furthermore, in older patients, the levels of plasma renin activity and serum aldosterone are reduced, and this could reduce the capacity of the kidney to retain sodium even more.[32] The critical effect of impaired sodium conservation in geriatric patients is that a 2-L diuresis induces a 24-mm Hg drop of systolic blood pressure in older subjects but not in young adults.[33] Therefore, the impaired ability to retain sodium may predispose geriatric patients to hemodynamic instability.

Potassium Balance

The excretion of potassium is derived from active transtubular transport in the distal nephron and collecting duct, which is linked to the reabsorption of sodium across the aldosterone-mediated Na-K ATPase transporters. Thus, impaired potassium secretion (and the corresponding impaired sodium reabsorption) may occur because of structural changes such as tubular atrophy, tubulointerstitial scarring due to ongoing glomerulosclerosis, or low levels of renin or aldosterone.[34] Furthermore, the prevalence of sodium and potassium disturbances increases with age and is asso-ciated with medication use.[35] Other studies in experimental animals have demon-strated that aging is characterized by impairment of the ability of renal tubules to adapt to a high potassium intake. This reduced efficiency of renal potassium excretion is associated with extrarenal impairment in potassium excretion, probably caused by a reduced activity of colon Na-K ATPase transporter.[36] These changes make older patients more likely to develop hyperkalemia, especially when given potassium supplements, potassium-sparing drugs such as spironolactone, or drugs that affect the renin-aldosterone system, such as angiotensin-converting enzyme inhibitors and angiotensin receptor blockers.

Renal Concentration and Dilution

Several studies have demonstrated an impaired renal concentrating ability in geriatric patients.[37,38] Studies in experimental animals have also demonstrated decreased responsiveness of renal tubules to arginine vasopressin (AVP), caused by a decrease in cyclic adenosine monophosphate generation and a lower expression of aquaporin-2 (AQP2).[39,40] These changes in renal concentration ability lead to hypernatremic dehydration in older patients. In addition, the renal diluting ability is also impaired in older subjects. In fact, after a water load, older subjects failed to reach the urine osmolality shown by younger subjects.[41] This impairment predisposes geriatric patients to hyponatremia, if excess fluid is administered.[42]

Other Physiologic Changes

Frassetto and colleagues[43] demonstrated that there is a progressive decline in plasma bicarbonate, with development of a moderate acidosis, in healthy older subjects with a steady state acid diet. The impairment of acid excretion may be due to a decrease in renal mass[44] or a reduction in ammonia production secondary to intrinsic tubular defect.[45] These changes make the older patient more likely to develop a metabolic acidosis, which can be a high anion gap and/or a normal anion gap acidosis. This acidosis can also cause hyperkalemia in these older patients.

In healthy subjects, the serum erythropoietin levels increase with increasing age.[46] However, the levels are unexpectedly lower in older anemic patients than in younger anemic patients, suggesting a blunted response to low hemoglobin levels.[47,48] Thus, it is more difficult for older patients to compensate for anemia and to respond to treatment of anemia.

HYPONATREMIA
Epidemiology

Hyponatremia, commonly defined as a serum sodium concentration less than 136 mEq/L (1 mEq/L = 1 mmol/L), is among the most common electrolyte abnormalities encountered in clinical practice.[49] In addition, patients with hyponatremia have a significantly increased risk of death during hospitalization and at 1 year and 5 years after admission.[50] However, in the emergency department (ED) study by Vroonhof and colleagues,[51] in patients visiting the ED, irrespective of the underlying condition, hyponatremia was not associated with an increase in mortality. As mentioned previously, the age-related changes and the effect of chronic diseases in the sensation of thirst, renal function, concentrating abilities, and hormonal modulators of sodium and water balance make geriatric patients more susceptible to impairment of water metabolism, which increases the risk of dehydration. Information on the frequency of hyponatremia in the ED setting is scarce. One study, reported by Lee and coworkers,[52] observed a 4% prevalence of hyponatremia (serum sodium levels <134 mEq/L) in an adult internal medicine patient population treated in the ED. Hypovolemic hyponatremia represents 65% of these cases, with the most common underlying disorders being those of the gastrointestinal system.[52] After adjusting for gender, increasing age (>30 years old) was independently associated with both hyponatremia at presentation and hospital-acquired hyponatremia (serum sodium levels <136 mEq/L) **(Fig. 1)**.[53]

In a study comparing the prevalence of hyponatremia in patients in nursing home with ambulatory geriatric patients, aged 60 years or older, the most recent serum sodium levels identified 18% of patients in the nursing home to be hyponatremic, compared with a prevalence of 8% in similarly aged ambulatory patients. In the nursing home population, 53% of the patients had at least 1 episode of hyponatremia in the previous 12 months. There was a high incidence of central nervous system (CNS) and spinal cord disease in the patients in the nursing home. Many episodes of hyponatremia were frequently associated with an increased intake of fluids, given either orally or intravenously or with tube feedings.[54]

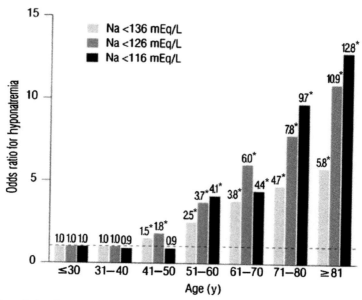

Fig. 1. Association between age and the odds of developing hospital-acquired hyponatremia at a large acute care hospital. Asterisk denotes $P<.05$ versus reference group (<30 years old). Analysis adjusted for sex. 1 mEq/L = 1 mmol/L. (*Data from* Hawkins RC. Age and gender as risk factors for hyponatremia and hypernatremia. Clin Chim Acta 2003;337:169–72.)

There are several risk factors for hyponatremia in the elderly. In a small sample of hospitalized Bronx adults, Choudhury and colleagues[55] identified some of the independent risk factors for hyponatremia at admission. Nursing home residents were 43-fold more likely to be hospitalized with hyponatremia (Na levels <135 mEq/L) and 16-fold more likely to be admitted with serum Na levels less than 125 mEq/L than were community patients. In addition, a declining serum Na level during hospitalization increased the risk of adverse outcome by fourfold. The drop in serum sodium levels during admission was strongly associated with increased length of stay, and this had been previously demonstrated by a cohort study in older patients admitted to 2 acute geriatric wards.[56]

Hyponatremia also increases the risk of large-bone (hip, pelvis, or femur) fractures in geriatric patients. Sandhu[57] demonstrated that the incidence of hyponatremia in geriatrics patients with fractures was more than double that of nonfracture patients. The degree of hyponatremia was noted to be mild to moderate. In the fracture group, 24.2% were taking antidepressants (3/4 of which were selective serotonin receptor inhibitors [SSRIs]), whereas there was no one taking these medications in the nonfracture group.[57] This result may indicate that administration of antidepressants is a probable risk factor for hyponatremia in geriatric patients. Increased fracture risk in hyponatremia also was independent of recent falls, pointing toward a possible adverse effect of hyponatremia on bone quality.[58]

Pathophysiology

Water homeostasis depends on an interaction between specialized sensors that translate the signals they receive (high serum osmolality, low effective circulating volume) to the central release of AVP (the antidiuretic hormone) into the circulation, which then stimulates water reabsorption in the renal collecting duct. Water balance regulation is primarily designed to maintain serum osmolality between 275 and 290 mOsm/kg and to a lesser extent, the blood volume (vasopressin levels start to increase after a 1% increment in serum osmolality vs a 5%–10% decrease in blood volume). The serum osmolality is sensed by osmoreceptors in several parts of the brain,[59] which stimulate the secretion of vasopressin into the bloodstream.[60] On the other hand, the carotid sinus baroreceptors sense a low effective circulating volume, and parasympathetic afferents transfer this signal to the vasomotor center, which increases the rate of vasopressin secretion by the cells in the paraventricular nuclei. Vasopressin stimulates an intracellular cascade in the renal tubular cells, which ultimately results in the insertion of AQP2 water channels in the apical membrane, which promotes water reabsorption.[61] The thirst stimulus (hypertonicity, hypovolemia, and other hormonal signals [eg, relaxin])[62] provides another crucial, but less-sensitive, means for the body to maintain water homeostasis by promoting oral intake of free water.[63] Thirst is decreased in older people as evidenced by response to water deprivation. Older persons, when compared with younger people, ingest smaller amounts of water during 24 hours of water deprivation.[64] A similar observation was made when older and younger persons were given hypertonic saline to induce hypertonicity. Older persons drank less water, when compared with their younger counterparts, after being given hypertonic saline.[64]

Dysregulation of AVP can be caused by both osmotic and nonosmotic mechanisms. Although osmotic regulation of AVP is more sensitive, nonosmotic stimulation is more potent. The presence of hyponatremia nearly always implies that vasopressin is released nonosmotically. Anderson and colleagues[49] showed that nonosmotic vasopressin secretion was present in 97% of hyponatremic patients studied. There are 4 mechanisms that result in abnormal vasopressin secretion during hyponatremia:

1. Nonosmotic vasopressin release caused by low effective circulating volume, several diseases, drugs, and nonspecific stimuli, such as anxiety, stress, pain, and nausea.
2. Ectopic vasopressin production (eg, small cell lung cancer).
3. Factors that may enhance the renal effects of vasopressin (eg, cyclophosphamide).
4. A vasopressin-like effect caused by an activating mutation of the vasopressin-2 receptor.[65]

There is increasing evidence for a relationship between high interleukin-6 levels and vasopressin release.[66] Furthermore, recently, a direct relationship was found between an increase in C-reactive protein levels and the development of hyponatremia, suggesting that the acute-phase response, perhaps mediated by interleukin-6, could explain the established relationship between certain infections and hyponatremia.[67]

Clinical Presentation

The signs and symptoms of hyponatremia depend not only on the absolute serum sodium level but also on the rate of serum sodium level decline. The symptoms are nonspecific and are related primarily to its effects on the CNS (**Fig. 2**). Mild hyponatremia (serum Na levels of 130–134 mmol/L) causes anorexia, cramping, nausea, vomiting, headache, and irritability. Moderate hyponatremia (serum Na levels of 125–129 mmol/L) causes disorientation, confusion, weakness, and lethargy. Acute severe hyponatremia is defined as the development of symptomatic hyponatremia of 125 mmol/L or less within 48 hours and can lead to seizures, coma, permanent brain damage, respiratory arrest, brainstem herniation, and death.[68]

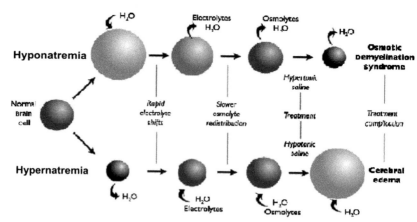

Fig. 2. Effects of transcellular fluid shifts on brain cells in hyponatremia and hypernatremia. Electrolytes and osmolytes shift in response to a hyposmolar and hyperosmolar extracellular environment, respectively, to preserve normal cellular volume. Overly aggressive fluid resuscitation can result in complications, such as osmotic demyelination syndrome and cerebral edema. (*From* Lin M, Liu SJ, Lim IT. Disorders of water imbalance. Emerg Med Clin North Am 2005;23:749–70; with permission.)

In chronic hyponatremia, symptoms are usually lacking, because of the adaptive mechanism of the brain in patients with sodium levels greater than 125 mEq/L, but when present, they may include subtle defects in gait and cognition.[69] Once serum sodium levels decrease below 125 mEq/L, neurologic symptoms become more profound and may include fatigue, memory impairment, vomiting, nausea, confusion, and seizures.

A careful review of recent events, medical history, medication changes, and social and psychiatric history is essential in ascertaining the cause of hyponatremia.

Physical examination should be focused on the assessment of the patient's neurologic status, including the level of consciousness, mental status assessed with the Mini-Mental Status Examination (MMSE), and volume status. In a study, geriatric patients with mild-to-moderate hyponatremia had significantly worse results in MMSE and other standardized tests of geriatric assessment compared with a normonatremic control group.[70] Major clinical indicators of hypervolemia include edema, rales, distended neck veins, and a third heart sound. The major clinical indicators of severe hypovolemia due to blood loss or severe dehydration include postural tachycardia, and severe postural dizziness. In patients with vomiting, diarrhea, or decreased oral intake, the presence of a dry axilla supports the diagnosis of hypovolemia (positive likelihood ratio of 2.8).[71] The hemodynamic response to extracellular fluid volume depletion seems to be dependent on the rate, magnitude, and source of fluid volume loss.[71] Therefore, clinical assessment of the extracellular fluid volume frequently yields misleading results in hyponatremic disorders. Chung and colleagues[72] demonstrated that clinical assessment correctly identified only 47% of hypovolemic patients with hyponatremia. Although the extracellular fluid volume should be routinely assessed in hyponatremic patients, it should be taken into consideration that misjudgment is common.

Tables 1 and **2** suggest some historical elements and some laboratory tests to help with the approach to hyponatremia.

Approach, Classification, and Causes

In the past, hyponatremia would always be classified initially based on the volume status. We find the following approach, which combines the volume status of the

Table 1
Some historical elements in hyponatremia

Category	Element
Current hospitalization	Recent surgery/trauma/pain IVF (hypotonic fluids) Irrigation with glycine (TURP, laparoscopy)
Medical history	Recent vomiting, diarrhea Diabetes mellitus, hyperglycemia Heart failure, edema, dyspnea Pulmonary disease or symptoms Renal disease Cirrhosis Hypothyroidism Adrenal insufficiency CNS disease or insult
Medicines	Medication changes Diuretics ACE inhibitors Medications associated with SIAD
Social history	Alcohol (beer potomania) Dietary history (Tea and toast diet)
Psychiatric history	Psychogenic polydipsia

Abbreviations: ACE, angiotensin-converting enzyme; IVF, intravenous fluids; SIAD, syndrome of inappropriate antidiuresis; TURP, transurethral resection of the prostate.
Data from Sra J, Repp AB. Hyponatremia. Hosp Med Clin 2012;1:2.

patient with some important laboratory values, to be very helpful in determining the cause of the hyponatremia and instituting correct management.

The initial approach to the hyponatremic patient is to measure the serum osmolality[73] or calculate it with the following formula:

$$\text{Plasma osmolality} = \left(2 \times \text{Na (mEq/L)} + \frac{\text{Glucose(mg/dL)}}{18} + \frac{\text{BUN(mg/dL)}}{2.8} \right)$$

where BUN denotes the blood urea nitrogen.

Although urea contributes to the absolute value of serum osmolality measured with an osmometer, it does not hold water within the extracellular space because of its membrane permeability. Urea is an ineffective osmole and does not contribute to

Table 2
Laboratory tests to help with the approach to hyponatremia

Initial test	Serum electrolytes Serum glucose, urea, creatinine, total protein Serum osmolality Urine osmolality and urine specific gravity Urine sodium and creatinine Calculation of FENa
Additional test	TSH Morning cortisol level Serum and urine uric acid Calculate FE_{urate}

Abbreviations: FEurate, fractional excretion of urate; FENa, fractional excretion of sodium; TSH, thyrotropin.

the effective serum osmolality (tonicity).[74] Based on effective serum tonicity (serum osmolality minus serum urea level), hyponatremia can be classified as hypertonic, isotonic, or hypotonic.

Hypertonic hyponatremia

Hyponatremia, with plasma osmolality exceeding 290 mOsm/kg (ie, hypertonic or hyperosmolar hyponatremia), suggests factitious hyponatremia secondary to hyperglycemia or administration of other osmotically active substances, such as mannitol.[75] Hyperglycemia generates a 1.6 to 2.4 mEq/L apparent decrease in plasma sodium for each 100-mg/dL increase in plasma glucose levels above 150 mg/dL.[76] Hillier and colleagues[77] have proposed that a correction factor of 2.4 mmol/L is a better overall estimate of the association between sodium and glucose levels.

Isotonic hyponatremia (pseudohyponatremia)

Hyponatremia with a normal plasma osmolality (275–290 mOsm/kg) is usually seen in patients with severe hypertriglyceridemia or paraproteinemia with serum lipids or protein level greater than 10 g/dL. Many laboratories now measure plasma sodium levels directly using ion-specific electrodes, thus eliminating this artifact.[78]

The 2 classifications mentioned above should be ruled out (by measuring the serum osmolality, lipid level, and protein level and managing accordingly) before treating hyponatremia.

Hypotonic hyponatremia

Most cases of hyponatremia are associated with a low osmolality (<275 mOsm/kg), reflecting a net gain of free water. The next step is measuring urine osmolality or specific gravity.[79] If the urine osmolality is less than 100 mOsm/kg, or if the specific gravity is 1.003 or less, then the urine is maximally dilute, which indicates that vasopressin secretion is completely and appropriately suppressed. This finding of hyponatremia and hyposmolar urine (<100 mOsm/kg) is seen in primary polydipsia or reset osmostat syndrome and is also observed in cases of extremely reduced solute intake as in "beer potomania syndrome."

Hyponatremia with hyposmolar urine (<100 mOsm/kg) Psychogenic polydipsia (primary polydipsia) occurs most frequently among schizophrenic patients and is characterized by excessive water intake, often in excess of 10 L/d.[80] Typical antipsychotics have been reported to worsen the polydipsia, favoring the use of atypical antipsychotics in these patients.[81]

Beer potomania is a rare cause of severe hyponatremia, and it is associated with a high rate of mortality and the osmotic demyelination syndrome (ODS).[82] The diagnosis is made based on the clinical history of heavy alcohol consumption in the setting of an otherwise poor nutritional intake and recognition of the low urine osmolality. Treatment of patients with beer potomania with isotonic or hypertonic saline causes brisk free-water diuresis, thereby increasing the risk of overly rapid sodium correction and ensuing osmotic demyelination. When serum sodium levels increase faster than 10 mEq/L in 24 hours or 18 mEq/L in 48 hours, dextrose 5% in water (D5W) should be infused at a rate to match the urine output (UO), and if needed, desmopressin may be used.[82,83]

Reset osmostat syndrome is a subset of the syndrome of inappropriate antidiuresis (SIAD) (formerly called syndrome of inappropriate antidiuretic hormone [SIADH]), which is often seen in elderly patients with pulmonary disease (eg, tuberculosis), and malnutrition.[84] When necessary, a water-loading test can be performed to distinguish reset osmostat syndrome from other patterns of AVP release.[85] When hyponatremia occurs because of "reset osmostat," renal concentrating and diluting capacities are normal but the regulation of AVP to maintain serum tonicity takes place at a lower osmolal threshold.

Hyponatremia with urine osmolality greater than 100 mOsm/kg If the urine osmolality is greater than 100 mOsm/kg, vasopressin-dependent impaired water excretion is indicated. The next step is to determine the urine sodium concentration, fractional excretion of sodium (FENa), and volume status. Urine sodium concentration less than 20mEq/L (ie, sodium conservation), and in older patients, levels of up to 30 mEq/L, are considered to indicate some degree of conservation of sodium.[30]

When the urine Na level is less than 30, the next step is to measure the volume status, which will be either hypovolemic or hypervolemic.

Hypovolemic hyponatremia with urine Na levels less than 30 mEq/L Hypovolemia with urine sodium levels less than 30 mEq/L or FENa less than 1% suggests active renal sodium retention to compensate for extrarenal losses that occur with gastrointestinal disorders with volume losses, due to vomiting, diarrhea, or third spacing; severe burns; or insensible losses. These patients represent the most common cause of hyponatremia found in patients in the ED (about 24.1%).[52] These patients need replacement of both volume and sodium.

Hypervolemic hyponatremia with urine Na levels less than 30 mEq/L Hyponatremia in the setting of an increased total body water (TBW) volume occurs in edematous states, such as congestive heart failure, liver failure, and nephrotic syndrome associated with a low effective arterial blood volume.[86] As a response to the reduced baroreceptor activity, the renin-angiotensin system is activated first, whereas the vasopressin axis is activated after a greater decrease in arterial filling. Recently, hyponatremia was also found to be a predictor of long-term mortality and admission for heart failure after hospital discharge in survivors of acute ST elevation myocardial infarction.[87]

A urine Na level greater than 30 mEq/L indicates that there is some sodium wasting, and the next step is to measure the volume status.

Hypovolemic hyponatremia with urine Na levels greater than 30 mEq/L This condition is seen in diuretics-induced hyponatremia. Although loop diuretics are more potent than thiazide diuretics, the latter are much more likely to cause hyponatremia. In cases of diuretic-induced hyponatremia, 73% was caused by thiazide diuretics alone, 20% by thiazide diuretics in combination with antikaliuretic agents, and only 8% was due to furosemide alone.[88] Thiazide-induced hyponatremia occurs most commonly in elderly women.

Other cause of hypovolemic hyponatremia with urine Na levels greater than 30 mEq/ L are salt-losing nephropathies, including renal tubular acidosis, polycystic kidney disease, and obstructive uropathy. Both type II renal tubular acidosis and metabolic alkalosis cause hyponatremia as a result of bicarbonaturia, which obligates sodium excretion.

Cerebral salt wasting syndrome (CSWS) has been described in patients with intracranial disease (mainly those with subarachnoid hemorrhage).[89] Although the exact mechanism of natriuresis is unknown, it has been suggested that a brain natriuretic peptide is released and causes an increase in sodium excretion and urine volume.[89] Volume status is a distinguishing feature, with euvolemia associated with SIADH and hypovolemia associated with CSWS. However, accurate determination of volume status under these conditions can be difficult.[90] Interestingly, the fractional excretion of urate (FE_{urate}) has been reported as a means of distinguishing these syndromes. In both SIADH and CSWS, FE_{urate} may increase more than 10%, but correction of hyponatremia normalizes FE_{urate} to less than 10% in SIADH, but not in CSWS.[91] Moreover, random urine sodium concentrations tend to exceed 100 mEq/L in CSWS, but rarely, if ever, in SIADH.

Euovolemic hyponatremia with urine Na levels greater than 20 mEq/L Hypothyroidism is a rare cause of euvolemic hypotonic hyponatremia that sometimes manifests as severe hyponatremia, and although the underlying mechanism is unclear, inappropriately elevated levels of circulating AVP is thought to be the cause of fluid retention.[92] Another endocrine disorder associated with hyponatremia is primary adrenal insufficiency, which is often missed, possibly because hyperkalemia is absent in one-third of the cases.[93] Hypopituitarism with secondary adrenal insufficiency is another overlooked cause of hyponatremia[94] and might be differentiated from SIAD by the presence of a compensated respiratory alkalosis with low plasma bicarbonate and low carbon dioxide levels.[95]

SIAD is a new terminology that is currently used, and it is a more generalized term than SIADH. In patients with euvolemic hyponatremia, several other clinical entities need to be excluded before making the diagnosis of SIAD. These include hypothyroidism, adrenal insufficiency, and hypopituitarism. There are specific criteria for diagnosis of SIAD. To be diagnosed with SIAD, patients must be euvolemic, have a urine osmolality greater than 100 mOsm/kg, and have a low effective plasma osmolality. Moreover, excessive water intake is necessary for hyponatremia to develop.[96] There are 4 patterns of SIAD. These patterns are unregulated vasopressin secretion, elevated basal secretion of vasopressin despite normal regulation by osmolarity, a reset osmostat syndrome, and nephrogenic SIAD,[97] which is characterized by undetectable vasopressin levels, unresponsiveness to vasopressin-receptor antagonists, and an abnormal response to a water-loading test. The causes of SIAD are myriad, and they are best classified into pulmonary disorders, malignant diseases, disorders of the nervous system, and drug-induced SIAD (**Table 3**). SSRI use poses a risk of development of hyponatremia, especially in patients who are older and have smaller body size.[98] Aging may be a risk factor for the development of SIAD-like hyponatremia in a subset of older patients who do not have an apparent underlying cause.[99] Patients with SIAD commonly exhibit low serum uric acid levels (<0.24 mmol/L), and it is associated with increased fractional excretion of urate (>10%).[100]

Fig. 3 shows an algorithm that can be used to differentiate the different causes of hyponatremia in older patients.

Management

Plasma osmolality provides the basis for an initial approach to management of hyponatremia. In hypertonic hyponatremia, treatment is directed at the underlying cause, for example, treating the hyperglycemia with fluids and insulin. No specific treatment is indicated for isotonic hyponatremia (ie, pseudohyponatremia) other than treating the underlying lipid disorder and investigating the protein disorder. Treatment of hypotonic hyponatremia is guided foremost by the presence or absence of symptoms and then by clinical volume status. Acute hyponatremia (occurring in <48 hours and more likely to be symptomatic) should be treated rapidly to prevent cerebral edema, whereas chronic hyponatremia (defined as present more than 48 hours) should be treated slowly to avoid OSD.[73] When the patient is severely symptomatic, for example, having seizures, severe altered mental status, or coma, aggressive therapy should be initiated. The treatment of choice is 3% hypertonic saline at 100 mL/h. For each 100 mL of 3% hypertonic saline, the serum sodium concentration increases by approximately 2 mmol/L. Hypertonic saline should not be used before laboratory

Table 3
Causes of syndrome of inappropriate antidiuresis (SIAD)

Central Nervous System Disorders	Neoplasms with Ectopic ADH Production	Pulmonary Disease	Drugs	Other
Vascular diseases (thrombosis, embolism, hemorrhage, vasculitis)	Small cell carcinoma of the lung	Pneumonia	CNS active drugs	Positive pressure ventilation
Trauma (subdural hematoma, subarachnoid or intracranial hemorrhage)	Pharyngeal carcinoma	Lung abscess	Antipsychotics	AIDS
Tumor	Pancreatic carcinoma	Bronchiectasis	Antidepressants (tricyclics, selective serotonin reuptake inhibitors)	Idiopathic SIAD of the elderly
Hydrocephalus	Thymoma	Tuberculosis	Anticonvulsants (carbamazepine)	
Infection (meningitis, encephalitis, brain abscess)	Lymphoma, Hodgkin disease, reticulum cell sarcoma		Narcotics	
Acute intermittent porphyria	Bladder carcinoma		Hallucinogenics (Ecstasy)	
Lupus erythematosus			ACE inhibitors	
Postoperative trans-sphenoidal hypophysectomy			Antineoplastic agents (vincristine, vinblastine, cyclophosphamide)	
Schizophrenia			Oxytocin	
			ADH analogs (desmopressin, lysine vasopressin)	
			Sulfonylureas (chlorpropamide)	
			Hypolipidemics (clofibrate)	

Abbreviations: ACE, angiotensin-converting enzyme; ADH, antidiuretic hormone; AIDS, acquired immune deficiency syndrome.
Modified from Miller M. Syndromes of excess antidiuretic hormone release. Crit Care Clin 2001;17:11–23.

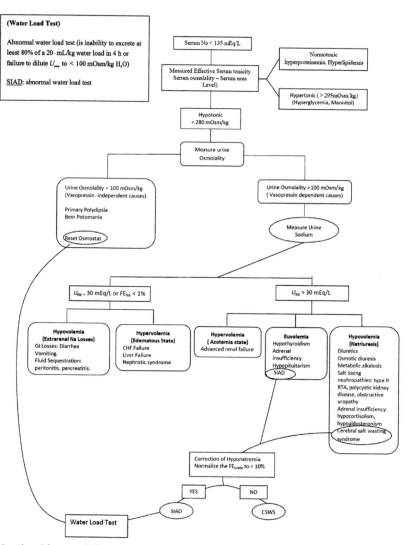

Fig. 3. Algorithm to differentiate the causes of hyponatremia. Gi, gastrointestinal; U_{osm}, urine osmolality; urine$_{Na}$, urine sodium; RTA, renal tubular acidosis.

confirmation of hyponatremia and should be used only in a closely monitored setting (ie, intensive care unit [ICU] or ED).[101] Duration of the hypertonic saline infusion is guided by the improvement of the patient's symptoms, or when the serum Na level reaches 120 mEq/L. The correction rate of acute hyponatremia should not exceed 8 to 10 mmol/L for the first 24 hours and 18 to 25 mmol/L for the first 48 hours.[101] In chronic hyponatremia, the correction goal is 6 mEq/L during the initial 24 hours.[102] The Adrogue–Madias formula[73] is the most widely used formula to predict the increment in serum sodium concentration after the infusion of either isotonic saline or hypertonic saline.[73] The use of this formula is demonstrated in **Table 4**.

For example, in a 80-kg elderly man who presents with significant altered mental status and a sodium concentration of 103 mEq/L, hypertonic saline should be instituted immediately in the ED. It is observed that 1 L of 3% saline (513 mEq/L sodium)

Table 4

$$\text{Change in plasma sodium} = \frac{(\text{Infusate sodium} - \text{plasma sodium})}{(\text{Total body water} + 1)}$$

Total Body Water = Weight(kg) × Correction Factor

Patient	Correction Factor
Male, elderly	0.5
Female, elderly	0.45

Na on the Infusate Solution	
IV Fluid	**Na (mEq/L)**
D5W	0
0.2% saline	34
0.45% saline	77
0.9% saline	154
3% saline	513

increases the serum sodium concentration by approximately 10 mEq/L, as calculated by (513 − 103)/([0.5 × 80] + 1). Thus, to increase the serum sodium concentration by 2 mEq/L in the first hour, one-fifth of a liter (200 mL) should be given.

The cornerstone of treatment of hypovolemic hypotonic hyponatremic patients is volume replacement with normal saline solutions. The elderly patient's vital signs and state of hydration (oxygen saturation by pulse oximeter, respiratory rate, and breath sounds) should be carefully monitored to ensure that the patient receives adequate volume replacement but does not become fluid overloaded. Also, any underlying cause of the patient's volume loss should be treated.

In asymptomatic patients with euvolemic (eg, SIAD) or hypervolemic hyponatremia (eg, cirrhosis with ascites and edema), fluid restriction is generally the treatment of choice. There are now nonpeptide antagonists to V2 vasopressin receptors, commonly referred to as "vaptans" or "aquaretics," which increase free water excretion and serum sodium concentration. One of these agents is conivaptan, which has been approved by the US Food and Drug Administration for intravenous use in the hospital to treat euvolemic and hypervolemic hyponatremia, specifically that due to SIAD and congestive heart failure (CHF).[101]

Treatment of SIAD can range from free-water restriction in asymptomatic patients to isotonic or hypertonic saline infusion in severely symptomatic patients. Hospitalized patients with symptomatic SIAD who do not respond to these treatments or who will not adhere to water restriction can be treated with either democycline or conivaptan. The dose of demeclocycline is 300–600 mg orally twice a day. It has an onset of action of 5–14 days. Conivaptan is administered as a loading dose of 20 mg intravenously, followed by a continuous intravenous infusion of 20–40 mg a day for no more than 4 days.[103] Corticosteroids can be used if hypocortisolism is suspected, and fludrocortisone can be used if hyponatremia is due to CSWS.[104]

In addition to directly treating the hyponatremia, it is very important to treat any underlying diseases that are causing or contributing to the hyponatremia, such as gastrointestinal, neurologic, cardiac, renal, pulmonary, psychiatric, and endocrine disorders. It is also very important to stop any medication that could be causing or aggravating the hyponatremia.

Osmotic demyelination syndrome

Osmotic demyelination syndrome is a well-recognized clinical entity and is a dreadful complication that classically occurs several days after aggressive rapid therapy for chronic hyponatremia. Osmotic demyelination syndrome includes central pontine myelinolysis (CPM) and extrapontine myelinolysis (EPM). CPM and EPM are the same disease, sharing the same conditions, associations, and time course but differing in clinical manifestations.[105] Different areas of the brain can be involved (**Box 1**).

The brain adaptation mechanism to hyponatremia begins shortly after an acute fall in serum sodium levels and is complete within 2 days. It is characterized initially by the loss of interstitial sodium and water into the cerebrospinal fluid because of increased hydraulic pressure and, within hours, by the loss of intracellular potassium, sodium, and organic solutes, called osmolytes (such as myoinositol, glutamate, and glutamine), from brain cells. This mechanism provides protection against cerebral edema. In chronic hyponatremia, this brain adaptation is already established, and these solutes cannot be as quickly replaced when the brain volume begins to shrink in response to correction of the hyponatremia. As a result, brain volume decreases from a value that is initially somewhat above normal to one below normal with rapid correction of hyponatremia, resulting in demyelination of areas of the brain. In contrast, overly rapid correction is not likely to induce ODS in patients with acute severe hyponatremia that has only been present for several hours, because the cerebral adaptation is at an early stage. The process by which demyelination occurs is not completely understood.[106] **Box 2** lists some of the risk factors for OSD.

The clinical features vary according to the site of involvement in the brain. The initial signs of CPM include dysarthria and dysphagia (secondary to corticobulbar fiber

---

Box 1
Areas of the brain that can be involved in CPM and EPM in descending order of frequency

- Pons
- Cerebellum
- Lateral geniculate body
- External capsule
- Extreme capsule
- Hippocampus
- Putamen
- Cerebral cortex/subcortex
- Thalamus
- Caudate nucleus

The following areas are involved in 10% or less cases:

- Claustrum
- Internal capsule
- Midbrain
- Internal medullary lamella
- Mamillary body
- Medulla oblongata

Data from Martin RJ. Central pontine and extrapontine myelinolysis: the osmotic demyelination syndromes. J Neurol Neurosurg Psychiatry 2004;75:22–8.

Box 2
Risk factors for osmotic demyelination syndrome

- Chronic hyponatremia
- Serum sodium concentration of 105 mEq/L or less
- Hypokalemia
- Alcoholism
- Malnutrition
- Liver disease

Data from Sterns R, Hix JK, Silver S. Treating profound hyponatremia: a strategy for controlled correction. Am J Kidney Dis 2010;56:774–9.

---

involvement) and a flaccid quadriparesis (from corticospinal tract involvement), which later becomes spastic, and all these are due to involvement of the base of the pons. If the lesion extends into the tegmentum of the pons, then pupillary and oculomotor abnormalities may occur. EPM is characterized by tremor and ataxia. In extreme cases, a "locked-in syndrome" may be present.[105] OSD can be seen on computed tomography (CT) or magnetic resonance imaging (MRI). MRI findings tend to lag behind the clinical features in some cases as much as by 1 to 2 weeks,[107] and if this diagnosis remains likely, a repeat imaging study at 10 to 14 days may reveal lesions not apparent on early scans. The management of patients with ODS is prolonged neurorehabilitation. There are case series about use of intravenous immunoglobulin[108] and reinduction of hyponatremia[109] with good outcomes. The prognosis is very difficult to be predicted. The outcome may be death, disability, or recovery.

Summary

Hyponatremia is more common in the older patients, because of the decreased ability and reserve to maintain homeostasis of fluids and electrolytes and the presence of more comorbidities.

Severe hyponatremia in geriatric patients has significant morbidity and mortality, because of neurologic complications, such as altered mental status, seizures, and coma.

When evaluating patients with hyponatremia, it is very important to classify what type of hyponatremia is present. Classification is based on the patient's volume status, serum osmolarity, specific gravity of urine, and sodium concentration.

Management is based on the type of hyponatremia the patient has and the patient's clinical status. For patients who have extremely low serum sodium levels and significant neurologic symptoms, such as seizures or altered mental status, treatment with hypertonic saline is the therapy of choice. Also, specific treatment for any underlying disorder should be given.

HYPERNATREMIA
Epidemiology

Hypernatremia is defined as a serum sodium concentration greater than 145 mEq/L. Hypernatremia invariably denotes hypertonic hyperosmolality and always causes cellular dehydration, even if just transiently. It is characterized by a deficit of TBW relative to total body sodium and can result either from net water loss, or, less commonly, from hypertonic sodium gain. The primary problem is inadequate water intake, secondary to a defective thirst mechanism due to aging or a lack of access to fluid.

The inpatient incidence of hypernatremia ranges from 0.3% to 1%.[110] Hypernatremia was reported in approximately 1% of hospitalized patients older than 60 years and up to 60% of febrile nursing home residents.[111]

The prevalence of hypernatremia in a study of 981 adults hospitalized in the ICU was 9% (2% had hypernatremia on admission and 7% developed hypernatremia during hospitalization).[112] In a retrospective survey, it was concluded that hypernatremia could potentially be used as an indicator of quality of care in the medical ICU.[113] The prevalence of hypernatremia in patients who present to the ED was 13%.[114] The presence of hypernatremia is associated with a mortality rate of more than 40%.[111] The change in the status of consciousness when hypernatremia was diagnosed was the single prognostic indicator associated with mortality.[115]

Pathophysiology

As mentioned earlier, with aging, urinary concentration ability in the elderly is diminished, which reflects diminished tubular function. A healthy young adult can achieve a maximum urinary concentration of 1200 mOsm/kg, whereas a healthy older person can often only achieve a urine osmolality of 700 to 800 mOsm/kg, thus increasing the risk of developing hypernatremia in the geriatric patients. Furthermore, the sensitivity of thirst in older patients is also diminished, which predisposes them to the development of hypernatremia.[64] In addition, the percentage of body water decreases with age, so equal volumes of fluid loss in older individuals may represent more severe dehydration than in younger individuals.[116]

Clinical Presentation

The presence of severe symptoms usually requires an acute and large elevation in the plasma sodium concentration to above 160 mEq/L.[117] Symptoms are usually nonspecific and include lethargy and weakness. Obtundation, stupor, coma, and seizures may accompany more severe hypernatremia.[118] Intense thirst may be present initially, but it dissipates as the disorder progresses and is absent in patients with hypodipsia.[111]

The following 4 signs were significantly and independently associated with hypernatremia in older adults: abnormal supraclavicular, skin turgor, abnormal thigh skin turgor, dry oral mucosa and recent change in consciousness. Abnormal skin turgor is defined as "tenting" lasting at least 3 seconds after 3 seconds of skin pinching.[115]

Serum glucose levels should be checked in all patients with these signs to rule out dehydration due to an osmotic diuresis caused by hyperglycemia. Serum creatinine, potassium, and calcium levels; osmolality; and BUN should be checked. Measurement of UO and urine osmolality helps in determining the cause. In a study, an elevated BUN/Cr ratio that coexisted with hypernatremia was sensitive in detecting patients with hypernatremic dehydration.[115]

Chronic hypernatremia is associated with milder symptoms because of the adaptive response that is initiated promptly and consists of solute gain by the brain that tends to restore the lost water and normalizes brain volume.[119]

CT scan of the brain is appropriate to evaluate patients with hypernatremia because acute brain shrinkage can induce vascular rupture with cerebral bleeding and subarachnoid hemorrhages.[120]

Box 3 mentions some factors that increase the risk of hypernatremia in elderly patients.[121,122]

> **Box 3**
> **Risk factors for hypernatremia in elderly patient**
>
> - Age greater than 85 years.
> - Female sec.
> - Having more than 4 chronic conditions.
> - Taking more than 4 medications.
> - Limited mobility.
> - Infections.
> - Altered mental status.
> - Hypertonic infusions.
> - Tube feedings.
> - Osmotic diuretics.
> - Laxatives.
> - Mechanical ventilation.

Causes and Approach

The cause of hypernatremia is typically evident from the routine history and physical examination; however, additional diagnostic tests of the AVP-renal axis may be needed to establish the diagnosis.

There are 4 major causes of hypernatremia: insufficient water intake, hypotonic fluid depletion, sodium overload, and transient transcellular water shift.

Insufficient water intake

Hypernatremia from inadequate water intake is usually a consequence of insufficient access to free water, an impaired or altered sensation of thirst, or neurologic injury with altered mental status.

Acquired hypothalamic structural lesions can result in a true defect of thirst and osmoregulation. This condition is called primary hypodipsia. Conditions that can cause primary hypodipsia include traumatic brain injury, brain tumors, granulomatous infiltration (ie, sarcoidosis), and vascular disease.[123] Furthermore, conditions that cause delirium, or that result in a significant neurologic injury (ie, stroke) aggravate age-related declines in thirst and hypodipsia caused by hypothalamic lesions. Essential hypernatremia is a variant of primary hypodipsia, in which the osmotic threshold for AVP and thirst has been reset to a higher level than the normal baseline.[124] The urine osmolality of these patients is elevated.

Hypotonic fluid depletion

In the setting of an elevated serum osmolality (>295 mOsm/kg H_2O), hypernatremia serum Na levels greater than 145 mmol/L with a urine osmolality of less than 800 mOsm/kg indicates a renal concentrating defect.

Renal loss of hypotonic fluid can be seen with an osmotic diuresis that is caused by an excess of urinary solute, typically nonreabsorbable, that induces polyuria and hypotonic fluid loss, as seen in hyperglycemia (ie, diabetic ketoacidosis) or with the use of mannitol.[125] The use of diuretics (ie, loop or thiazide diuretics) is also common in critically ill patients and can contribute to hypotonic urinary fluid losses. The relief of complete postrenal urinary obstruction can initially be associated with a large diuresis that may result in hypernatremia.[126] In cases of renal loss of hypotonic fluid, the urinary sodium concentration is usually greater than 20 mEq/L and the urine osmolality is less than 700 mOsm/kg.

Fluid losses from the gastrointestinal tract are generally hypotonic to serum, and, consequently, lead to hypernatremia if not replaced. These losses can occur from vomiting, nasogastric drainage, enterocutaneous fistulas, diarrhea, or the use of osmotic cathartic agents (ie, lactulose).

Insensible fluid losses from the skin (ie, sweat) and the respiratory tract (ie, evaporation) are generally hypotonic to serum; hypernatremia ensues in circumstances of increased insensible fluid loss, such as fever, diaphoresis, or tachypnea. Febrile illness in elderly individuals with decreased sensorium is the most common cause of hypernatremia.[116] Upper respiratory tract, lung, and urinary tract infections are the most common causes for the fever.[127] It has been suggested that in elderly patients with acute febrile disease, temporary hypernatremia may reflect an inadequate vasopressin response to the hyperosmolar state.[128] In all cases of extrarenal fluid loss, the urinary sodium concentration is less than 20 mEq/L and the urine osmolality is greater than 700 mOsm/kg).

Diabetes insipidus (DI) is a condition that is characterized by the excretion of large amounts of severely diluted urine (<700 mOsm/kg and often <200 mOsm/kg). There are 2 types of DI: central DI (a consequence of a deficiency of AVP secretion) and nephrogenic DI (due to AVP resistance at the collecting tubules). These 2 types can be distinguished by administering exogenous AVP (dDAVP, 10 mcg intranasal, or vasopressin, 5 units subcutaneous). Urine osmolality increases by 50% in central DI, whereas no significant change occurs in nephrogenic DI. Even in the most severe forms of DI, hypernatremia does not develop unless there is a concomitant defect in thirst or restricted access to water.[129]

Central DI is uncommon, and most cases can be linked to lesions or injury to the hypothalamus after pituitary surgery,[130] traumatic brain injury,[131] and subarachnoid hemorrhage[132] as well as with tumors,[133] granulomatous infiltration,[134] or autoimmune disease.[135]

Nephrogenic DI can result from drugs, acute and chronic renal failure, obstructive uropathy, hypercalcemia, hypokalemia, and sickle cell disease.[136] Lithium is the most common cause of drug-induced nephrogenic DI, followed by foscarnet and clozapine. Lithium causes nephrogenic DI by downregulation of AVP-2 receptors and/or reduced expression of AQP2 channels.[137]

Sodium overload

Hypernatremia from pure sodium overload is rare and frequently iatrogenic. This condition is seen in excessive sodium bicarbonate administration during cardiopulmonary resuscitation, overcorrection of hyponatremia with hypertonic saline, hypertonic dialysate in peritoneal dialysis (PD) and hemodialysis (HD), and hypertonic enteral or parenteral hyperalimentation. Noniatrogenic causes include primary hyperaldosteronism and Cushing syndrome.

Transient water shift into cells

Transient hypernatremia is induced by intense exercise or prolonged convulsive seizure activity. This phenomenon typically occurs in the context of marked lactic acidosis and can transiently raise the serum sodium concentration by 10 to 15 mEq/L, which returns to normal within 10 to 15 minutes.[138]

Treatment

The treatment of hypernatremia consists of addressing the underlying causes (eg, fever, diuretic use and so on) and correcting the hypernatremia. When hypernatremia is associated with extra-cellular fluid (ECF) depletion that causes hemodynamic compromise, isotonic saline should be administrated initially to improve blood pressure and end-organ perfusion.

Serum electrolytes should be monitored at least daily, and more frequently (every 4 to 6 hours) if the patient is severely ill, so adjustments in therapy can be made accordingly. In addition, frequent neurologic examinations, assessment of mental status, pupil examination, and examination of motor strength and reflexes should be performed to assess for clinical deterioration because transient improvement followed by deterioration in the neurologic status suggests the development of iatrogenic cerebral edema.

The preferred route for administering fluids is the oral route or a feeding tube; if this is not feasible, fluids should be given intravenously. Only hypotonic fluid should be used to correct the hypernatremia, the choice includes pure water, ¼ isotonic saline (0.2% NaCl), and ½ isotonic saline (0.45% NaCl) with or without 5% dextrose. The more hypotonic the infusate, the lower the infusion rate that is required. The risk of cerebral edema increases with the volume of the infusate. The sodium concentration should be corrected with a rate of 0.5 to 1 mEq/L/h, with a maximum decrease of 10 mEq/L per 24-hour period.

Even in hypernatremia, the Adrogue formula[118] can be used to predict the effect of 1000 mL of an infusate

$$\text{Change in plasma sodium} = \frac{(\text{Infusate sodium} - \text{Plasma sodium})}{(\text{Total body water} + 1)}$$

For example, in a 68-kg elderly man who presents with severe obtundation and a sodium concentration of 168 mEq/L 1 L of D5W (0 mEq/L sodium) decreases the serum sodium concentration by approximately 4.8 mEq/L, as calculated by $(0 - 168)/([0.5 \times 68] + 1)$. The goal is to reduce the sodium concentration by 10 mEq/L over a 24-hour period, and to do this we need 2.1 L of D5W (10/4.8). Furthermore, we should add 1.5 L to compensate for average obligatory water losses over the 24-hour period, therefore a total of 3.6 L should be administered for the next 24 hours at a rate of 150 mL/h.

Correction of hypernatremia in hospitalized adults within 4 days was associated with a higher frequency of improvement in the level of consciousness. Correction that extended over more than 4 days was associated with a tendency toward permanent loss of cognitive function.[117]

There is also an association between hypokalemia and hypernatremia.[117] The correction of hypokalemia is important because it reverses the defect in the concentrating ability of the kidney and thus improves water conservation.[139]

In patients with central DI with altered mental status or lacking access to water, the polyuria can usually be controlled by hormone replacement with AVP analogs such as desmopressin (dDAVP). In nephrogenic DI, the offending drug should be discontinued and the hypercalcemia and hypokalemia should be corrected. A low-salt and low-protein diet can also help, and thiazides with or without amiloride and nonsteroidal anti-inflammatory drugs (NSAIDs) have been demonstrated to be useful.[140]

In patients with sodium overload, a combination of furosemide and free water such as D5W can be tried. Furosemide alone should not be given because it will exacerbate hypernatremia by causing the excretion of hypotonic urine. Patients may need dialysis if severe renal failure is present.[140]

Summary

Hypernatremia is common in older patients, especially those who are frail, bedridden, and febrile. Hypernatremia often presents in geriatric patients as dehydration and altered mental status. Initially, very hypernatremic dehydrated older patients need normal saline to correct severe hypovolemia; however, once they are hemodynamically stable, they require hypotonic fluids. The hypernatremia should be corrected slowly to avoid cerebral edema. Underlying causes should also be promptly identified and managed appropriately.

HYPERCALCEMIA
Introduction

Hypercalcemia is a very important and relatively frequent problem, especially in older patients. If not recognized and treated expeditiously, patients with hypercalcemia can have significant mortality and morbidity. The normal level of serum calcium is 8.7 to 10.4 mg/dL (2.12–2.55 mmol/L). Mild hypercalcemia is when the serum calcium levels are 10.5 to 12 mg/dL (2.55–3 mmol/L), and in moderate hypercalcemia, the serum calcium level is 12 to 14 mg/dL (2.55–3.0 mmol/L).

Severe hypercalcemia is defined as calcium levels greater than 14 mg/dL (>3.5 mmol/L)[141] and always requires emergency management.[142] However, it must be emphasized that the level of calcium alone does not determine the severity of symptoms. Severe symptoms requiring emergency management may occur even at lower levels of calcium (12–14 mg/dL) in geriatric patients and in patients who have rapidly rising levels of calcium.[143,144] The term hypercalcemic crisis is often used for patients who require emergency management of their elevated calcium levels.

When evaluating an abnormal calcium level, it is important to measure the patient's albumin as well as the serum calcium levels because about 40% of serum calcium is protein bound, mainly with albumin; 50% is in the active ionized form; and 10% is bound to other anions. Low serum albumin levels can give falsely low serum calcium levels, and high serum albumin levels can give falsely high serum calcium levels. The following equations can be very useful in correcting the serum calcium level when serum albumin levels are abnormal:

For values in mg/dL: Corrected Ca = Measured total Ca + 0.8 × (4.5 − albumin)

For values in mmol/L: Corrected Ca = Measured total Ca + 0.02 × (40 − albumin)

Measuring the ionized calcium levels directly when available can sometimes be very useful, especially in acutely ill older patients who often are hypoalbuminemic. This measurement avoids errors related to abnormal albumin levels.[145] Normal ionized serum calcium levels range from 4 to 5.6 mg/dL (1–1.4 mmol/L).

Epidemiology

Hypercalcemia is a fairly frequent problem. Severe hypercalcemia accounts for more than 3% of hospital admissions from the ED. More than 90% of cases are due to either primary hyperparathyroidism or malignancy.[146] In the United States, 25 per 100,000 persons in the general population have primary hyperparathyroidism, which is the most frequent cause of mild hypercalcemia.[147] The occurrence of primary hyperparathyroidism increases with age, and its incidence in older women is 250 per 100,000. Malignancy-related hypercalcemia is the most common cause of hypercalcemic crisis. More than 20% of patients with cancer develop hypercalcemia during the course of their disease.[148,149] The mortality rate of patients with hypercalcemia because of malignancy is very high.[148,149] Because the incidence of malignancy increases with age, the incidence of malignancy-associated hypercalcemia also increases with age. In the Netherlands, the overall incidence of hypercalcemia in elderly women is 3%.[150]

Other causes of hypercalcemia are also present in geriatric patients, but are much less common. Immobilization can cause hypercalcemia, which is usually mild, but it can rarely cause severe hypercalcemia and can also exacerbate the hypercalcemia associated with hyperparathyroidism and malignancy.[151] Medications, especially thiazides, have been noted to cause hypercalcemia, in older patients, and also worsen the hypercalcemia associated with other causes, especially primary hyperparathyroidism.[150–152] Other medications that can cause and/or exacerbate hypercalcemia because of other causes in geriatric patients are vitamin D,[153] vitamin A,[154] retinoic acid,[155] lithium,[156] calcium carbonate causing the milk-alkali syndrome,[157] and tamoxifen.[158] In addition to hyperparathyroidism, other endocrine diseases have been noted to cause hypercalcemia, most prominently hyperthyroidism.[159] Other illnesses that have been reported as causing hypercalcemia in older patients are granulomatous diseases, especially sarcoidosis,[160,161] renal-disease-related secondary and tertiary hyperparathyroidism, and Paget disease.[152]

Pathophysiology

Hypercalcemia occurs when the amount of calcium entering the body via the small intestine exceeds the amount of calcium being excreted through the kidney and being deposited in bones. Hypercalcemia can occur when an excess of calcium is absorbed through the intestine, when there is an increase in bone resorption, or when the excretion of calcium through the kidney is decreased. More than one of these mechanisms acting in concert may cause hypercalcemia.

Serum calcium levels are regulated by the action of 3 hormones: parathyroid hormone (PTH), 1,25-dihydroxyvitamin D (calcitriol), and calcitonin. There is feedback between these hormones that normally keeps serum calcium levels within the normal range. Hypercalcemia occurs when this regulatory system becomes overwhelmed by an excess of PTH; the secretion by tumor of a parathyroid-hormone-related protein (PTHrP), which has the same effects as PTH; an excess of calcitriol, which primarily increases absorption of calcium in the gastrointestinal tract; an increase in local bone resorption; a decrease in the excretion of calcium through the kidney; or an increased amount of calcium being ingested and absorbed in the gastrointestinal tract.

In older patients, the ability to respond to an excess of calcium and maintain homeostasis is much less than in younger patients and the incidence of the 2 most common diseases that cause hypercalcemia, that is, hyperparathyroidism and malignancy, is greater.[148,150,162] Therefore, it is not surprising that severe hypercalcemia is much more common in older patients.[150] **Box 4** demonstrates why older patients are more likely to develop severe hypercalcemia.

Box 4
Reasons for increased severe hypercalcemia in older patients

Increased incidence of malignancy

Increased ingestion of drugs that increase calcium

Decreased renal clearance of calcium

Increased absorption of calcium in the gastrointestinal tract

Increased incidence of hyperparathyroidism

More immobility

Increased incidence of dehydration because of comorbidities

Increased resorption of bone

Most cases of primary hyperparathyroidism in geriatric patients are due to parathyroid adenomas, and most of these patients have only mild elevations of their serum calcium levels and are relatively asymptomatic. However, some of these elderly patients eventually become symptomatic and therefore need to be closely followed up.[162] Hyperparathyroidism increases serum calcium levels by increasing calcitriol production, which increases gastrointestinal absorption. An excess of PTH also increases calcium absorption in the distal renal tubules and increases resorption of bone, although this effect is opposed by deposition of excess calcium in the bone because of the action of calcitonin, which also opposes the action of PTH on the kidney. Also, some parathyroid adenomas may decrease their secretion of PTH in response to the hypercalcemia.[162] This response may explain why very high levels of calcium (>14 mg/dL, >3.5 mmol/L) are not usually found in isolated primary hyperparathyroidism. When severe hypercalcemia is found in a patient with primary hyperparathyroidism, something that exacerbates the effects of the hyperparathyroidism, such as the ingestion of thiazides, calcium carbonate, excessive vitamin D, or immobilization, should be considered.

Hypercalcemia associated with malignancy is usually more severe than that due to primary hyperparathyroidism. Hypercalcemia associated with malignancy is most commonly caused by multiple myeloma, metastatic breast cancer, or metastatic lung cancer and is due to increased local osteoclastic activity in the involved bone.[163] Metastatic invasion of bone by solid tumors, lymphomas, and leukemias causes hypercalcemia by increasing the local osteoclastic activity. Nonmetastatic solid tumors usually cause hypercalcemia by the secretion of PTHrP.[164] Lymphomas can also cause hypercalcemia by increased levels of calcitriol produced by macrophages. Ghazi reported the case of an older patient with lymphoma caused by both tumor secretion of PTHrP and calcitriol.[165]

Hyperthyroidism causes hypercalcemia that is usually mild by increasing resorption of bone.[150,159] Granulomatous diseases, such as sarcoidosis, can cause hypercalcemia by increasing the level of calcitriol and thereby increasing calcium absorption in the small intestine.[161] Thiazides increase serum calcium levels by decreasing the urinary excretion of calcium. Lithium increases calcium levels by increasing the set point of PTH.[166] Vitamin A causes hypercalcemia by increasing bone resorption.[152]

Clinical Effects of Hypercalcemia

Hypercalcemia causes hyperpolarization of cell membranes. Patients with mild elevations of calcium levels (10.5–12 mg/dL) are often asymptomatic.[167] When the serum calcium level becomes higher than this, multiple organ systems can be involved and cause a multitude of symptoms. The classical mnemonic "stones, bones, moans, and groans" refers to pain from renal stones; bone pain; moans because of abdominal pain, which may be caused by peptic ulcer disease or pancreatitis; and psychic moans because of altered mental status, all of which may be seen with hypercalcemia, especially when caused by primary hyperparathyroidism.[152] However, in older patients, symptoms may not be "classical" and may be "nonspecific."[168] The diagnosis of hypercalcemia should be strongly considered whenever an older patient presents with altered mental status or new-onset psychiatric symptoms and/or vague gastrointestinal symptoms, especially if there is a history of carcinoma.[150]

Neuromuscular and neuropsychiatric symptoms include impaired concentration, anxiety, depression, confusion, altered mental status, fatigue, and muscle weakness.[169] More severe symptoms, such as lethargy, stupor, and coma may occur with very high levels of serum calcium and are more common in geriatric patients.[142]

Gastrointestinal symptoms, especially anorexia, nausea, vomiting, and constipation, are common. Abdominal pain, peptic ulcer disease, and pancreatitis occur, but are less common.[170,171]

Important renal manifestations are polyuria, nephrolithiasis, and acute and chronic renal failure, which may result from nephrocalcinosis. Hypercalcemia causes a nephrogenic DI syndrome that interferes with the ability to concentrate urine.[152] The ensuing polyuria, along with the gastrointestinal symptoms of hypercalcemia, can cause severe dehydration. This dehydration and the subsequent fall in GFR lead to decreased excretion of calcium and worsening of the hypercalcemia and its symptoms. A vicious cycle of worsening dehydration and hypercalcemia results from this.

Bone pain is commonly seen with both hyperparathyroidism and malignancy. Severe osteoporosis and cystic lesions of bone more commonly occur with primary hyperparathyroidism.[172]

Hypercalcemia can have adverse cardiovascular effects. Acute severe hypercalcemia causes a short QT interval because of shortening of the action potential of the heart.[173] However, rare cardiac arrhythmias have occurred in patients with acute severe hypercalcemia, including ventricular fibrillation, bradycardia, and conduction defects.[174] Also, ST elevation mimicking an acute myocardial infarction has been noted in patients with acute severe hypercalcemia.[175] Chronic effects of hypercalcemia, such as calcification of heart valves, coronary arteries, and myocardial fibers; cardiomyopathy; and hypertension have been described in patients with hyperparathyroidism.[176]

Clinical Evaluation

The possibility of severe hypercalcemia must be considered in any older patient who presents with acutely altered mental status.[150] Initially, clinicians should use focused history, physical examination, and laboratory evaluations to evaluate for other causes of altered mental status in geriatric patients, including infection, adverse drug reactions, hypoglycemia, hyperglycemia, dehydration, hyponatremia, and acute neurologic, cardiac, or pulmonary events.[177]

When the initial elevated serum calcium level returns, establishing the diagnosis of hypercalcemia, a thorough history and physical examination should be performed looking for the clinical effects of hypercalcemia and their severity and clues to the various causes of hypercalcemia. These causes include malignancies, hyperparathyroidism, medications (thiazides, lithium, vitamin D, vitamin A, calcium carbonate, tamoxifen, and theophylline), hyperthyroidism, immobilization, Paget disease, and granulomatous diseases (sarcoidosis and tuberculosis). On physical examination, findings that should be looked for are abnormal mental status, muscle weakness, signs of dehydration, corneal calcifications, neck masses, lymphadenopathy, and other signs of malignancy.

Laboratory Evaluation

Measurement of serum calcium levels should be repeated for confirmation and to monitor the effects of therapy. As noted previously, serum calcium levels should be corrected for any abnormality of the patient's serum albumin levels. Several authorities prefer to follow ionized calcium levels to avoid this problem.[145] Once the diagnosis of hypercalcemia has been confirmed, tests should be performed to confirm the cause of the hypercalcemia. Tests should be performed to differentiate between malignancy and hyperparathyroidism, the 2 most common causes of hypercalcemia in the elderly.

PTH levels should be checked. Elevated PTH levels in the face of hypercalcemia confirm the diagnosis of hyperparathyroidism. Other laboratory clues that point to hyperparathyroidism are low serum phosphate and high serum chloride levels. Imaging studies of the head and neck may be needed to further delineate the exact cause of the hyperparathyroidism before surgery. PTHrP secretion by many solid tumors can cause hypercalcemia, and its levels can be measured.[178] Appropriate imaging should be done to diagnose suspected malignancy.

Thyroid function tests should be sent if hyperthyroidism is suspected as a possible cause of the hypercalcemia.

Hypercalcemia caused by overdosing vitamin D supplements can be diagnosed by measuring 25-hydroxyvitamin D levels. Granulomatous diseases, such as sarcoidosis, and Hodgkin lymphoma can cause hypercalcemia by increasing 1,25-dihdroxyvitamin D (calcitriol) levels, and this can be measured.[152] These entities usually have both high serum calcium and phosphate levels.

Table 5 gives a diagnostic approach for the evaluation of hypercalcemia in geriatric patients.

Management of Severe Hypercalcemia in Older Patients

Patients with severe hypercalcemia, which is defined as calcium levels greater than 14 mg/dL, and patients with mental status changes and calcium levels greater than 12 mg/dL require acute management in the ED and admission.[142] The goals of management are resuscitating the patient as needed, improving symptoms by expeditiously lowering serum calcium levels, and treating the underlying cause. As always, airway, breathing, and circulation need to be evaluated and supported as required. Severe hypercalcemia can cause coma that could adversely affect the airway and breathing. Hypercalcemic crisis often causes severe hypovolemia, requiring aggressive fluid resuscitation. Severe hypercalcemia can occasionally cause arrhythmias, and therefore, these patients should have cardiac monitoring.

The best way to rapidly lower calcium levels is hydration with normal saline, intravenous bisphosphonates, and parenteral calcitonin. Hydration with intravenous normal saline should be the initial treatment given in the ED.[179] The amount and rate of intravenous saline given to a particular patient depends on the patient's initial volume status, the serum calcium level, and comorbidities, such as congestive heart failure and renal failure. Older patients are less likely to tolerate overhydration and must be

Table 5	
Evaluation for hypercalcemia in older patients	
Cause of Hypercalcemia	**Appropriate Diagnostic Tests**
All causes	Directed history: history of malignancy, comorbidities, bone pain, immobilization, medications
All causes	Directed physical examination: vital signs, signs of dehydration, neck masses, lymphadenopathy, signs of malignancy
Hyperparathyroidism	PTH level and if high, imaging of neck
Malignancy	PTHrp level, malignancy workup with appropriate imaging, serum and urine protein electrophoresis, biopsy as appropriate
Hyperthyroidism	Thyroid function tests
Granulomatous disease	Chest radiograph, ACE, lymph node biopsy, calcitriol level
Vitamin D intoxication	25-hydroxyvitamin D level
Renal disease	BUN, creatinine, urine pH, and electrolytes
Paget disease	Bone radiographs

Abbreviation: ACE, angiotensin-converting enzyme.

closely monitored for signs of fluid overload. In special situations, central venous pressure monitoring may be useful. The aim of saline hydration is to restore the normal intravascular volume and promote good UO. In most cases, it is recommended to start with a rate of 200 to 300 mL/h and then adjust the rate to maintain a UO of 100 to 150 mL/h, once the patient is euvolemic.[180] If the patient develops signs of fluid overload, furosemide can be used. The routine use of massive saline infusion and furosemide are no longer recommended.[181]

Bisphosphonates, which act by inhibiting bone resorption by osteoclasts, have become a mainstay in the treatment of moderate and severe hypercalcemia, especially when caused by malignancies.[182] Intravenous zoledronic acid (ZA), 4 mg, given over 15 minutes and intravenous pamidronate, 60 to 90 mg, given over 2 hours are the bisphosphonates available for the treatment of severe hypercalcemia. ZA is preferred by many experts because it is more potent, it is given more easily, and its effect on serum calcium lasts longer than that of pamidronate.[183]

Both medications require dosage adjustment in patients with renal disease. Because both drugs take 2 to 4 days to show their maximum effect, patients with severe hypercalcemia are also treated with hydration and calcitonin, which work faster. Salmon calcitonin, which works by both increasing urinary excretion of calcium and decreasing bone resorption, has a fairly rapid onset of action (4–6 hours), but its therapeutic effect only lasts for 48 hours. Therefore, it is mainly used for treating severe hypercalcemia to gain time until the more sustained action of the bisphosphonates can take effect.[184] Salmon calcitonin is given as a dose of 4 IU/kg intramuscularly or subcutaneously every 12 hours for 3 doses.

Treatment of Specific Causes and Special Situations

Medications that cause hypercalcemia should be stopped. Glucocorticoids are used to treat hypercalcemia caused by excessive intake of vitamin D or the overproduction of calcitriol that occurs in patients with granulomatous diseases, Hodgkin lymphoma, and multiple myeloma.[152] Prednisone is usually given at a dose of 40 mg/d.

Cinacalcet, a calcimimetic drug, is used to treat severe hypercalcemia in patients with parathyroid carcinoma and patients undergoing dialysis with secondary hyperparathyroidism. The starting dose is 30 mg orally once a day, and it is titrated up by 30 mg/d every 2 to 4 weeks depending on the calcium and PTH levels. Gallium nitrate and cisplatin have been used to treat hypercalcemia due to malignancy that is refractory to treatment with bisphosphonates.[185,186] Patients with primary hyperparathyroidism and severe hypercalcemia should have urgent parathyroid surgery once their condition has been stabilized.[162,163]

Dialysis, especially HD with no calcium in the dialysis fluid, can be used for severe hypercalcemia resistant to other therapies and in patients with fluid overload due to congestive heart failure or renal failure, in which hydration cannot be used.[187]

Summary

Hypercalcemia in geriatric patients is relatively common, and has significant morbidity and mortality. Common clinical manifestations of hypercalcemia in older patients are altered mental status, gastrointestinal complaints, bone pain, and dehydration. Important causes of hypercalcemia to consider in older patients are malignancy, hyperparathyroidism, hyperthyroidism, medications, granulomatous diseases, and immobilization. Management of severe hypercalcemia in geriatric patients should consist of hydration with normal saline, intravenous bisphosphonates, and calcitonin and treating the underlying cause.

ACUTE RENAL FAILURE IN GERIATRIC PATIENTS
Introduction and Epidemiology

Acute renal failure, now referred to as AKI, is much more common in the older popu-lation, a trend compounded by the fact that older people are rapidly becoming a bigger percentage of the population. Overall, AKI is becoming more common.[188] Old age seems to be a risk factor for AKI.[188,189] In a recent study, the frequency of AKI and acute on chronic failure were much higher than they were previously thought with an incidence of 1.811 per million population and 336 per million population, respec-tively. The median age of the patients who developed AKI was 76 years and that of the patients who developed acute on chronic renal failure was 80.5 years.[190] There-fore, AKI is largely a geriatric disease.

In addition to a new name, there are also new classification systems for AKI, with the most commonly used system being the risk, injury, failure, loss, and ESRD (RIFLE) classification.[191] This classification is based on an increase in serum creatinine level, a decrease in GFR, or a decrease in UO as follows:

1. Risk: Increase in serum creatinine level × 1.5, decrease in GFR by 25%, or UO less than 0.5 mL/kg/h for 6 hours.
2. Injury: Increase in serum creatinine level × 2, decrease in GFR by 50%, or UO less than 0.5 mL/kg/h for 12 hours.
3. Failure: Increase in serum creatinine level × 3; decrease in GFR by 75%, or serum creatinine level of 4 mg/dL or more, with an acute increase of more than 0.5 mg/dL; UO less than 0.3 mL/kg/h for 24 hours, or anuria for 12 hours.
4. Loss: Persistent acute renal failure (ARF), complete loss of kidney function for more than 4 weeks.
5. End-stage renal disease: Loss of kidney function for more than 3 months.

AKI has a very poor prognosis in older patients, especially when it is associated with sepsis, and/or multiorgan failure,[192] with mortality rates as high as 75%.[193] Older patients are not only more likely to develop AKI, with the associated increased mortality and morbidity, but also more likely to have impaired recovery of renal func-tion.[194] They are also more likely to develop chronic renal disease and ESRD from AKI.[195] Therefore, it is imperative that steps be taken in older patients to prevent AKI, to look for it and diagnose it early, and to treat it expeditiously when it occurs.[196]

Pathophysiology and Causes

Structural and functional changes occur with aging that make the kidney more susceptible to AKI.[197] These changes have been previously described in this article.

In addition to these changes in the kidney, older patients also have age-related changes in the cardiovascular and immunologic systems that make them more prone to AKI.[198] The elderly are more likely to have comorbidities that are important risk factors for the development of AKI, including chronic kidney disease, diabetes, hyper-tension, coronary artery disease, congestive heart failure, and atheroembolic disease.[195,196,198,199] Recently, "cardiorenal syndrome" has been recognized as an important entity. Cardiorenal syndrome is a disorder of the heart and kidney whereby acute or chronic dysfunction of one organ causes or exacerbates acute dysfunction of the other organ and increases the overall mortality and morbidity.[200] Patients with congestive heart failure who have a significant acute decrease in renal function have a 3 times greater mortality rate than those who have normal renal function.[200]

Important causes of AKI in the older patients are sepsis, hypovolemia, medications, vascular disease, and urinary obstruction. These causes are very important to consider because they are potentially reversible if found early and treated appropriately and expeditiously.[193] The cause of AKI is often multifactorial in geriatric adults.[193]

Owing to changes in the immune system with aging, older patients have an increased susceptibility to serious infections.[201] Often, these infections present atypically in geriatric adults and are undetected until late in the disease course. Because sepsis is a leading cause of AKI and a prominent source of morbidity and mortality in older patients, it is imperative that physicians consider and look for occult infections in acutely ill older patients.[202]

The cause of AKI is commonly classified into 3 categories: prerenal (33% of cases in older adults), intrinsic (58% of cases in older adults), and postrenal (9% of cases in older adults). Prerenal AKI, usually due to hypovolemia, is the second most common cause of acute renal failure in geriatric patients.[193] As noted previously, older patients are much more likely to become dehydrated than younger adults. If these patients are allowed to become significantly hypovolemic, the kidneys become ischemic, and unless this situation is detected early and the patient treated aggressively with fluids, irreversible intrinsic renal failure due to acute tubular necrosis (ATN) occurs, which increases morbidity and mortality. For example, older surgical patients, who became hypovolemic in the perioperative period, are more likely to develop acute renal failure postoperatively, with significant complications related to the AKI.[203] In fact, surgery puts older patients at risk for AKI, and any factor, such as hypovolemia, infection, and nephrotoxic medications, that further adds to this risk should be avoided, monitored, and corrected, if found.[203,204]

Intrinsic AKI, particularly ATN, is the most common type of acute renal failure in geriatric patients and usually occurs after an ischemic or toxic event.[193] Nephrotoxic medications, especially NSAIDs, loop diuretic, laxatives, radiocontrast dyes, and antibiotics, such as aminoglycosides, are common causes of this type of AKI in geriatric patients.[205] Older patients are more likely to have nephrotoxic reactions to medications than younger patients, because the older adults are more likely to be on more medications and have more difficulty in metabolizing and excreting medications because of preexisting comorbidities.[206,207] Therefore, all physicians must be very careful when prescribing medications to older patients. Potentially nephrotoxic medications should be avoided when possible, and proper dosing should be checked when prescribing new medications to geriatric patients. "Start low and go slow" is a good general rule to follow when prescribing new medications in older patients.

Vasculitis is another important cause of intrinsic acute renal failure in older patients that should be looked for because it not only can be life threatening but also can be treated if detected early.[193,208]

Postrenal AKI, caused by urinary tract obstruction, is almost exclusively seen in older patients. There are really no good studies to show how common urinary obstruction is in the general population; however, surveys in older men showed that 20% to 35% of older men had moderate symptoms of urinary obstruction.[209] Autopsy studies showed that the incidence of hydronephrosis was 3.8% in adults and 2% in children.[209] Although most commonly seen in older men with benign prostatic hypertrophy or prostatic cancer, urinary tract obstruction can also be seen in older women and is caused by pelvic malignancy, uterine prolapse, hypotonic bladder, or medications, such as anticholinergics and narcotics.[193] Urinary tract obstruction is another very important cause of AKI not to miss because it can sometimes be easily treated by relieving the obstruction early before significant permanent kidney damage has occurred. With complete obstruction, renal damage can be seen in 12 to 24 hours; however, the amount of permanent damage and recovery of renal function depends on the duration and level of obstruction, preexisting renal function, and the presence of comorbidities or infection.[210] Once the diagnosis of urinary obstruction is considered, a transurethral catheter should be placed into the bladder. This procedure should be performed in a sterile manner. Plenty of lubricant should be used. Usually, in an adult, a 16-French Foley catheter can be used. If this catheter cannot be passed because of a urethral stricture or an enlarged prostate, a smaller-sized catheter can be tried. If this catheter also cannot be passed, then a Crudet catheter can be tried, either by the emergency physician or the urologist, depending on the emergency physician's level of skill and comfort with this procedure. If this procedure is unsuccessful, then urology should be consulted, and then the consultant can try filiform catheters or can perform a suprapubic cystotomy. Once the obstruction is relieved, the bladder should be completely drained, and clamping of the catheter is not necessary.[211] Postobstructive diuresis is an uncommon complication of relieving urinary obstruction. It is recognized when the patient continues to pass more than 200 mL/h for more than 2 hours. Urinary losses should be replaced with intravenous half-normal or normal saline, and electrolytes, such as potassium and magnesium, should be monitored and replaced as needed.[211]

Box 5, Table 6 show the common causes of AKI in geriatric patients.

Clinical Manifestations and Evaluation

A comprehensive history, including medication history, and physical examination should be done.[193] Clinicians should evaluate for symptoms and signs of uremia, such as weakness, anorexia, vomiting, altered mental status, seizures, signs of fluid overload, and pericarditis. However, these are late findings, and any very ill elderly patients should have appropriate laboratory testing to evaluate renal function. The history and physical examination should also focus on finding possible causes of the AKI, as noted earlier, that may be treatable if found early.[212] The most important symptoms and signs to note are evidence of dehydration, infection, drug toxicity, urinary tract obstruction, cardiovascular disease, or vasculitis. It is very important to note these signs and symptoms, because they point to underlying causes that if treated appropriately early on, may prevent ongoing AKI and decrease subsequent morbidity and mortality. Special attention should be given to the vital signs and to the volume status of the patient, noting signs of dehydration or fluid overload.[193,212]

Box 5
Common causes of acute kidney injury in older patient

Sepsis/Infection

Medications

Renal ischemia & renal vascular complications

Peri/Post-operative complications

Acute cardiac complications

Dehydration

Contrast dye

Vasculitis

Urinary obstruction

Toxins (myoglobin, hemoglobin, etc.)

Table 6	
Causes of acute kidney injury in older patients	
Causes of AKI in Older Patients	Percentage of Cases
Prerenal	33
Intrinsic	58
Postrenal	9

Laboratory Evaluation

Laboratory evaluation is used to make the diagnosis of AKI, to help differentiate between the various causes of AKI, and to look for complications of AKI. As per the RIFLE criteria, an acute increase in serum creatinine levels, a decrease in the GFR, and/or a decrease in urinary output are now the standards for making the diagnosis of AKI.[191] Unfortunately, the level of serum creatinine is not a very accurate marker for AKI in the elderly, because it increases relatively late, is influenced by muscle mass and the hydration status of the patient, and tends to be "falsely" low in older patients.[213] Although not currently available for general use, several biomarkers have been proposed to more accurately diagnose acute renal failure in older patients, especially cystatin C.[214] Cystatin C is a nonglycosylated 13-kDa protein, which is believed to be more accurate in estimating GFR than creatinine levels because it seems to be less influenced by the muscle mass and diet. GFR decreases with age, and cystatin C may better estimate true renal function than creatinine in older patients because it is not affected by muscle mass. Cystatin C levels have been shown to increase about 1 to 2 days earlier than the serum creatinine level in patients developing AKI. Cystatin C thus seems to be a much better biomarker for detecting AKI in older patients than the serum creatinine.

Several laboratory tests may help in differentiating and diagnosing the different causes of AKI, especially between prerenal and intrinsic acute renal failure. A high BUN/serum creatinine ratio (>20) suggests a prerenal cause of the AKI; however, the sensitivity and specificity is not very good and other entities, such as gastrointestinal bleeding and the use of the sulfonylurea class of drugs, can cause an elevated BUN/creatinine ratio.[215] A low fractional excretion of sodium (<1%), low urine sodium concentration (<20 mEq/L), and high urine osmolality (>500 mOsmol/kg) all suggest a prerenal cause for the AKI, rather than ATN. However, because of the frequent use of diuretics in geriatric patients, and the increased possibility of chronic renal disease in older patients, these findings are not always accurate in older patients.[193,216] Urinalysis should be done to look for leukocytes, hematuria, protein, and casts to help in diagnosing infection, glomerulonephritis, and ATN. The presence of white blood cells (WBCs) and WBC casts would suggest the diagnosis of urinary tract infection or acute interstitial nephritis. Positive result of nitrite test is very specific for infection, but unfortunately not sensitive. Presence of bacteria on an unspun specimen of urine indicates infection. The presence of red cell casts would suggest the diagnosis of glomerulonephritis. The presence of granular cell casts, tubular cells, or tubular cell casts would suggest the diagnosis of ATN.[217] If the urine dipstick tests positive for blood but no red cells are seen on microscopic examination, either rhabdomyolysis or hemolysis is indicated. The serum creatinine kinase level would be very high with rhabdomyolysis. UO should be closely followed. Ultrasonography should be performed to look for urinary obstruction, which is much more common in older patients. CT scan can be performed to look for renal stones and obstruction if clinically suspected, but intravenous contrast should not be used.

Complications of severe AKI should be looked for, including hyperkalemia, metabolic acidosis, fluid overload, and pericarditis. The diagnosis of fluid overload is made clinically. The patient may complain of shortness of breath and swelling of the extremities. On examination, the clinician may find tachypnea, tachycardia, jugular venous distention, rales, and peripheral edema. A chest radiograph may show signs of vascular congestion and also helps diagnose other causes of shortness of breath, such as pneumonia, if present. B-type natriuretic peptide BNP levels are elevated in renal disease, as well as in patients with congestive heart failure. Very high levels of BNP may indicate the presence of concomitant CHF in patients with renal failure, but the clinical usefulness of BNP in the setting of renal failure is still unclear.[218,219] Acute uremic pericarditis is also mainly a clinical diagnosis. Patients complain of sharp chest pain that is often pleuritic and may be worse on lying down. A pericardial friction rub may sometimes be heard, but it is transient and usually disappears as pericardial fluid accumulates. Electrocardiogram (ECG) early on may show diffuse ST elevations, but as fluid accumulates in the pericardial sac, these changes disappear and low voltage and electrical alternans may be seen. Bedside ultrasonography can be very useful in diagnosing pericardial effusion and pericardial tamponade. In acute severe AKI, as compared with ESRD that has occurred from progression of chronic renal failure, complications such as uremic symptoms, hyperkalemia, and metabolic acidosis often occur at relatively lower levels of creatinine and BUN. Although, patients with AKI are at risk for developing ESRD, not all patients do so, and some recover partially or even completely and do not require lifetime dialysis like the ESRD patients do.[220,221] It is therefore very important to aggressively look for and treat the underlying causes and acute complications of AKI.

Management

In the ED, management priorities emphasize the treatment of life-threatening complications of renal failure, such as respiratory failure, pulmonary edema, hyperkalemia, and metabolic acidosis.[193]

"An ounce of prevention is worth a pound of cure" when it comes to managing acute renal failure in older patients.[222] Steps must be taken to prevent the AKI from getting worse because older patients have high mortality and morbidity with acute renal failure. Unless there is obvious evidence of fluid overload, these patients should be given intravenous volume replacement, but they must be carefully monitored because older patients are more prone to become fluid-overloaded, with resultant increased morbidity.[223] Nephrotoxic drugs must be stopped, and any new drug that is given must be given in renal appropriate doses. If there is any evidence of urinary obstruction, it must be relieved. A urinary catheter should be placed to relieve the obstruction, and the UO should be followed. Urology consultation may sometimes be required. As noted earlier, permanent kidney damage can occur within 12 to 24 hours after acute complete urinary tract obstruction occurs. Therefore, if urgent urologic consultation is not available, steps should be taken to relieve bladder obstruction by passing a urinary catheter into the bladder. Special techniques such as using a Crudet catheter can be tried. As previously noted, specific underlying causes, such as sepsis and vasculitis, should be looked for and appropriately treated.

Complications of acute renal failure, such as hyperkalemia and fluid overload, must be treated. Severe hyperkalemia, which is defined as serum potassium levels greater than 7 mEq/L, if not rapidly treated has a mortality of 67%.[224] However, it should be noted that it is not only the absolute level of serum potassium that matters but also the rate of increase of the serum potassium levels. The faster the increase of the serum potassium levels, the more is one likely to have symptoms and signs of hyperkalemia.[224] Severe hyperkalemia may manifest itself on the ECG as QRS widening, disappearance of the P wave, and arrhythmias,[225,226] but there have reports of severe hyperkalemia with minimal ECG changes.[227] Until dialysis can be instituted, life-threatening hyperkalemia can be treated with calcium,[228] insulin and glucose,[229] and sodium bicarbonate, although it seems to work well only when the patient has significant metabolic acidosis[230] and albuterol nebulization.[231] Although ion exchange resins, such as kayexalate with sorbitol, are commonly used, there is no good evidence that they really work, and they may cause severe gastrointestinal problems.[232] Vasodilators and loop diuretics may be effective to treat fluid overload until dialysis is available, but often, furosemide does not work in the setting of acute renal failure. There is no evidence that giving furosemide to patients with AKI and oliguria improves the prognosis and giving furosemide to patients who are not fluid overloaded may actually worsen morbidity and mortality.[233] In one recent study of very elderly Chinese patients who developed AKI in the hospital, the use of α-keto acid seemed to be a protective factor and seemed to improve the prognosis of AKI (odds ratio = 0.656).[234] However, more research needs to be done on the use of this agent before its use can be recommended.

Emergency renal replacement therapy (RRT), for example, HD, is indicated for pulmonary edema, severe uremic symptoms such as encephalopathy, severe hyperkalemia, severe metabolic acidosis, and pericarditis.[212] Some studies showed that instituting dialysis prophylactically, for example, when the BUN was 100 or more, before the onset of life-threatening symptoms improved the outcome in these patients. Data from the Program to Improve Care in Acute Renal disease showed that the relative risk for death for patients who had RRT initiated at higher BUN values was 1.85.[235] However, this result is still controversial because it was not supported by the results of other studies, and an adequately prospective randomized clinical trial is needed.[236,237] Although older patients may have more complications with RRT, such as hypotension, bleeding, and dysequilibrium, than younger patients, they generally tolerate this procedure. In general, HD is preferred to PD because PD can have complications such as catheter leaks, peritonitis, and loss of serum albumin. Also, HD corrects acid–base and solute status faster in critically ill patients and causes less mortality when compared with PD.[238] However, PD is usually effective and is less costly and complex than HD. PD is also less likely to cause hypotension than HD and does not require anticoagulation like HD does. Therefore, PD can be very useful as an alternative to HD in certain patients.[238] There are some special regimens that have been used in unstable older patients, such as continuous RRT, but at present, there is insufficient evidence that these regimens are superior to the usual HD regimens.[239] Sometimes, ethical considerations regarding instituting RRT in frail elderly patients arise, and the wishes of the patients and their family, not just the medical indications, must be taken into consideration.[240]

Table 7 summarizes the important steps that should be taken in evaluating and treating older patients with AKI.

Summary

Acute renal failure is more common and has a worse prognosis in older patients. Underlying causes, such as sepsis, hypovolemia, drug toxicity, and urinary obstruction, must be looked for and treated expeditiously. Life-threatening complications, such as hyperkalemia and pulmonary edema, should be watched for and treated. The best treatment for the complications of AKI is RRT.

Table 7
Evaluation and management of AKI in older patients

Evaluation	Management
Evaluate airway, breathing, and circulation	Resuscitate as needed
Evaluate volume status	Hydrate with IV fluids as needed
Review all medications	DC all renal toxic medications and adjust doses of other medications
Look for underlying causes: infection, urinary obstruction, renal ischemia, cardiac disease, vasculitis, rhabdomyelisis, etc.	Treat any underlying causes, antibiotics for infection, relieve urinary obstruction, etc. Insert urinary catheter to relieve bladder obstruction
Monitor creatinine, BUN, electrolytes, urinary output	Treat fluid and electrolyte abnormalities as needed. Insert urinary catheter to follow output. Consider "early dialysis" for creatinine levels >10 or BUN >100 (controversial)
Look for life-threatening complications of AKI: hyperkalemia, fluid overload, CNS uremic symptoms, metabolic acidosis, pericarditis	Start renal replacement therapy (dialysis) for life-threatening complications. Temporizing measures can be tried pending dialysis: Hyperkalemia: calcium, $NaHCO_3$, insulin + glucose, albuterol, kayexalate? Fluid overload: vasodilators, furosemide Acidosis: $NaHCO_3$ Pericardiocentesis or window for tamponade

Abbreviation: DC, discontinue.

CONCLUDING REMARKS

Older patients are at high risk for renal and electrolyte emergencies. Practitioners who take care of the geriatric patients must know how to evaluate for and manage these emergencies, including AKI, hyponatremia, hypernatremia, and hypercalcemia.

REFERENCES

RENAL AGING

1. CDC. The State of Aging and Health in America 2007. Centers for disease Control and Prevention and the Merck Company Foundation. Whitehouse Station, NJ: The Merck Company Foundation; 2007.
2. USRDS. USRDS 2007 annual data report: atlas of chronic kidney disease and end-stage renal disease in the United States, vol. 2007. Bethesda (MD): National Institutes of Health, National Institute of Diabetes and Digestive and Kidney Diseases; 2007.
3. Zou XJ, Saxena R, Liu Z, et al. Renal senescence in 2008: progress and challenges. Int Urol Nephrol 2008;40:823–39.
4. Zhou XJ, Laszik ZG, Silva FG. Anatomical changes in the aging kidney. In: Macias-Nunez JF, Cameron JS, Oreopoulos DG, editors. The aging kidney in health and disease. New York: Springer; 2007. p. 39–54.
5. Silva FG. The aging kidney: a review – part I. Int Urol Nephrol 2005;37:185–205.
6. Takazakura E, Sawabu N, Handa A, et al. Intrarenal vascular changes with age and disease. Kidney Int 1972;2:224–30.

7. Schlanger L. Chapter 4: Kidney senescence, Proceedings of the American Society of Nephrology, Geriatric Nephrology Curriculum 2009. American Society of Nephrology: P3–4.

8. Nyengaard JR, Bendtsen TF. Glomerular number and size in relation to age, kidney weight and body surface in normal man. Anat Rec 1992;232:194–201.

9. Kasiske BL. Relationship between vascular disease and age-associated changes in the human kidney. Kidney Int 1987;31:1153–9.

10. Kaplan C, Pasternack B, Shah H, et al. Age-related incidence of sclerotic glomeruli in human kidneys. Am J Pathol 1975;80:227–34.

11. Smith SM, Hoy WE, Cobb L. Low incidence of glomerulosclerosis in normal kidneys. Arch Pathol Lab Med 1989;118:1253–5.

12. McLachlan MS. The ageing kidney. Lancet 1978;2:143–6.

13. Weinstein JR, Anderson S. The aging kidney: physiological changes. Adv Chronic Kidney Dis 2010;17(4):302–7.

14. Silva FG. The ageing kidney: a review - part II. Int Urol Nephrol 2005;37:419–32.

15. Baert L, Steg A. Is the diverticulum of the distal and collecting tubules a preliminary stage of the simple cyst in the adult? J Urol 1977;118:707–10.

16. Tada S, Yamagishi J, Kobayashi H, et al. The incidence of simple renal cyst by computed tomography. Clin Radiol 1983;34:437–9.

17. Goldring W, Chasis H, Ranges HA, et al. Relations of effective renal blood flow and glomerular filtration to tubular excretory mass in normal man. J Clin Invest 1940;19:739–50.

18. Davies DF, Shock NW. Age changes in glomerular filtration rate, effective renal plasma flow and tubular excretory capacity in adult males. J Clin Invest 1950; 29:496–507.

19. Watkin DM, Shock NW. Age-wise standard value for Cin, CPAH, and TmPAH in adult males. J Clin Invest 1955;34:969–77.

20. Wesson LG. Renal hemodynamics in physiological states. In: Wesson LG, editor. Physiology of the human kidney. New York: Grune & Stratton; 1969. p. 96–116.

21. Hollenberg NK, Adams DF, Solomon HS, et al. Senescence and the renal vasculature in normal man. Circ Res 1974;34:309–16.

22. Fuiano G, Sund S, Mazza G, et al. Renal hemodynamic response to maximal vasodilating stimulus in healthy older subjects. Kidney Int 2001;59:1052–8.

23. Esposito C, Plati A, Mazzullo T, et al. Renal function and functional reserve in healthy elderly individuals. J Nephrol 2007;20:617–25.

24. Rowe JW, Andres R, Tobin JD, et al. The effect of age on creatinine clearance in men: a cross-sectional and longitudinal study. J Gerontol 1976;31:155–63.

25. Berg UB. Differences in decline in GFR with age between males and females: reference data on clearances of inulin and PAH in potential kidney donors. Nephrol Dial Transplant 2006;21:2577–82.

26. Pendse S, Singh A. Approach to patients with chronic kidney disease, stages 1–4. In: Daugirdas J, Blake P, Ing T, editors. Dialysis handbook. Philadelphia: Kluwer; 2008. p. 4–13.

27. Kimmel PL, Lew SQ, Bosch JP. Nutrition, ageing and GFR: is age associated decline inevitable? Nephrol Dial Transplant 1996;11(Suppl 9):85–8.

28. Berman N, Hostetter TH. Comparing the Cockcroft-Gault and MDRD equations for calculation of GFR and drug doses in the elderly. Nat Clin Pract Nephrol 2007;3:644–5.

29. Gill J, Malyuk R, Djurdjev O, et al. Use of GFR equations to adjust drug doses in an elderly multi-ethnic group a cautionary tale. Nephrol Dial Transplant 2007;22: 2894–9.

30. Epstein M, Hollenberg NK. Age as a determinant of renal sodium conservation in normal man. J Lab Clin Med 1976;87:411–7.
31. Luft FC, Grim CE, Fineberg N, et al. Effects of volume expansion and contraction in normotensive whites, blacks and subjects of different ages. Circulation 1979; 59:644–55.
32. Bauer J. Age-related changes in the renin-aldosterone system. Drugs Aging 1993;3:238–45.
33. Shannon RP, Wei JY, Rosa RM, et al. The effect of age and sodium depletion on cardiovascular response to orthostasis. Hypertension 1986;8:438–43.
34. Perazella MA, Mahnensmith RL. Hyperkalemia in the elderly: drugs exacerbate impaired potassium homeostasis. J Gen Intern Med 1997;12:646–56.
35. Passare G, Viitanen M, Torring O, et al. Sodium and potassium disturbances in the elderly: prevalence and association with drug use. Clin Drug Investig 2004; 24:535–44.
36. Bengele H, Mathias R, Perkins JH, et al. Impaired renal and extrarenal potassium adaptation in old rats. Kidney Int 1983;23:684–90.
37. Rowe J, Shock N, De Fronzo R. The influence of age on the renal response to water deprivation in man. Nephron 1976;17:270–8.
38. Lindeman RD, Van Buren H, Maisz L. Osmolar renal concentrating ability in healthy young men and hospitalized patients without renal disease. N Engl J Med 1960;262:1306–9.
39. Beck N, Yu B. Effect of aging on urinary concentrating mechanism and vasopressin-dependent cAMP in rats. Am J Physiol 1982;243:F121–5.
40. Terashima Y, Kondo K, Inagaki A, et al. Age-associated decrease in response of rat aquaporin-2 gene expression to dehydration. Life Sci 1998;62:873–82.
41. Crowe MJ, Forsling ML, Rolls BJ, et al. Altered water excretion in healthy elderly man. Age Ageing 1987;16:285–93.
42. Faull CM, Holmes C, Baylis PH. Water balance in elderly people: is there a deficiency of vasopressin? Age Ageing 1993;22:114–20.
43. Frassetto L, Morris RC, Sebastian A. Effect of age on blood acid-base composition in adult human: role of age-related renal functional decline. Am J Physiol 1996;271:1112–4.
44. Adler S, Lindeman RD, Yiengst MJ, et al. Effect of acute acid loading on urinary acid excretion by the aging human kidney. J Lab Clin Med 1968;72:278–89.
45. Agarwal BN, Cabebe FG. Renal acidification in elderly subjects. Nephron 1980; 26:291–5.
46. Ershler WB, Sheng S, McKelvey J, et al. Serum erythropoietin and aging: a longitudinal analysis. J Am Geriatr Soc 2005;53:1360–5.
47. Carpenter MA, Kendall RG, O'Brien AE, et al. Reduced erythropoietin response to anaemia in elderly patients with normocytic anaemia. Eur J Haematol 1992;49: 119–21.
48. Ferrucci L, Guralnik JM, Bandinelli S, et al. Unexplained anaemia in older persons is characterized by low erythropoietin and low levels of pro-inflammatory markers. Br J Haematol 2007;136:849–55.

HYPONATREMIA

49. Anderson RJ, Chung HM, Kluge R, et al. Hyponatremia: a prospective analysis of its epidemiology and the pathogenetic role of vasopressin. Ann Intern Med 1985; 102:164–8.

50. Waikar SS, Mount DB, Curhan G. Mortality after hospitalization with mild, moderate, and severe hyponatremia. Am J Med 2009;122(9):857.

51. Vroonhof K, Van Solinge WW, Rovers MM, et al. Differences in mortality on the basis of laboratory parameters in an unselected population at the emergency department. Clin Chem Lab Med 2005;43(5):536–41.

52. Lee CT, Guo HR, Chen JB. Hyponatremia in the emergency department. Am J Emerg Med 2000;18:264–8.

53. Hawkins RC. Age and gender as risk factors for hyponatremia and hypernatremia. Clin Chim Acta 2003;337:169–72.

54. Miller M, Morley JE, Rubenstein LZ. Hyponatremia. J Am Geriatr Soc 1995;12:1410–3.

55. Choudhury M, Aparanji K, Norkus EP, et al. Hyponatremia in hospitalized nursing home residents and outcome: minimize hospitalization and keep the stay short! J Am Med Dir Assoc 2012;13(1):8–9.

56. Chua M, Hoyle GE, Soiza RL. Prognostic implications of hyponatremia in elderly hospitalized patients. Arch Gerontol Geriatr 2007;45(3):253–8.

57. Sandhu HS. Hyponatremia associated with large-bone fracture in elderly patients. Int Urol Nephrol 2009;41(3):733–7.

58. Hoorn EJ. Mild hyponatremia as a risk factor for fractures: the Rotterdam study. J Bone Miner Res 2011;26(8):1822–8.

59. Bourque CW, Oliet SH. Osmoreceptors in the central nervous system. Annu Rev Physiol 1997;59:601–19.

60. Burbach JP, Luckman SM, Murphy D, et al. Gene regulation in the magnocellular hypothalamo-neurohypophysial system. Physiol Rev 2001;81:1197–267.

61. Nielsen S, Frokiaer J, Marples D, et al. Aquaporins in the kidney: from molecules to medicine. Physiol Rev 2002;82:205–44.

62. McKinley MJ, Johnson AK. The physiological regulation of thirst and fluid intake. News Physiol Sci 2004;19(1):1–6.

63. Zerbe RL, Robertson GL. Osmoregulation of thirst and vasopressin secretion in human subjects: effect of various solutes. Am J Physiol 1983;244(6):E607–14.

64. Dyke MM, Daxis KM, Clark BA, et al. Effects of hypertonicity on water intake in the elderly: an age related failure. Geriatr Nephrol Urol 1997;7:11–6.

65. Patel GP, Balk RA. Recognition and treatment of hyponatremia in acutely ill hospitalized patients. Clin Ther 2007;29:211–29.

66. Papanicolaou DA, Wilder RL, Manolagas SC, et al. The pathophysiologic roles of interleukin-6 in human disease. Ann Intern Med 1998;128:127–37.

67. Beukhof CM, Hoorn EJ, Lindemans J, et al. Novel risk factors for hospital-acquired hyponatraemia: a matched case-control study. Clin Endocrinol (Oxf) 2007;66:367–72.

68. Ellis SJ. Severe hyponatraemia: complications and treatment. QJM 1995;88:905–9.

69. Renneboog B, Musch W, Vandemergel X, et al. Mild chronic hyponatremia is associated with falls, unsteadiness, and attention deficits. Am J Med 2006;119(1):71.e1–8.

70. Gosch M, Joosten-Gstrein B, Heppner HJ, et al. Hyponatremia in geriatric in-hospital patients: effects on results of a comprehensive geriatric assessment. Gerontology 2012;58(5):430–40.

71. McGee S, Abernethy WB 3rd, Simel DL. The rational clinical examination. Is this patient hypovolemic? JAMA 1999;281(11):1022–9.

72. Chung HM, Kluge R, Schrier RW, et al. Clinical assessment of extracellular fluid volume in hyponatremia. Am J Med 1987;83:905–8.

73. Adrogue HJ, Madias NE. Hyponatremia. N Engl J Med 2000;342:1581–9.
74. Abramow M, Beauwens R, Cogan E. Cellular events in vasopressin action. Kidney Int Suppl 1987;21:S56–66.
75. Yun JJ, Cheong I. Mannitol-induced hyperosmolal hyponatraemia. Intern Med J 2008;38:73.
76. Katz MA. Hyperglycemia-induced hyponatremia–calculation of expected serum sodium depression. N Engl J Med 1973;289(16):843–4.
77. Hillier TA, Abbott RD, Barrett EJ. Hyponatremia: evaluating the correction factor for hyperglycemia. Am J Med 1999;106:399–403.
78. Maas AH, Siggaard-Andersen O, Weisberg HF, et al. Ion-selective electrodes for sodium and potassium: a new problem of what is measured and what should be reported. Clin Chem 1985;31:482–5.
79. Rose BD. Hypoosmolal states — hyponatremia. In: Rose BD, Post TW, editors. Clinical physiology of acid-base and electrolyte disorders. 5th edition. New York: MacGraw Hill; 2001. p. 696–745.
80. Dundas B, Harris M, Narasimhan M. Psychogenic polydipsia review: etiology, differential, and treatment. Curr Psychiatry Rep 2007;9:236–41.
81. Bersani G, Pesaresi L, Orlandi V, et al. Atypical antipsychotics and polydipsia: a cause or a treatment? Hum Psychopharmacol 2007;22:103–7.
82. Fenves AZ, Thomas S, Knochel JP. Beer potomania: two cases and review of the literature. Clin Nephrol 1996;45(1):61–4.
83. Sanghvi SR, Kellerman PS, Nanovic L. Beer potomania: an unusual cause of hyponatremia at high risk of complications from rapid correction. Am J Kidney Dis 2007;50(4):673–80.
84. Chen LK, Lin MH, Hwang SJ, et al. Hyponatremia among the institutionalized elderly in 2 long-term care facilities in Taipei. J Chin Med Assoc 2006;69: 115–9.
85. Saghafi D. Water loading test in the reset osmostat variant of SIADH [letter]. Am J Med 1993;95:343.
86. Schrier RW. Pathogenesis of sodium and water retention in high-output and low-output cardiac failure, nephrotic syndrome, cirrhosis, and pregnancy. N Engl J Med 1988;319:1065–72.
87. Goldberg A, Hammerman H, Petcherski S, et al. Hyponatremia and long-term mortality in survivors of acute ST-elevation myocardial infarction. Arch Intern Med 2006;166:781–6.
88. Sonnenblick M, Friedlander Y, Rosin AJ. Diuretic-induced severe hyponatremia. Review and analysis of 129 reported patients. Chest 1993;103:601–6.
89. Palmer BF. Hyponatraemia in a neurosurgical patient: syndrome of inappropriate antidiuretic hormone secretion versus cerebral salt wasting. Nephrol Dial Transplant 2000;15:262–8.
90. Sterns RH, Silver SM. Cerebral salt wasting versus SIADH: what difference? J Am Soc Nephrol 2008;19:194–6.
91. Maesaka JK, Gupta S, Fishbane S. Cerebral salt-wasting syndrome: does it exist? Nephron 1999;82:100–9.
92. Kimura T. Potential mechanisms of hypothyroidism-induced hyponatremia [editorial]. Intern Med 2000;39:1002–3.
93. Gagnon RF, Halperin ML. Possible mechanisms to explain the absence of hyperkalaemia in Addison's disease. Nephrol Dial Transplant 2001;16:1280–4.
94. Diederich S, Franzen NF, Bahr V, et al. Severe hyponatremia due to hypopituitarism with adrenal insufficiency: report on 28 cases. Eur J Endocrinol 2003;148: 609–17.

95. Decaux G, Musch W, Penninckx R, et al. Low plasma bicarbonate level in hyponatremia related to adrenocorticotropin deficiency. J Clin Endocrinol Metab 2003; 88:5255–7.

96. Ellison DH, Berl T. Clinical practice. The syndrome of inappropriate antidiuresis. N Engl J Med 2007;356:2064–72.

97. Robertson GL. Regulation of arginine vasopressin in the syndrome of inappropriate antidiuresis. Am J Med 2006;119(Suppl 1):S36–42.

98. Fabian TJ, Amico JA, Kroboth PD, et al. Paroxetine-induced hyponatremia in older adults. A 12-week prospective study. Arch Intern Med 2004;164:327–32.

99. Miller M, Hecker MS, Friedlander DA, et al. Apparent idiopathic hyponatremia in an ambulatory geriatric population. J Am Geriatr Soc 1996;44(4):404–8.

100. Maesaka JK. An expanded view of SIADH, hyponatremia and hypouricemia. Clin Nephrol 1996;46:79–83.

101. Verbalis JG, Goldsmith SR, Greenberg A, et al. Hyponatremia treatment guidelines 2007: expert panel recommendations. Am J Med 2007;120(11 Suppl 1):S1–21.

102. Sterns R, Hix JK, Silver S. Treating profound hyponatremia: a strategy for controlled correction. Am J Kidney Dis 2010;56:774–9.

103. Vaidya C, Ho W, Freda BJ. Management of hyponatremia: providing treatment and avoiding harm. Cleve Clin J Med 2010;77(10):715–26.

104. Lee P, Jones GR, Center JR. Successful treatment of adult cerebral salt wasting with fludrocortisone. Arch Intern Med 2008;168:325–6.

105. Martin RJ. Central pontine and extrapontine myelinolysis: the osmotic demyelination syndromes. J Neurol Neurosurg Psychiatry 2004;75:22–8.

106. Sterns R. Osmotic demyelination syndrome and overly rapid correction of hyponatremia. In: Uptodate. 2012. Available at: http://www.uptodate.com/contents/osmotic-demyelination-syndrome-and-overly-rapid-correction-of-hyponatremia?source=search_result&search=osmotic+demyelination+syndrome&selectedTitle=1%7E35. Accessed September 29, 2012.

107. Kumar SR, Mone AP, Gray LC, et al. Central pontine myelinolysis: delayed changes on neuroimaging. J Neuroimaging 2000;10:169–72.

108. Finsterer J, Engelmayar E, Trnka E, et al. Immunoglobulins are effective in pontine myelinolysis. Clin Neuropharmacol 2000;23:110–3.

109. Oya S, Tsutsumi K, Ueki K, et al. Reinduction of hyponatraemia to treat central pontine myelinolysis. Neurology 2001;57:1931–2.

HYPERNATREMIA

110. Long CA, Marin P, Bayer AJ, et al. Hypernatremia in an adult in-patient population. Postgrad Med J 1991;67(789):643–5.

111. Lindner G, Funk GC, Schwarz C, et al. Hypernatremia in the critically ill is an independent risk factor for mortality. Am J Kidney Dis 2007;50:952.

112. Polderman KH, Schreuder WO, Strack van Schijndel RJ, et al. Hypernatremia in the intensive care unit: an indicator of quality of care? Crit Care Med 1999;27(6): 1105–8.

113. Arampatzis S, Exadaktylos A, Buhl D, et al. Dysnatraemias in the emergency room: undetected, untreated, unknown? Wien Klin Wochenschr 2012;124(5–6): 181–3.

114. Snyder NA, Feigal DW, Arieff AL. Hypematremia in elderly patients. A heterogeneous, morbid and iatrogenic entity. Ann Intern Med 1987;107:309–19.

115. Chassagne P, Druesne L, Capet C, et al. Clinical presentation of hypernatremia in elderly patients: a case control study. J Am Geriatr Soc 2006;54:1225–30.

116. Phillips PA, Rolls BJ, Ledingham JG, et al. Reduced thirst after water deprivation in healthy elderly men. N Engl J Med 1984;311:753–9.
117. Borra SI, Beredo R, Kleinfeld M. Hypernatremia in the aging: causes, manifestations, and outcome. J Natl Med Assoc 1995;87(3):220–4.
118. Adrogue HJ, Madias NE. Hypernatraemia. N Engl J Med 2000;342:1493–9.
119. Lien YH, Shapiro JI, Chan L. Effects of hypernatremia on organic brain osmoles. J Clin Invest 1990;85:1427–35.
120. Simmons M, Adcock EW III, Bard H, et al. Hypernatremia and intracranial hemorrhage in infants. N Engl J Med 1974;291:6.
121. Lavizzo-Mourey R, Johnson J, Stolley P. Risk factors for dehydration among elderly nursing home residents. J Am Geriatr Soc 1988;36:213–8.
122. Kumar S, Berl T. Sodium. Lancet 1998;352(9123):220–8.
123. Robertson GL. Abnormalities of thirst regulation. Kidney Int 1984;25:460–9.
124. DeRubertis FR, Michelis MF, Davis BB. Essential hypernatremia. Report of three cases and review of the literature. Arch Intern Med 1974;134(5):889–95.
125. Gennari FJ, Kassirer JP. Osmotic diuresis. N Engl J Med 1977;291(14):714–20.
126. Craig JC, Grigor WG, Knight JF. Acute obstructive uropathy a rare complication of circumcision. Eur J Pediatr 1994;153(5):369–71.
127. Arinzona Z, Feldmanc J, Peisakhb A, et al. Water and sodium disturbances predict prognosis of acute disease in long term cared frail elderly. Arch Gerontol Geriatr 2005;40:317–26.
128. Sonnenblick M, Algur N. Hypernatremia in the acutely ill elderly patients: role of impaired arginine-vasopressin secretion. Miner Electrolyte Metab 1993;19(1):32–5.
129. Lin M, Liu SJ, Lim IT. Disorders of water imbalance. Emerg Med Clin North Am 2005;23:749–70.
130. Nemergut EC, Zuo Z, Jane JA Jr, et al. Predictors of diabetes insipidus after transsphenoidal surgery: a review of 881 patients. J Neurosurg 2005;103(3):448.
131. Hadjizacharia P, Beale EO, Inaba K, et al. Acute diabetes insipidus in severe head injury: a prospective study. J Am Coll Surg 2008;207(4):477.
132. Aimaretti G, Ambrosio MR, Di Somma C, et al. Traumatic brain injury and subarachnoid haemorrhage are conditions at high risk for hypopituitarism: screening study at 3 months after the brain injury. Clin Endocrinol (Oxf) 2004;61(3):320–6.
133. Kimmel DW, O'Neil BP. Systemic cancer presenting as diabetes insipidus clinical and radiographic features of 11 patients with review of metastatic-induced diabetes insipidus. Cancer 1983;52(12):2355.
134. Stuart CA, Neelon FA, Lebovitz HE. Disordered control of thirst in hypothalamic-pituitary sarcoidosis. N Engl J Med 1980;303(19):1078.
135. Thodou E, Asa SL, Kontogeorgos G, et al. Clinical case seminar: lymphocytic hypophysitis: clinicopathological findings. J Clin Endocrinol Metab 1995;80(8):2303.
136. Holtzman EJ, Ausiello DA. Nephrogenic diabetes insipidus: causes revealed. Hosp Pract 1994;29(3):89–93.
137. Bendz H, Aurell M. Drug-induced diabetes insipidus: incidence, prevention and management. Drug Saf 1999;21(6):449–56.
138. Felig P, Johnson C, Levitt M, et al. Hypernatremia induced by maximal exercise. JAMA 1982;248:1209–11.
139. Manitius A, Levitin H, Beck D, et al. On the mechanism of impairment of renal concentrating ability in potassium deficiency. J Clin Invest 1960;39:684–92.
140. Agrawal V, Agarwal M, Joshi S, et al. Hyponatremia and hypernatremia: disorder of water balance. J Assoc Physicians India 2008;56:956–64.

HYPERCALCEMIA

141. Shane E, Dinaz I. Hypercalcemia: pathogenesis, clinical manifestations, differential diagnosis, and management. In: Favus MJ, editor. Primer on the metabolic bone diseases and disorders of mineral metabolism, vol. 26, 6th edition. Philadelphia: Lippincott, Williams, and Wilkins; 2006. p. 176.
142. Bilezikian JP. Management of acute hypercalcemia. N Engl J Med 1992;326: 1196.
143. Inzucchi SE. Understanding hypercalcemia. Its metabolic basis, signs and symptoms. Postgrad Med 2004;115:69.
144. Ohrvall U, Akerstrom G, Ljunghall S, et al. Surgery for sporadic primary hyperparathyroidism in the elderly. World J Surg 1994;18:612.
145. French S, Subauste J, Geraci S. Calcium abnormalities in hospitalized patients. South Med J 2012;105(4):231–7.
146. Lafferty FW. Differential diagnosis of hypercalcemia. J Bone Miner Res 1991; 6(Suppl 2):S51.
147. Dent DM, Miller JL, Klaff L, et al. The incidence and causes of hypercalcaemia. Postgrad Med J 1987;63(743):745–50.
148. Mundy GR, Guise TA. Hypercalcemia of malignancy. Am J Med 1997;103(2): 134–45.
149. Edelson GW, Kleerekoper M. Hypercalcemic crisis. Med Clin North Am 1995;79: 79–92.
150. Raymakers JA. Hypercalcemia in the elderly. Tijdschr Gerontol Geriatr 1990; 21(1):11–6 [in Dutch].
151. Wick JY. Immobilization hypercalcemia in the elderly. Consult Pharm 2007; 22(11):892–905.
152. Carroll MF, Schade DS. A practical approach to hypercalcemia. Am Fam Physician 2003;67:1959–66.
153. Parfitt AM, Gallagher JC, Hearney RP, et al. Vitamin D and bone health in the elderly. Am J Clin Nutr 1982;36(Suppl 5):1014–31.
154. Fishbane S, Frei GL, Finger M, et al. Hypervitaminosis A in two hemodialysis patients. Am J Kidney Dis 1995;25:346.
155. Niesvizky R, Siegel DS, Busquets X, et al. Hypercalcaemia and increased serum interleukin-6 levels induced by all-trans retinoic acid in patients with multiple myeloma. Br J Haematol 1995;89:217.
156. Khairallah W, Fawaz A, Brown EM, et al. Hypercalcemia and diabetes insipidus in a patient previously treated with lithium. Nat Clin Pract Nephrol 2007; 3:397.
157. Abreo K, Adiakha A, Kilpatrick S, et al. The milk-alkali syndrome. A reversible form of acute renal failure. Arch Intern Med 1993;153:1005.
158. Legha SS, Powell K, Buzdar AU, et al. Tamoxifen-induced hypercalcemia in breast cancer. Cancer 1981;47:2803.
159. Kikuchi R, Mochizuli S, Shimizu M, et al. Elderly patient presenting with severe thyrotoxic hpercalcemia. Geriatr Gerontol Int 2000;6:270–3.
160. Jamie S, Tyler CV, Parambil JG. Sarcoidosis presenting as symptomatic hypercalcemia in octogenarian. Clin Geriatr 2011;19(14):43–6.
161. Ianuzzi MC, Fontana JR. Sarcoidosis: clinical presentation, immunopathogenesis and treatment. JAMA 2011;305(4):391–9.
162. Boonen S, Vanderschueren D, Pelemans W, et al. Primary hyperparathyroidism: diagnosis and management in the older individual. Eur J Endocrinol 2004; 151(3):297–304.

163. Blomquist CP. Malignant hypercalcemia: a hospital survey. Acta Med Scand 1986;220(5):455–63.
164. Bollanti L, Rindino G, Strollo F. Endocrine paraneoplastic syndromes with special reference to the elderly. Endocrine 2001;14(2):151–7.
165. Ghazi AA, Attarian H, Attarian S, et al. Hypercalcemia and huge splenomegaly presenting in an elderly patient with B-cell non-Hodgkin's lymphoma. J Med Case Rep 2010;4:330.
166. Mallette LE, Eichhorn E. Effects of lithium carbonate on human calcium metabolism. Arch Intern Med 1986;146:770–6.
167. Aryan CE, Sosa JA. Assessment and management of patients with abnormal calcium. Crit Care Med 2004;32(Suppl 4):745–50.
168. Verges B. Hypercalemia in the eldely. Presse Med 2001;30(7):313–6 [in French].
169. Solomon BL, Schaaf M, Smallridge RC. Psychologic symptoms before and after parathyroid surgery. Am J Med 1994;96:101–6.
170. Gardner EC Jr, Hersh T. Primary hyperparathyroidism and the gastrointestinal tract. South Med J 1981;74:197.
171. Wynn D, Everett GD, Boothby RA. Small cell carcinoma of the ovary with hypercalcemia causes severe pancreatitis and altered mental status. Gynecol Oncol 2004;95:716.
172. Abelhadi M, Nordenstrom J. Bone mineral recovery after parathyroidectomy in primary and renal hyperparathyroidism. J Clin Endocrinol Metab 1998;83:3845–51.
173. Ahmed R, Hashiba K. Reliability of QT intervals as indicators of clinical hypercalcemia. Clin Cardiol 1988;11:395.
174. Diercks DB, Shumaik GM, Harrigan RA, et al. Electrocardiographic manifestations: electrolyte abnormalities. J Emerg Med 2004;27:153.
175. Nishi SP, Barbagelata NA, Atar S, et al. Hypercalcemia-induced ST-segment elevation mimicking acute myocardial infarction. J Electrocardiol 2006;39:298.
176. Roberts WC, Waller BF. Effect of chronic hypercalcemia on the heart. An analysis of 18 necropsy patients. Am J Med 1981;71:371.
177. Okeefe KP, Sanson TG. Elderly patients with altered mental status. Emerg Med Clin North Am 1998;16(4):701–15, v.
178. Grill V, Ho P, Brody JJ, et al. Partathyroid hormone-related protein: elevated levels in both humoral hypercalcemia of malignancy and hypercalcemia complicating metastatic breast cancer. J Clin Endocrinol Metab 1991;73(6):1309–15.
179. Hosking DJ, Cowley A, Bucknall CA. Rehydration in the treatment of severe hypercalcemia. Q J Med 1981;50:473–81.
180. Body JJ. Hypercalcemia of malignancy. Semin Nephrol 2004;24:48.
181. Legrand SB, Leskuski D, Zama I. Narrative review: furosemide for hyprcalcemia: an unproven yet common practice. Ann Intern Med 2008;149:259.
182. Stewart AF. Clinical practice. Hypercalcemia associated with cancer. N Engl J Med 2005;352:373.
183. Major P, Lortholary A, Hon J, et al. Zoledronic acid is superior to pamidronate in the treatment of hypercalcemia of malignancy: a pooled analysis of two randomized, controlled clinical trials. J Clin Oncol 2001;19:558.
184. Wisneski LA. Salmon calcitonin in the acute management of hypercalcemia. Calcif Tissue Int 1990;46(Suppl):S26.
185. Chitambar CR. Gallium nitrate revisited. Semin Oncol 2003;30:1.
186. Lin PH, Chiu CF, Lu YS. Cisplatin as an active treatment of zoledronate-refractory hypercalcemia. Ann Oncol 2011;22(5):1244–6.

187. Koo WS, Jeon DS, Ahn SJ, et al. Calcium-free hemodialysis for the management of hypercalcemia. Nephron 1996;72:424.

ACUTE RENAL FAILURE

188. Coca SG. Acute kidney injury in elderly persons. Am J Kidney Dis 2010;56(1): 122–31.
189. Baraldi A, Ballestri M, Rapana R, et al. Acute renal failure of medical type in an elderly population. Nephrol Dial Transplant 1998;13(Suppl 7):S25–9.
190. Ali T, Khan I, Simpson W, et al. Incidence and outcomes in acute kidney injury: a comprehensive population-based study. J Am Soc Nephrol 2007;18:1292–8.
191. Rizzi Z, Cruz D, Ronco C. The RIFLE criteria and mortality in acute kidney injury: a systematic review. Kidney Int 2008;73:538–46.
192. Neild GH. Multi-organ renal failure in the elderly. Int Urol Nephrol 2001;32(4): 559–65.
193. Cheung CM, Ponnusamy A, Anderton JG. Management of acute renal failure in the elderly patient: a clinician's guide. Drugs Aging 2008;25(6):455–76.
194. Schmitt R, Coca S, Kanbay ME, et al. Recovery of kidney function after acute kidney injury in the elderly: a systematic review and meta-analysis. Am J Kidney Dis 2008;52(2):262–71.
195. Coca SG, Cho KC, Hsu CY. Acute kidney injury in the elderly: predisposition to chronic kidney disease and vice versa. Nephron Clin Pract 2011;119(Suppl 1): c19–24.
196. Chronopoulos A, Rosner MH, Cruz DN, et al. Acute kidney injury in the elderly: a review. Contrib Nephrol 2010;165:315–21.
197. Martin JE, Scheaff MT. Renal ageing. J Pathol 2007;211:198–205.
198. Chronopoulos A, Cruz DN, Ronco C. Hospital acquired kidney injury in the elderly. Nat Rev Nephrol 2010;6(3):141–9.
199. Pascual J, Liano F, Ortuno J. The elderly patient with acute renal failure. J Am Soc Nephrol 1995;6:144–53.
200. Ronco C, Haapio M, House AA, et al. Cardiorenal syndrome. J Am Coll Cardiol 2008;52:1527–39.
201. Schmitt R, Cantley LG. The impact of aging on kidney repair. Am J Physiol Renal Physiol 2008;294:F1265–72.
202. Bagshaw SM, George C, Bellomo R, et al. Early acute kidney injury and sepsis: a multicenter evaluation. Crit Care 2008;12:R47.
203. Noor S, Usmani A. Post operative renal failure. Clin Geriatr Med 2008;24:721–9.
204. Kishen R. Acute kidney injury in the elderly: a review. Indian Anesthetists Forum. 2011.
205. Jerkic M, Volvodic S, Lopez-Novoa JM. The mechanism of increased renal susceptibility to toxic substances in the elderly. Part1. The role of increased vasoconstriction. Int Urol Nephrol 2001;32(4):539–47.
206. Sweleh W, Sawalha A, Al-Jaba S, et al. Discharge medications among ischemic stroke survivors. J Stroke Cerebrovasc Dis 2009;18:97–102.
207. Kohli HS, Bhaskaran MC, Muthukumar T, et al. Treatment-related acute renal failure in the elderly: a hospital based prospective study. Nephrol Dial Transplant 2000;15:212–7.
208. Serra A, Romero R. Acute kidney failure in systemic vasculitis associated with antineutrophil cytoplasmic antibodies (ANCA) in aged patients. Nefrologia 2001;21(1):1–8.
209. Becker A, Buam M. Obstructive uropathy. Early Hum Dev 2006;82(1):15–22.

210. Christensan J, Ostri P, Frimodt-Moller C, et al. Intravesical pressure changes during bladder drainage in patients with acute urinary retention. Urol Int 1987; 42(3):181–4.

211. Zeidel ML, Pirtskhalaishvili G. Urinary tract obstruction. In: Brenner BM, editor. Brenner and Rector's The Kidney. 8th edition. Philadelphia, PA: Saunders Elsevier; 2007. Chap. 35.

212. Abdel-Kadar K, Palevsky P. Acute kidney injury in the elderly. Clin Geriatr Med 2008;25(3):331–58.

213. Haase M, Story DA, Hasse-Fielitz A. Renal injury in the elderly: diagnosis, biomarkers and prevention. Best Pract Res Clin Anaesthesiol 2011;25(3):401–12.

214. Fliser D, Ritz E. Serum cystatin C concentration as a marker of renal dysfunction in the elderly. Am J Kidney Dis 2001;37:79–83.

215. Thomas DR, Cote TR, Lawhorne L, et al. Understanding clinical dehydration and its treatment. J Am Med Dir Assoc 2008;9:292–301.

216. Musso CG, Liakopoulos V, Ioannidis I, et al. Acute renal failure in the elderly: particular characteristics. Int Urol Nephrol 2006;38(3–4):787–93.

217. Schrier RW, Wang W, Poole B, et al. Acute renal failure: definitions, diagnosis, pathogenesis, and therapy. J Clin Invest 2004;114(1):5–14.

218. McCullough PA, Sandberg KR. B-type naturetic peptide and renal disease. Heart Fail Rev 2003;8:355–8.

219. Srisawasdi P, Vanavanan S, Charoenpanichkit C, et al. The effect of renal dysfunction on BNP, NT-proBNP, and their ratio. Am J Clin Pathol 2010;133: 14–23.

220. Macedo E, Bouchard J, Mehta RL. Renal recovery following acute kidney injury. Curr Opin Crit Care 2008;14:660–6.

221. Ishani A, Xue JL, Himmelfarb J, et al. Acute kidney injury increases the risk of ESRD among elderly. J Am Soc Nephrol 2009;20:223–8.

222. Stallone G, Infante B, Grandaliano G. Acute kidney injury in the elderly population. J Nephrol 2012;25(Suppl 19):58–66. http://dx.doi.org/10.5301/jn.5000140.

223. Anderson S, Eldadah B, Halter JB, et al. Acute kidney injury in older adults. J Am Soc Nephrol 2011;22(1):28–38.

224. Weisberg LS. Management of severe hyperkalemia. Crit Care Med 2008;36(12): 3246–51.

225. Khanna A, White WB. The management of hyperkalemia in patients with cardiovascular disease. Am J Med 2009;1223(3):215–21.

226. Mattu A, Brady WJ, Robinson DA. Electrocardiographic manifestations of hyperkalemia. Am J Emerg Med 2000;18(6):721–9.

227. Martinez-Vea A, Bardaji A, Garcia C, et al. Severe hyperkalemia with minimal electrocardiographic manifestations: a report of seven cases. J Electrocardiol 1999;32(1):45–9.

228. Kim HJ, Han SW. Therapeutic approach to hyperkalemia. Nephron 2002; 92(Suppl 1):33–40.

229. Ahee P, Crowe AC. The management of hyperkalaemia in the emergency department. J Accid Emerg Med 2000;17:188–91.

230. Kim HJ. Combined effect of bicarbonate and insulin with glucose in acute therapy of hyperkalemia in end-stage renal disease patients. Nephron 1996; 72:476–82.

231. Allon M, Dunlay R, Copkney C. Nebulized albuterol for acute hyperkalemia in patients on hemodialysis. Ann Intern Med 1989;110:426–9.

232. Sterns RH, Rojas M, Bernstein P, et al. Ion-exchange resins for the treatment of hyperkalemia, are they safe and effective? J Am Soc Nephrol 2010;21:733–5.

233. Kleinknecht D, Ganeval D, Gonzalez-Duque LA, et al. Furosemide in acute oliguric renal failure: a controlled trial. Nephron 1976;17:51–8.
234. Wen J, Cheng Q, Zhao J, et al. Hospital-acquired acute kidney injury in Chinese very elderly persons. J Nephrol 2012. http://dx.doi.org/10.5301/jn.5000182.
235. Liu KD, Himmelfarb J, Paganini E, et al. Timing of initiation of dialysis in critically ill patients with acute kidney injury. Clin J Am Soc Nephrol 2006;1:915.
236. Seabra VF, Balk EM, Liangos O, et al. Timing of renal replacement therapy initiation in acute renal failure: a meta-analysis. Am J Kidney Dis 2008;52(2):272–84.
237. Palevsky PM. Renal replacement therapy I: indications and timing. Crit Care Clin 2005;21:347–56.
238. Techan GS, Llangos O, Jaber BL. Update on dialytic management of acute renal failure. J Intensive Care Med 2003;18:130–8.
239. Van de noortgate N, Verbeke F, Dhondt A, et al. The dialytic management of acute renal failure in the elderly. Semin Dial 2002;15(2):127–32.
240. Somogyi-zalud E, Zhong Z, Hamel MB, et al. The use of life-sustaining treatments in hospitalized persons aged 80 and older. J Am Geriatr Soc 2002;50: 930–4.

Index

Note: Page numbers of article titles are in **boldface** type.

Clin Geriatr Med 29 (2013) 321–328
http://dx.doi.org/10.1016/S0749-0690(12)00122-X
0749-0690/13/$ – see front matter © 2013 Elsevier Inc. All rights reserved.

geriatric.theclinics.com

Moving?

Make sure your subscription moves with you!

To notify us of your new address, find your **Clinics Account Number** (located on your mailing label above your name), and contact customer service at:

Email: journalscustomerservice-usa@elsevier.com

800-654-2452 (subscribers in the U.S. & Canada)
314-447-8871 (subscribers outside of the U.S. & Canada)

Fax number: 314-447-8029

Elsevier Health Sciences Division
Subscription Customer Service
3251 Riverport Lane
Maryland Heights, MO 63043

*To ensure uninterrupted delivery of your subscription, please notify us at least 4 weeks in advance of move.